Atlas of Disease Mortalities in Hong Kong

Atlas of Disease Mortalities in Hong Kong for the Three Five-year Periods in 1979–93

Owen Llewelyn LLOYD

WONG Tze-wai

WONG Siu-lan

YU Tak-sun Ignatius

The Chinese University Press

ISBN: 962–201–732–0

Cartographic Consultant: Fung Tung
Statistical Computation Consultant: Luo Fu-tian
Maps Production Assistant: Aprille Sham

THE CHINESE UNIVERSITY PRESS,
The Chinese University of Hong Kong,
Sha Tin, N.T., Hong Kong.
Fax: +852 2603 6692/7355
E-mail: cup@cuhk.edu.hk
Web-site: http://www.cuhk.edu.hk/cupress/w1.htm

Printed in Hong Kong

Contents

Maps, Tables and Graphs

Foreword

Professor Arthur K.C. Li
Vice Chancellor, The Chinese University of Hong Kong

Over the past two decades, atlases of mortality have been published for most developed countries of the world, particularly in Europe and North America. In 1979, a new cancer atlas for the People's Republic of China was applauded not only for its scientific qualities but also for the artistic beauty of its maps. Hong Kong did not appear in that atlas. With the coming union between Mainland China and Hong Kong, it is fitting that an atlas for Hong Kong, produced by the Faculty of Medicine of The Chinese University of Hong Kong and published by its University Press, has completed the epidemiological picture.

But — why bother mapping diseases at all? Just over one and a half centuries ago, it was through case-mapping that the aetiology of the cholera epidemic in London was found, enabling the effective responses of preventive medicine to control the disease. By answering the question "where?", those maps had pointed the way to answering the questions "why?" and "what then?". Since that time, our knowledge of disease causations has been accelerating, often through the clues provided by disease mapping, not only for infectious diseases but also for the modern plagues of cancer and degenerative diseases. Disease maps illustrate the success or failure with which man has tried to adapt to his environment, the degree of balance and harmony existing between humanity (and its artificial environments) and nature.

The Taoist sages and other wise men of ancient China perceived the value to health from living in harmony with nature. They saw ecological harmony as a virtue, with benefits through preventive medicine which far outweighed those from curative medicine: "If one wants a kettle of soup to stop boiling, one must take away the fire from underneath. As for all these leeches and physicians, with their drugs and potions supposed to expel diseases ..., the wise men of old esteemed such men but little, considering that they deal with the branch and not with the root." [*Master Lu's Spring and Autumn Annals*《吕氏春秋》, 239 B.C.]

Nowadays, threats to the public's health can still strike down victims in corners of one's own backyard, as these mortality maps for Hong Kong show clearly. Further towards the horizon, one sees an approaching epidemic of potential threats: from resurgent (old) and surgent (new) infections — cholera, plague, malaria, tuberculosis and AIDS — and from diseases caused by the increasingly complex industrial chemicals which incessantly infiltrate our environments.

The disease maps in this atlas for Hong Kong constitute reader-friendly baseline parameters for the public's health, indicating the localities where preventive medicine and its allies among town planners, hospital administrators, factory inspectors, environmental health officers and others still have substantial work to do to improve those parameters. And the continued monitoring of mortality, by means of disease mapping planned for current and future years, will provide an early warning system alerting us to new threats to our health, as we struggle to adapt ourselves and our environments in a way which is harmonious with nature's ecological balances. Perhaps, therefore, if we in Hong Kong can learn from the modern-sounding concepts of our sage Chinese traditions, preventible diseases here eventually will become largely prevented.

Foreword

Dr Margaret Chan
Director of Health, Hong Kong Government

Hong Kong has made remarkable achievements in health care and our disease surveillance system has provided a rich collection of health information and epidemiological data awaiting the astute medical researcher. However, the paucity of locally published medical books is especially noticeable in the field of public health. Professor Owen Lloyd and his team of researchers have made a timely and important contribution to public health by publishing this *Atlas of Disease Mortalities in Hong Kong*, the first local text on medical geography. This atlas deals with "time" and "place", two of the three "magic words" — "time", "place" and "person" in descriptive epidemiology. By presenting the distribution of major disease mortalities in maps and comparing the changes in three five-year periods, the authors have provided the essential ingredient in the generation of hypotheses in disease aetiology. The atlas also provides the reader with a concise yet well written overview of the epidemiology of major diseases, ranging from common cancers to major degenerative diseases of the heart and lung. It will be an important reference book for health planners, administrators and researchers in public health and epidemiology.

Medical geography is an old science, but is rapidly rejuvenating and developing, thanks to recent advances in epidemiological and statistical methods. This atlas represents an important step forwards by local researchers in this exciting discipline, and I warmly recommend it to all public health workers. It is also gratifying to know that further research by this team on cancer incidence is making good progress.

Preface

The Atlas, *from genesis to revelation*

Taking a plan along the voyage from conception to destination can prove a long, arduous and frustrating expedition. It can also be a total waste of time and energy, for many an excellently conceived and scientifically valuable plan sinks without trace *en route*, through simply bad luck or through a lack of supporters to convoy it safely through the circumstantial squalls and doldrums of the voyage.

The idea of an atlas of mortality for Hong Kong was conceived in 1991 in the Department of Community and Family Medicine at The Chinese University of Hong Kong. A pilot study of the medical geography of Hong Kong proved the scientific validity of the idea, underlining the immense potential value of disease mapping for the surveillance and improvement of the health of Hong Kong people. So, with the advice and assistance of the Department of Geography and of the Chinese University Press, the *Atlas* as a project was launched the following year. However, the huge scale of the project soon brought home to the original "crew" the need for further outside help. And had it not been for the moral and financial support generously emanating from so many directions in response to appeals for help, the *Atlas* project might well have foundered *en voyage* or been becalmed into a state of irrelevance. The many sources of support include: the provision of the mortality and census data from the Commissioner of Census and Statistics Department; the Vice-Chancellor's grant from Professor Charles Kao, former Vice Chancellor of The Chinese University of Hong Kong, which enabled the publication of the *Atlas* and also the extension of the study period to cover fifteen years of mortality experience in place of the original ten years; the warm and practical encouragement from the Faculty of Medicine of The Chinese University of Hong Kong through its successive Deans, Professor Teik Oh, Professor Arthur Li and Professor Joseph Lee; the support from successive Directors of Health, Dr S.H. Lee and Dr Margaret Chan; the generosity of Sun Yat-sen University of Medical Sciences in Guangdong in "lending" Dr Luo Fu-tian, who assisted in much of the statistical computation, to the team. Also, Ms Aprille Sham of the Department of Community and Family Medicine contributed towards the production of the maps; Professor Fung Tung of the Department of Geography was our cartographic consultant; Dr Freda Yeang helped in the data preparation. Thus the project became *en route* a truly collaborative enterprise. We are deeply grateful to all our helpers.

The *Atlas* has now reached the haven of its publication. But that cannot be seen as the final outcome. For the information on board is there to be unloaded, applied and, if possible, developed during the coming years. Many of the patterns of mortality will be of value for health care planners and administrators, by indicating where the local demands for particular types of treatment and care will be most pressing. Many other of the patterns cry out for further investigations: are the inequalities or mortality "real" or merely the result of some cryptic artefact? If real, what has caused them? And how can the "hot spots" of diseases be eliminated and the low rates seen in some areas be extended to cover the whole Territory, thereby maximizing "Health for All by the Year 2000"? So the publication of the *Atlas*, major achievement though it may be, would fail in its purpose if it were seen as having reached the destination. Let us hope, therefore, that it will prove a useful stepping stone towards the real goal: further collaborative achievement in the continuing fight against disease and premature death in Hong Kong.

Owen L. Lloyd, Wong Tze-wai, Wong Siu-lan & Yu Tak-sun

About the Authors

Professor Owen Llewelyn Lloyd, MA, MBCh, MD, BSCHons, PhD, DipComMed, DipEd, FFPHM, FFOM, FRCP(Edin), FHKAM, MREHIS

After tertiary education at Edinburgh University, Owen Lloyd spent six years in the Department of Physiology at Edinburgh University as MRC Fellow and Lecturer researching into the central nervous system. The challenges of public health and environmental health led him to the Lothian Health Board in Edinburgh, then for 13 years to Dundee University as senior lecturer and honorary consultant in Occupational and Environmental Health (a product of this period was the *Scottish Atlas of Mortality* published by Croom Helm in 1986), and finally to the west of Scotland as consultant and part-time senior lecturer at the University of Glasgow. In 1991, he became chairman of the Department of Community and Family Medicine at The Chinese University of Hong Kong, and moved to the United Arab Emirates around three years later. Over these years and in the varied environments, his professional concerns and researches have continued to focus on the increasingly evident connections between environmental pollution and health and on the application of disease mapping to uncovering those connections.

Professor Wong Tze-wai, MBBS, MSc, MFPHM, FAFOM, FAMS, MACE, FHKCCM, FHKAM

A medical graduate of The University of Hong Kong, Wong Tze-wai started his career in public health as health officer in Hong Kong Government for seven years. His interest in teaching and research transformed his career in the next 12 years into an academic, initially in the National University of Singapore and then in the Department of Community and Family Medicine of The Chinese University of Hong Kong, where he is currently professor. His research interest is broad, ranging from the epidemiology of hantaviruses, traffic and industrial accidents, environmental pollution, occupational diseases to traditional Chinese medicine. Inspired by Professor Lloyd's enthusiasm in disease mapping, he became a core member of the research team and took up the leadership of the project when Professor Lloyd left Hong Kong.

Dr Wong Siu-lan, MB, MPhil

Wong Siu-lan obtained her medical qualification in Beijing Medical University in 1955. An expert medical statistician for over 40 years, she has acquired extensive experience in cancer research, in particular, the epidemiology of nasopharyngeal cancer. She was former professor and consultant in medical statistics in the Sun Yat-sen University of Medical Sciences. After obtaining an MPhil (Statistics) in The University of Hong Kong, she joined the Department of Community and Family Medicine of The Chinese University of Hong Kong in 1987. She is the statistical consultant of this research team and her research interest includes environmental health, time trend of disease mortalities and geographical analyses of mortality and morbidity.

Professor Yu Tak-sun Ignatius, MBBS, MPH, FAFOM, FHKCCM, FHKAM

Yu Tak-sun, a graduate from the Medical School of the University of Hong Kong, started his career in community health and occupational medicine. After being a front-line health care worker for over ten years, he joined the Department of Community and Family Medicine of The Chinese University of Hong Kong where he is currently associate professor. His research interest is mainly in occupational and environmental health. His involvement in the latter field has prompted him to participate in this disease mapping project.

Introduction

That the environment can influence the patterns of disease has been evident since the beginnings of rational medicine. In the 4th century B.C., Hippocrates, the Father of Western Medicine, in his treatise, "On Airs, Water and Places", advised those wishing "to investigate medicine properly" that pleurisy and tonsillitis were usually more frequent in inhabitants of north-facing cities, because of the persistence of fogs and mists in those situations. The beneficial or harmful qualities of various types of water were also noted.[1] Similar observations were also voiced in ancient China. *Master Lu's Spring and Autumn Annals* (《吕氏春秋》) advised around 239 B.C. that "in places with too much light water there is found baldness and goitre; much heavy water brings a high incidence of swellings and dropsies ...; where sweet waters abound there will be healthy people, but much acrid water brings skin infections ...; bitter waters bring ulcers and rickets ..."[2–3] So even in those earliest times, links between environment and disease were recognized.

Mapping of the environment itself was practised around 2000 years ago by the early Greeks and the ancient Chinese, for both theoretical and practical purposes. So why was it that medical geography, the visual demonstration of the relationships between health and the environment, was so slow to develop, only surfacing during the past 200 years?[4] The disintegration of the Roman Empire and the consequent fragmentation of Europe during the Dark Ages not only scattered or destroyed scholarship but also inhibited long-distance travelling. What maps there were in Europe served only allegorical or religious purposes; so the science of mapping the general environment died. It was the resurgence of exploration and commerce during the Middle Ages and subsequent European Renaissance which revived again the need for maps: thence first the rebirth of cartography in general and then the subsequent birth of medical geography in particular. During its emergence, medical geography received powerful assistance from two Germans.[5] Johann Peter Frank (1745–1821), a professor at five universities including those of Paris and Vienna, used his appointments at the courts of German principalities to advocate medical geography to all "humane physicians". Leonhard Ludwig Finke (1747–1828), whose medical functions included environmental health and general public health in Germany's Westphalia, produced in 1792 the first comprehensive book on medical geography — a literary landmark in the subject.

Medical geography's pictorial representation, disease mapping, began in the early 19th century.[6] It was the methodological response by medical scientists to those population-scything epidemics of infectious disease of which yellow fever and cholera were such fearsome examples.[1] Thus, in 1820 a spot-map of yellow fever in New York resulted from the attempt of Pascalis-Ouviere to grapple with its cryptic causation there. Six years later, the patterns on a disease map of a district in Mississippi were combined with the then-fashionable miasmatic theory of disease to explain the causation: "A damp climate, an eighty-degree temperature ... combined with the special effluvia of rotting pork and oysters to envelop the community in a sort of pathogenic mist. The inevitable consequence was widespread yellow fever." And so, when the Asiatic cholera — cause and prevention hitherto unknown — began to scourge Europe towards the middle of the 19th century, disease mapping was applied with fresh vigour, and with successful consequences for disease prevention. In 1833, the report of the Board of Health of Leeds (in England) included a map showing the districts badly smitten with cholera, noting "... how exceedingly the disease has prevailed in those parts of the town where there is a deficiency ... of sewage, drainage and paving." During the subsequent cholera outbreak in 1848, a book appeared containing maps of the locations of cholera deaths in Exeter between 1832 and 1834, together with a description of environments considered of potential relevance, such as the sites where infected clothes were destroyed and the locations of the victims' graveyards, of chemists' premises and of the soup kitchens; the maps pointed to the vulnerability of the low-lying, poorly drained districts of the old walled city. That such disease mapping clearly had an auspicious future was the prophesy in 1840 in the precursor journal to the *British Medical Journal*: "It is from the well-arranged medico-statistical and topographical inquiries that we are ultimately to expect a vast increase to our knowledge of the remote causes of diseases ..."[4]

This prophesy was to be proved accurate in 1854 by John Snow's justly celebrated maps of the contemporaneous cholera epidemics in London. These maps showed two outstanding spatial patterns.[1, 6] The first was a highly-suspicious clustering of cases around the water pump in Broad Street; and the removal of the pump's handle prevented a secondary recurrence of the epidemic. The second was the clear demarcation of cholera by water supply: in the households supplied with polluted, estuarine Thames water by the Southwark and Vauxhall Company, the rates were far higher than in the neighbouring households supplied with cleaner river water by the Lambeth Company. These simple maps conveyed the strong association of guilt between a polluted water supply and cholera. And almost 50 years on, the celebrated bacteriologist Robert Koch used the same simple mapping techniques to convey the same clear lesson to the hygienically-feckless, epidemiologically-ignorant, cholera-ravaged citizenry of the German port of Hamburg.

The latter part of the 19th century saw the study of the environmental causes of acute infections taking firm root with the founding of the Epidemiological Society of London in 1850 and the appearance of John Parkin's "Epidemiology; or the Remote Cause of Epidemic Disease in the Animal and in the Vegetable Creation" in 1873. Yet it was only towards the end of the 19th century that the chronic infectious and non-communicable diseases began to receive epidemiological attention. Of the 58 chapters in which Hirsch described in 1864 the extent of epidemiological knowledge at that time, only 20 dealt with non-infectious diseases. However, an advance in epidemiological and cartographic analysis of the less dramatic maladies was made in 1875 with the publication by a London surgeon named Alfred Haviland of a book containing maps of heart disease, dropsy, female cancer and female tuberculosis — his attempt to explain the patterns of those diseases by the geophysics of the environment.[4] Shortly after, research sponsored by the British Medical Association yielded maps showing areas of Great Britain with high and low frequencies of rickets, cancer, rheumatism, chorea and urinary calculus.[7] Although many patterns remained inexplicable, the high endemicity of rickets coincided clearly with the urban areas gloomily shouldering their grimy shrouds of industrial and domestic smoke.[1] And now we know the pathologic links: in those urban areas, the polluted air intervened between the sky's ultraviolet light and the skins of the residents, the synthesis of vitamin D precursors in those tissues was reduced, and hundreds of malnourished children with vitamin D-deficient diets developed rickets.

During the past century, disease mapping has continued to stride forward, both technologically and in the successful exploration of disease causations. The 1930s saw the publication for the British Empire Cancer Campaign of Percy Stocks' cancer maps in England and Wales. During the 1960s, the geographer Melvyn Howe produced his *National Atlas of Disease Mortality* in the United Kingdom, covering the two periods of 1954–58 and 1959–63.[8] From the 1980s onwards, disease mapping benefited from computer-graphic innovations to become a new form of publishing epidemic, with most developed countries producing their own atlases of mortality.[9–11] It might be asked: what use do they serve? One answer can be given by referring to the *Scottish Atlas of Mortality* in which an epidemiological anomaly stood out clearly — an epidemic of lung cancer which suddenly struck the small industrial town of Armadale in central Scotland between 1968 and 1975.[12] Concurrent mapping of disease and air pollution within that town showed the strong geographical association between the cancer cluster and metal pollution from the steel foundry there; the causal nature of this association was supported by its replication in a nearby town and also by the subsequent linked disappearance of both the pollution and the cancer cluster after filters had been applied to the foundry's fumestack.[13–15] In the Asian region, the magnificent mortality atlases recently produced for the People's Republic of China and for Taiwan have gained worldwide acclaim, in turn stimulating the search for new causal agents in those countries.[16–18] Thus, disease maps point out public health problems and often indicate their causes.

But what about Hong Kong? Here we have a population which presents great challenges to the would-be disease mapper. Its population is substantial and spatially confined, but internally mobile and multi-ethnic; and its aqueous and atmospheric environments are full of the pollution, both chemical and microbiological, generated by most countries during the first dizzy ascent of their economic balloons. Do these features of Hong Kong, while undoubtedly fascinating, present an insuperably hostile ecology for the would-be medical geographer? Our preliminary studies (using relatively large districts) have already given grounds for cautious optimism on the answer to that question.[19–20] The patterns of many diseases were found to be stable over time, male and female patterns often coincided where biologically plausible, and the associations between the patterns of different diseases often replicated those described for other countries with stabler populations. These early studies, however, utilized the 26 modified electoral districts as units for analysis because the demographic and mortality data for those units were readily available. But those districts were rather large and heterogeneous in socio-economic quality, so that "hot spots" of disease linked with one geographical locality or with a specific attribute of one of those socio-economic components were liable to remain submerged under the clutter of confounding variables. We decided, therefore, to re-analyze the population of Hong Kong, amalgamating the smallest population subunits available to produce larger communities which were more numerous and more socio-economically homogeneous than those of the electoral districts used in the preliminary studies. The maps in this atlas are the result.

Nowadays, doctors undertaking disease mapping in the furtherance of preventive medicine no longer need feel isolated, eccentric and defensive. The concept is widely-applied and well-established. Its achievements in the detection of causal mechanisms of disease and acknowledged benefits in the allocation of health care resources are beyond dispute. So we hope that some of the disease patterns in our *Atlas of Disease Mortalities in Hong Kong* will stimulate a sense first of puzzlement and then of tenacious enquiry amongst Hong Kong physicians and members of allied professions such as environmental health — and indeed amongst all concerned members of the educated public of the Territory. For it is the sharp observations, profound background knowledge and motivated deductions of all members of Hong Kong's society which will pave the preventive medicine pathway towards the reduction or elimination of the "hot spots" of disease which appear in the following pages.

Methods

Data Sources

Death records for the period 1979–93, held on computer tapes by the Census and Statistics Department of Hong Kong, provided the following details: sex, age, year of death, code number of the certified underlying cause of death according to the 9th revision of the International Classification of Disease (ICD 9), and the place of residence at time of death by Tertiary Planning Unit (TPU) code; the TPU was the smallest area identified on tape.

Reports of the 1981 Census, the 1986 By-census and the 1991 Census provided the demographic details for each TPU on the numbers by sex and five-year age-group, and the frequency distributions of details such as monthly household income, educational attainment and occupation.

Mortality Data

The causes of death selected comprised nine cancers (only seven for males) and six non-malignant diseases. The cancers were of the following sites: nasopharynx (ICD 147), oesophagus (ICD 150), stomach (ICD 151), colon and rectum, rectosigmoid junction and anus (ICD 153–54), liver and intrahepatic bile ducts (ICD 155), trachea, bronchus and lung (ICD 162), female breast (ICD 174) and cervix uteri (ICD 180), and leukaemia (ICD 204–8). The non-malignant diseases were: tuberculosis [TB] (ICD 010–18), hypertension [HBP] (ICD 401–4), ischaemic heart disease [IHD] (ICD 410–14), cerebrovascular disease [CVA] (ICD 430–38), pneumonia (ICD 480–86) and chronic obstructive airways disease [COAD] (ICD 490–96). The width of the categories of disease described under these headings in the ICD provided the following advantages: the numbers of deaths in the defined areas were increased, facilitating the interpretation of the mortality results in the small areas; the difficulties arising from diagnostic change over time — partly the result of modifications to ICD categories — were lessened; and the risks of artefactual distortion of results through diagnostic or clerical misclassification were minimized.

Although SMRs are sometimes based on truncated age-rates because deaths in the older age groups are more likely to have inaccurate diagnoses, mortality at all ages was used in this study for the following reasons: experience elsewhere has indicated that truncation may not alter greatly the spatial patterns of diseases;[12, 21] and truncation also removes the large numbers in the older age-groups from the analysis.

When comparing the mortality data and the demographic data, a major problem was that different versions of TPU codes had been used for compiling the data: TPU codes for the 1976 By-census had been used for the death data during 1979–93, whereas the 1981 Census, the 1986 By-census and the 1991 Census versions of the TPU codes had been used for the demographic data. The boundaries of some TPUs had changed since 1976 with the development of new towns in the New Territories, so that the 219 TPUs (from the 1976 Census) used for the death data contrasted with the 253, 239 and 274 TPUs (from the 1981 Census, the 1986 By-census and the 1991 Census respectively) used for the demographic data. This problem was resolved by amalgamating many of the (over 200) original TPUs to provide 65 larger communities which were compatible between the censuses (Appendix 1); thus, 65 was the highest number of localities compatible with the data in both the death and the demographic sources during the period studied. Deaths were excluded from the study if the place of normal residence was unknown or outside Hong Kong. The marine population was also excluded.

Changes in population structure during the inter-census years and fluctuations of the mortality rates during the period of study can distort the distributions of diseases, particularly for rare diseases in small communities. The effects of such changes were minimized by dividing the data for the 15 years into three consecutive quinquennia (1979–83, 1984–88 and 1989–93), each centred on a Census or By-census year.[12] The total numbers of available deaths in the three quinquennia were 123,061, 129,208 and 145,306.

Reliability of Mortality and Population Data

In Hong Kong, it is a statutory requirement for the documentation of the cause of death in the death certificate to be provided by a registered medical practitioner. Hence, the reliability of the mortality data was considered acceptable, with no reason to suspect major regional differences of diagnostic classification. In our previous study (1980–82), it was found that 80% of all deaths occurred in hospitals and 99.9% of the deaths had been certified by medical practitioners.[22] From 1989 to 93, 81.8% of deaths occurred in hospital and 99.98% of death certificates were issued by medical doctors. The percentages of deaths diagnosed as ill-defined and with unknown causes of morbidity and mortality (ICD code 797–99) among all deaths were 4.6, 2.5 and 2.4 for the three quinquennia respectively. The figures for unknown place of residence were 1.3%, 2.4% and 1.3% respectively.

The five years population of each community was estimated from the Census or By-census data. The calculating procedures used for community "HK1" (women only) are shown in the following table:

Age (1)	Person-years for Hong Kong 1979–83 (2)	Population of Hong Kong in 1981 Census (3)	Population of HK1 1981 (4)	Person-years estimated of HK1 (5)=(4)*(2)/(3)
0–4	1,005,600	185,733	2,973	16,118
5–9	1,000,900	196,537	2,988	15,217
	.	.	.	.
	.	.	.	.
Total	12,292,200	2,382,392	39,915	206,056

Because the estimated person-years of each community was

based on the population of that community in 1981, differences would have arisen in some communities between their estimated and their actual person-years during the period, particularly in the New Territories as a result of the development of large new towns.

The Comparison of Mortalities

The parameter used to represent the mortality level for each cause of death in the communities was the Standardized Mortality Ratio (SMR). The mortality rates by age, sex and cause of death of the whole Hong Kong population in 1979–83, 1984–88 and 1989–93 were used as the standard rates for the respective quinquennia. The expected numbers of deaths (E) during the quinquennia were derived from the products of the appropriate standard cause-specific death rates (by five-year group by sex and age) and the relevant populations (person-years) of each community. The observed numbers of deaths in each quinquennium were the total numbers of deaths during those periods in each community. The SMR is the ratio of the observed deaths to the expected deaths multiplied by 100. If a community has an SMR less than 100, its age-standardized mortality rate is lower than the figure for Hong Kong as a whole, and vice versa. The confidence intervals for SMRs are usually calculated on the assumption that the numbers of observed deaths within a community follow a Poisson distribution; however, when the number of observed deaths is large, the normal approximation is valid. In this study, therefore, when the observed numbers of deaths were equal to or larger than 25, the confidence intervals were estimated by the following equation:

$$SMR \pm 1.96(SMR/E)^{1/2}$$

If the expected numbers of deaths were less than 25, the assumption of the normal approximation is invalid. Bailar's table with 95% significance factor for the SMR was used.[23] For example, in 1979–83, the SMR of leukaemia for males in community "HK1" was 143.3 based on 11 observed deaths. According to Bailar's table, 95% lower and upper significance factors were 0.559 and 2.0 when observed deaths equal 11. Then,

the 95% confidence lower limit of that SMR = 143.3/2.0
= 71.65, and

the 95% confidence upper limit of that SMR = 143.3/0.559
= 256.35

Since 100 is included in the 95% confidence interval (71.65–256.35), the SMR (143.3) was not considered to differ statistically significantly from the value for the whole of Hong Kong at the 5% level of significance.

The Use of the Standardized Mortality Ratio (SMR)

The advantages of using the SMR as a summary index are that it has been widely used, is easy to compute and is readily understood. Kilpatrick, in comparing four different techniques for producing an age-adjusted index, concluded that the SMR was the most appropriate and efficient index to use for general purposes.[24–26] One problem with the use and interpretation of the SMR was the choice of the standard population. In our computation of SMRs, the Hong Kong Census and By-census populations were used as standards for the three quinquennia respectively. The differences in the proportion of the elderly population among the 65 communities in Hong Kong were relatively small, further justifying our use of the SMR for geographical comparison within Hong Kong itself. Despite its acknowledged limitations, therefore, we followed the practice adopted in most disease atlases in using the SMR. Nevertheless, the inherent limitations mean that aberrant values of the SMR cannot be accepted uncritically; in such cases, further, usually *ad hoc*, studies are needed to obtain and assess the age-specific rates before suspicions about the causal factors can be entertained seriously.

Index of Socio-economic Status

The variables used to describe the socio-economic status of a community, obtained from the 1981 Census, the 1986 By-census and the 1991 Census, were the percentages of the populations within the following socio-economic parameters:

(1) with no schooling in 1981 and no or lower primary schooling in 1986 and 1991;
(2) with tertiary and higher education;
(3) production workers;
(4) administrative and professional workers;
(5) with lower incomes (household monthly income below HK$2,000 in 1981, HK$3,000 in 1986 and HK$6,000 in 1991, i.e. around the 25th percentile);
(6) with higher incomes (household monthly income equal or over HK$5,000 in 1981, HK$9,000 in 1986 and HK$20,000 in 1991, i.e. around the 75th percentile).

Most of the variables were highly correlated. In 1979–83, for example, nine out of the fifteen correlation coefficients were either higher than 0.70 or less than –0.70. Therefore, factor analysis was used to combine these six variables in the various communities into one or two conceptually meaningful and relatively independent factors.[27] Factor scores (F-scores) for communities were derived to indicate their socio-economic status: the higher the F-score of a community, the higher its socio-economic status. In this study, only a single factor was found to account for 74% of total variance in 1981, 70% in 1986 and 85.2% in 1991.

Mortality Maps

Areas on each map were given one of seven types of colour-shading. Three different densities of red represented areas with three different criteria for high SMR, and three densities of green represented areas within different categories of low SMR. The criteria for colour-shading were:

(1) dark red: SMR greater than 100, in the top 20% of the 65 communities and with statistical significance at $p < 0.05$;
(2) red: SMR greater than 100, with statistical significance, but not in the top 20% of the 65 communities;
(3) pink: SMR greater than 100, in the top 20%, but not statistically significant;
(4) light green: SMR less than 100, in the lowest 20%, but not statistically significant;
(5) green: SMR less than 100, with statistical significance, but not in the lowest 20%;

(6) dark green: SMR less than 100, in the lowest 20%, and with statistical significance at $p < 0.05$;

(7) yellow: the remaining communities, with SMRs which did not satisfy the above criteria or where the observed and expected numbers of deaths from a particular cause during the five years were fewer than four, even if the SMR was in the highest 20% or in the lowest 20%. This exclusion was intended to reduce the epidemiological distraction caused by communities with small populations where the SMRs are less reliable than those based on larger populations.

The maps were produced at the Department of Community & Family Medicine and the Department of Geography of The Chinese University of Hong Kong, using the "Atlas Pro" programme on the Macintosh IIsi computer.

For each cause of death, the maps are followed by four summary tables and one graph containing the numbers of deaths and the SMRs for each of the communities, the age-sex-specific mortality rates, the number of communities on the maps by category based on SMR and values of the SMR which divide the 65 communities into quintiles. A map of the 65 communities is shown.

Maps of the Socio-economic and Physical Environment

Population densities and percentages of old age populations (aged 65 and over) in 1981, 1986 and 1991, the change in population in the 65 communities, the F-score in 1981, 1986 and 1991 and land use data are provided.

Cautions on Interpretation

(1) **Ecological fallacies**[28–29]

Ecological studies are more prone to the problems of confounding and more subject to bias by systematic errors in exposure measurement. The presence of potential confounding factors and their effects have to be considered carefully. The greatest weakness of ecological studies is that, for reasons of unavailability of data, one is often unable to assess the effects of confounding factors. Associations that occur in aggregated data might be spurious and may be subject to considerable confounding. However, they are less affected by random errors.

(2) **Problems with mapping communities with small numbers of deaths.**

When few deaths are reported in a district, the resultant SMR is highly unstable. The maps have allowed those districts with very small numbers of deaths (i.e., less than four) to be identified by their yellow colour. The risk of making epidemiological interpretations from SMRs based on small numbers is well known, and must be borne in mind when viewing these maps. The reader is advised to check the legend of the maps for the correct interpretation of the colour codes and refer to the tables following the maps for the numbers of deaths and the confidence intervals of the SMRs in the communities.

Description of Maps

Commentary

The presentation of data (whether as tables or maps) accompanied by speculation and informed comment is a tradition started by the pioneers of epidemiology and medical mapping, such as John Graunt, William Farr and John Snow — a tradition continued by modern successors including Melvyn Howe, Fraentzel-Beyme, Martin Gardner and McGlashan.[8–11] Such commentaries have proposed causal hypotheses, many of which were later proved correct; but even those ultimately abandoned were creative through their challenge to other epidemiologists to develop more plausible hypotheses of causation; such devil's advocacy, as by Mephistopheles in Goethe's *Faust*, "must, like a devil, be creative". In seeking to continue this tradition of intellectual adventure through this *Atlas*, nevertheless, readers must also maintain the parallel tradition of exercising both vigilance and caution: vigilance to detect the unexpected or previously undetected pattern of possible biological importance, and caution in remembering the scope for epidemiological artefact (such as from migration, misdiagnosis or clerical error) and for the "ecological fallacy";[28] for deaths from a disease in an area are not necessarily the result of the current environment. Indeed they may be from a minority group atypical of the broad social and ethnic categories of that area's population. These cautions underlie the present commentary, in which we outline the ecologies of the diseases as found elsewhere and ask the reader's opinion on whether or not those patterns and causal "risk factors" might explain some of the map patterns in Hong Kong. We hope the commentaries will stimulate widespread interest; for suggestions from Hong Kong residents with detailed background knowledge of some of the districts could help preventive medicine to uncover and eliminate causal factors in the Territory.

Population Changes

The maps for total population change between 1981–86 and between 1986–91 show many similarities and some differences (Pages 47–48). On Hong Kong Island, for example, populations in the Mid-levels and the Southern Districts generally rise in both periods, whereas those in the districts along the north coast decline. However, Quarry Bay (HK15) shows a decline in the earlier period but a substantial growth in the later, whereas Tai Hang/North Point (HK10) shows the opposite; Aberdeen (HK20) shows a substantial increase in the earlier period, but the growth in the later period is markedly smaller. In Kowloon, most districts show a decline in both periods; in the New Territories, by contrast, most populations grow in both periods, with the consistent exceptions of some districts of Tsuen Wan (NT2, 5 & 6), part of Fanling (NT14) and Islands (NT19).

During the three quinquennia, more districts show relatively large proportions of elderly people (11%+, aged 65 and over), particularly between the last two censuses: 2 in 1981, 5 in 1986, 17 in 1991 (Pages 44–46). Nevertheless, the general pattern remains relatively constant. The "mortality hot spot" of Wan Chai southern (HK5) and its neighbour with relatively normal mortality (HK4) share similar proportions at the three censuses — a phenomenon ripe for epidemiological investigation. The increasing concentrations of districts in northern Kowloon with high proportions have obvious implications for health care planning, as has the high proportion on the less accessible Island (NT18 & 19).

F-Score

The maps for 1981, 1986 and 1991 are broadly similar, indicating stability of socio-economic geography. Hong Kong Island generally has affluent districts, the most affluent occupying a central axis running west/east. The poor districts are Aberdeen (HK20) and Chai Wan south (HK17). In Kowloon, the axis of affluence runs vertically from Tsim Sha Tsui (KL1) to Kowloon Tong (KL17), with an isolated district on the extreme west (KL11). In the New Territories, only part of Tsuen Wan (NT1) falls into the affluent category, in both 1986 and 1991; the more southerly districts (NT2–3, 5–6 & 16–17) are intermediate; and the least affluent districts are in the central and northern locations, but include Islands and Cheung Chau (NT18 & 19).

Nasopharyngeal Cancer (NPC)

The global pattern is highly relevant to Hong Kong,[18, 30–32] located almost centrally in this cancer's hyperendemic heartland of the Pacific Pool territories, where the age-specific rates rise steeply after the age of twenty years to peak at the late 50s. Elsewhere, notably, high rates are also found in Africa and amongst native tribes of northern North America which also experience high rates of primary liver cancer, another cancer burden for Hong Kong. The environmental causation of NPC is betrayed by the tell-tale epidemiological signs: migrants from high-risk areas who adopt the lifestyles of low-risk countries show declining rates; conversely, high rates develop among individuals of European (low risk) origin when they live in high-risk areas and are reared according to the habits of their adopted countries. Causal factors proposed include the Epstein-Barr (EB) virus infection, salted fish consumed during early childhood, dietary lack of fresh vegetables and fruit with a consequent deficiency of vitamin C, industrial or domestic air pollutants and a genetic component. Although DNA from the EB virus, which is widespread in Southeast Asia, has been found in NPC cells, high NPC rates do not always accompany that finding. So whether the virus forms part of a causal mechanism or is merely coincidental is still unclear. For the salted fish hypothesis,[31] high-risk groups such as those in Hong Kong (particularly boat-dwellers) and southern China are known to feed salted fish with rice porridge (congee) to their babies during and after weaning, probably with little fresh fruit and vegetables. So the causal sequence might be: a deficiency of vitamin C allows nitrosation of amines in the upper bowel; the carcinogenic nitrosamines are circulated from there to the nasopharyngeal tissues, peculiarly sensitive to chemicals amongst the young; there they sensitize the tissues to the effects of some further carcinogen (tumour promoter or cocarcinogen) — perhaps the EB virus or some chemical pollutant — in inhaled air; and NPC starts to develop. But it remains unclear why male rates are nearly twice those of females, unless male babies are fed more of the dietary carcinogen or have a sex-linked vulnerability to the carcinogens.

In Hong Kong as elsewhere, the cancer affects males much more frequently than females. Encouragingly, the incidence and mortality rates for both sexes have fallen sharply during recent decades: indoor pollution from cooking stoves may have declined during this time, but it is perhaps less likely that traditional religious practices such as incense burning have also done so; however, the traditional diet of salted fish given to young children in Hong Kong may have become less common as a result of the rising costs of that food. In all three periods, the patterns partly resemble those of liver cancer in sparing the affluent areas. Thus, relatively few areas of high mortality are found on Hong Kong Island. This congruence between the mortality patterns of both cancers possibly indicates a common predisposing role for poor hygiene. During the first two periods, high rates are present frequently in poor or traditional districts such as Aberdeen (HK20) on Hong Kong Island and Cheung Chau (NT18) in the New Territories. However, by the last period the pattern has altered substantially, with only Cheung Chau showing persistently high mortality. For the New Territories, a distinctive feature is the many districts with elevated rates in the first period, the near-elimination of such rates in the second period, and the resurgence of a few higher rates in the last period; this phenomenon is difficult to explain through the hypothesis of dramatic changes in indoor pollution from cooking, in salted fish eating or in incense burning. Indeed, studies in Hong Kong have not as yet demonstrated any risk from indoor air pollution by the incense from joss sticks or by fumes from cooking stoves or oil lamps, although a Buddhist or ancestor-worship religious background and the presence of a religious altar in the house have been noted as (not necessarily causal) associations. So the patterns remain unexplained.

Oesophageal Cancer

The global pattern shows intriguing differences in rates between adjacent countries. In Latin America, high male rates are found in a cluster of Latin American countries including Chile, Argentina, Uruguay and Paraguay which contrast with low rates in neighbouring countries; and in the Old World, a band of countries with high rates extends from East Africa through the Middle East, south of the Caspian Sea and through Afghanistan to western China.[33] In the USA, the highest rate for black males in Washington DC was twice the national rate for male Afro-Americans and seven times higher than that of Caucasian Americans.[34] These patterns have incriminated a variety of agents, possibly sometimes working together: apple brandy in northwest France, dietary factors (low vitamin C, low molybdenum, pickled vegetables and dietary nitrosamines) in parts of China,[35–38] and tobacco, opium, vitamin A and C deficiencies, and iron deficiency elsewhere. Nevertheless, it must be remembered that most data on this cancer do not allow the numbers or rates of squamous carcinomas to be distinguished from those of adenocarcinomas, which have different aetiologies.[39]

Hong Kong's male and female rates have ranked high internationally. It is around the fifth commonest cause of cancer deaths in males, with its rate remaining stable; in females, it is less common and is declining. On Hong Kong Island, high rates are found more than once in Chai Wan (HK17) and in Aberdeen (HK20), a district beset with high rates for many other diseases. However, the outstanding feature of the maps is a huge, persistent cluster of high rates in districts in northeast Kowloon, some with high proportions of people originating from the Shantou (汕頭) area of China, itself notorious for high rates for this cancer.[40–42] This clustering in Kowloon persists throughout the three periods for males, but diminishes rapidly for females. In the New Territories, districts in Tsuen Wan (NT2 & 4), Tuen Mun (NT8) and Yuen Long (NT11) show elevated rates more than once. Dietary habits appear the most probable cause of these patterns, particularly in northeast Kowloon; nevertheless, it is difficult to interpret the discrepancy between the evolving male and female patterns according to that hypothesis unless the food eaten by men and by women differs in some important component.

Gastric Cancer

The global map shows huge differences in mortality rates: those in Japan around three- to four-fold higher than those in Canada for both sexes; low rates consistently in India and in sub-Saharan Africa; and in Mainland China, high rates particularly in coastal and northern regions.[43–45] Environmental causation is clear, because when ethnic groups migrate, their risks change. Amongst Japanese migrants to the USA, for instance, mortality in the first generation falls by 28%, and in the second generation by 62%. Genetic factors have a minor influence in modulating vulnerability to gastric cancer, as suggested by its link with blood group A.[46] From studies of geographic patterns, the diet is now recognized as the main influence. Suspect components include a high concentration of nitrates in drinking water and foods rich in nitrosamines, often preserved by salt, pickling or smoke-curing; protection may be given by fruit, fresh vegetables and dairy products, with their vitamins A, C and E.[47–50] The hypothesis is that salted or pickled foods generate atrophic gastritis; the associated high pH promotes the proliferation of bacterial flora within the bowel which convert the dietary nitrate first to nitrite and then to carcinogenic N-nitroso compounds. This hypothesis is consistent with the declining rates in Western countries, where food conservation has moved from chemical preservatives to refrigeration, and where food industries have organized the pan-seasonal and widespread availability of fresh fruit and vegetables at low cost. As yet unknown carcinogens in occupational environments must underlie the high rates of gastric cancer in workforces such as ceramic, stone and textile workers, miners, fishermen, clerical workers, printers, painters and workers in the metal, construction and chemical industries.[26] Lastly, infection with the bacterium *Helicobacter pylori* has been implicated in the causal mechanism.[51–52]

In Hong Kong, the mortality rates follow the international trend in showing a male predominance and in declining during recent decades. Being the second commonest cause of cancer death in both sexes in the 1960s, it had fallen to around the fifth place for both sexes by 1989. However, the incidence for both sexes has risen recently. The maps show that the strong link with poverty, noted in the West, does not hold consistently between periods and between sexes in Hong Kong. One district in the southwest of Hong Kong Island must generate particular concern: Aberdeen (HK20), with its badly polluted harbour, has high rates in males in all three periods, but in females only in the second period; the same district shows high rates also for NPC, liver cancer and (to a lesser degree) oesophageal cancer. Why? Elsewhere, the high rates in Chai Wan (HK17) are present in both sexes in the first period only, and in eastern Kowloon (KL25) and Islands (NT19) in males in the first and third periods respectively. The strong epidemiological links found elsewhere between gastric cancer and a fish diet containing potential carcinogens suggest similar links for populations of Hong Kong. Their diets and the concentrations of pollutants in their fish diets merit investigation, not least to explain why the incidence rates should have risen recently and why the male rates should be substantially higher than those of the females.

Colorectal Cancer

(Colon and rectal cancers are often considered together: the two bowel segments are difficult to demarcate anatomically, and many cancers arise from the disputed area; their international mortality rates are correlated positively; and many causal factors are common to both cancers.[9, 43, 53])

Globally, high mortality rates affect affluent populations such as in the United Kingdom and Western Europe, Australia, New Zealand and North America (Caucasians) but are rare in the poorer, more traditional regions such as Africa and Asia. The evidence for environmental causes is strong: the rates for migrants shift from the values in their home countries to those of their adopted lands, as they abandon their traditional diets. Of causal importance are diets rich in animal fats and low in vegetables and other high residue foods. The affluent Western diet may activate the following sequence: an altered bowel flora synthesizing carcinogens from faecal residues; an increased substrate of metabolites from the fatty diet enhancing this synthesis of carcinogens; less dilution of faecal carcinogens; and intestinal sluggishness increasing the contact time between faecal carcinogens and bowel mucosa. The geographical and social class patterns support this causal hypothesis: wealthy groups with their richer diets have a higher mortality. Occupational factors, such as textiles, leather, metals and acrylonitrile used in the production of plastic and synthetic fibres, have also been proposed.[26] Diseases associated with this cancer include cancers of the breast (possibly through the same dietary mechanisms), uterus and ovary, and ulcerative colitis and Crohn's disease.[43] A small genetic component for colorectal cancer is shown by its link with diseases such as familial polyposis coli.[54–55]

Within Hong Kong, the steady increase in mortality and incidence in both sexes is consistent with a known change in dietary practice from the traditional meals rich in vegetable fibre to the more Western diets, as the population has become wealthier and more exposed to international influences. This interpretation is supported by the maps: generally lower rates in the poorer and more traditional areas of the New Territories (where few "hot spots" are found during the three periods) score low values consistently; and higher rates on the northern districts of the Island — a pattern seen more strongly with breast cancer, also linked with unhealthy diets. However, in the most affluent parts of Kowloon (e.g. KL17) the males show consistently high rates, whereas the males in some of the wealthy districts of Hong Kong Island (e.g. HK21) are spared. Females in these districts have high rates in both the first and third period. Occupational risk factors cannot be discerned in these patterns.

Liver Cancer

(Hepatocellular carcinoma, the most common type of primary liver cancer is described.)

This cancer[43, 56–57] is a particular scourge in Southeast Asia (particularly Hong Kong, Taiwan and southeast coastal China), southern and eastern Europe, and sub-Saharan Africa where it can be the commonest male cancer. Within the Asian countries of the Pacific Basin, however, Caucasian residents have low rates. Male victims usually predominate, possibly reflecting the role of endogenous androgens. Migration studies incriminate environmental causes: migrants from high-risk to low-risk areas adapt their rates to their new environments: for example, male and female Chinese immigrants in the USA have incidence rates eleven and five times respectively those of their white US counterparts, whereas the US-born offspring of those Chinese immigrants have rates only two- to three-fold higher. And the carcinogens? In warm, humid climates of Africa and Asia, foods such as groundnuts and cereal can become heavily contaminated by carcinogenic aflatoxin from fungi; in China, the highest rates (up to 70% and 57% of all male and female cancers respectively) are in warm, humid coastal areas and in the southeast, notably along the Yangtze delta. The hepatitis B virus (HBV) has also been incriminated as an important cause in Africa and Asia: the cancer and the HBV carriage rates are far higher on the Asian coast of the Pacific Basin than on the American coast; familial clustering of the carrier state and of the cancer has been reported in several countries, with infection of the children both vertically from a "carrier" mother around birth and laterally from other children during early childhood.[58] Nevertheless, some localities have a high infection rate but a low cancer rate, and so other factors must contribute to the causal sequence. The better food hygiene in urban populations may protect them from the higher rates usually in rural areas. Other lifestyle factors implicated include alcoholism, tobacco, nitrosamines, and occupational exposure to organic chemicals. Environmental and lifestyle factors may interact to enhance their causal potencies.

The male predominance of liver cancer found elsewhere is also present in Hong Kong, where for years it has been the second commonest cancer in males but only the fourth in females. The incidence and mortality rates have changed little during recent years, but in both sexes the rates for those below 50 years have been falling. The maps show low rates quite consistently in the affluent, urbanized districts, where people are probably more hygiene-conscious. Conversely, high rates are found in densely crowded areas, but also notably in the New Territories where a relatively high frequency of "hot spots" is seen in the more traditional and rural districts such as Tai Po (NT15), Sai Kung (NT17), Tsing Yi Island (NT7), Tsuen Wan New Town (NT5) and Cheung Chau (NT18). On Hong Kong Island, high rates appear frequently in Aberdeen (HK20) and Shau Kei Wan (HK16) during the two earlier periods, and in southern Wan Chai (HK5) in the first and third period; in Kowloon they appear frequently in Kowloon City/Wong Tai Sin central (KL21 & 23), Sham Shui Po (KL16), Cheung Sha Wan south (KL15) and Yau Ma Tei (KL5) in different periods. This spatial pattern, mostly associated with dense crowding and urbanization or with poorer coastal or fishing communities, may be linked with the state of general environmental hygiene, possibly linked with fishing or sea water pollution and food hygiene.

Lung Cancer

This disease has followed a slow but massive global epidemic from early this century, when its textbook description was "among the rarest forms of disease",[59] to its current eminence as the commonest cancer in men and women in many developed countries. In the UK where the Industrial Revolution began, the rates rose early;[25,43,45,60] other Western countries followed after some decades, and in later-industrialized countries, such as Japan, Taiwan and Mainland China, the rates increased only comparatively recently. Mortality rates can differ substantially between nations even where these have comparable cultures or genetics: in the UK they are about twice those in Australia and New Zealand or in Denmark and France. Migration studies have confirmed environmental factors as causes, of which the most widespread globally is tobacco smoke from direct inhalation or "passive smoking";[61–65] poorer people usually show higher rates because they smoke more. However, the urban-rural gradient seen in many countries and similar to that for chronic bronchitis may reflect not only different tobacco habits but greater exposure to carcinogens in polluted urban air.[12–15,34,66] In parts of Asia, indoor pollution from cooking stoves has been blamed[41,67] for the high female rates which cause the sex ratios of mortality (male divided by female) to fall as low as 2.16 in China, in contrast to the high ratios (ranging between 6 and 12) in the West. Occupational causes include radon, carcinogenic metals and asbestos in mines and factories.[26,34]

In Hong Kong, lung cancer is the commonest cancer for both males and females; its rates have been rising steeply for both sexes; and females in particular have high rates on the international scale. The maps illustrate the patterns related to social class seen elsewhere, generally with affluent areas spared and high rates in the poor areas on Hong Kong Island and Kowloon; inexplicably as yet, high rates only appear widely in the New Territories in the last period when a large number of districts emerge with high mortality for males only. High rates appear frequently in many districts. On Hong Kong Island they are found in Aberdeen (HK20) in the earlier two periods, in southern Wan Chai (HK5), which also has high rates for liver cancer, cerebrovascular accidents, ischaemic heart disease and pneumonia, Shau Kei Wan (HK16), Chai Wan (HK17) and southern Pokfulam (HK19) in several periods, and in West/Sheung Wan (HK2) (females only) and Tai Hang (HK11) in the two earlier periods. In Kowloon, high rates are seen repeatedly in southern Cheung Sha Wan (KL15), Sham Shui Po (KL16) and southern Kowloon City/Wong Tai Sin (KL23). In the New Territories, high rates are seen in Shatin (NT16) in all periods; and also, though less consistently, on Tsing Yi and Cheung Chau Islands (NT7 & 18). These patterns may result from several causes, of which fumes from tobacco, industrial pollution and indoor cooking are the most obvious suspects. Other factors cannot be excluded, however, such as radon from buildings.

Breast Cancer

This disease is feared in the affluent West where it is often the commonest female cancer; women in poorer countries in Asia, Africa and elsewhere are usually spared.[43, 45, 68] However, migrants from poor to affluent countries show mortality rates slowly rising towards the high values in their host countries: for example, black Africans in Africa have rates only 15% of the rates of US Caucasians, whereas the comparable figure for US blacks is 75%. These findings implicate environmental risk factors.[69–76] The most important type of factor arises from the metabolism of endogenous sex hormones, expressed as early menarche, short ovulatory cycles, nulliparity, late first full-term pregnancy, late menopause and raised post-menopausal weight; exogenous sex hormones, for example for contraception, may be carcinogenic at the extremes of reproductive life. The second type of risk factor, particularly for older cases, is a dietary excess of animal fats. The two types may interact: a fatty diet enhancing the synthesis and secretion of bile acids, and finally the conversion of these acids by bowel microbes into oestrogenic compounds; and obesity itself can promote the production of oestrogens by adipose tissues. Ionizing radiation and tobacco are also incriminated.[43, 77] Other causes, as yet undetected, in urban environments are suggested by their higher rates in the urbanized areas of many countries including China.[16, 41] Breast and colorectal cancers share the unusual social class gradient where higher classes have higher risks, perhaps through the dietary mechanism. A genetic influence has been shown by family histories and twin studies.[43, 78]

In Hong Kong, it is the third most frequent female cancer but contributes less than 10% to total cancer. Mortality and incidence rates have changed little recently; so Hong Kong, despite its new affluence, is not yet following the Western trend of a slow increase. The map patterns are as predicted from international studies in general, but not in detail. For example, high rates affect frequently the more affluent Hong Kong Island along or near the north coast but also, sporadically, inland; but they spare not only its poor districts but also many of its most affluent ones; Kowloon, with its fewer affluent districts, has few high rates, but these affect sporadically both poor and affluent districts (that of southern Kowloon City/Wong Tai Sin (KL23) being consistent but unexplained), and most of its wealthiest districts are spared; and the poorer districts of the New Territories are almost totally spared, striking exceptions being the poor districts of Cheung Chau and Island (NT18 & 19) in the first and last periods. Nevertheless, these patterns, despite the exceptions, may suggest that generally the traditional lifestyles in the poor areas of the New Territories, Kowloon and the Island are maintaining their protective effects, that the wealthiest communities know the risks of affluent lifestyles and how to combat them, but that some "transitional" communities have neither form of protection.

Cancer of the Cervix Uteri (Cervical Cancer)

The global pattern contains intriguing contrasts:[43, 79] generally high in Latin America (Chile, Costa Rica and Venezuela) but low in Argentina and Dominica; generally intermediate in Europe although high in Portugal but low in Spain, high in Denmark and West Germany but low in nearby countries, and high in Romania but low in Bulgaria; and generally low in the Far East and Australia. While some of these contrasts may arise from differences in diagnostic fashions, they may also result from differences in ethnic customs: in the USA, for example, women of African origin have higher rates than Caucasians. Different degrees of access to health care may also contribute to the patterns, as within China, where rural death rates generally exceed those of cities.[40] Although in most countries the rates have been falling for many decades, rising rates have been noted for the youngest age-groups. The risk factors are linked with sexual behaviour: early marriage and childbearing, multiparity, early sexual activity with multiple partners, a history of infection with sexually transmitted disease, and avoidance of barrier contraception;[80–81] nuns have very low rates. The herpes simplex virus and the human papilloma virus have been implicated.[79]

In Hong Kong, by contrast with breast cancer, the mortality and incidence rates for this cancer have fallen steadily during recent decades. The maps may support the sex-related aetiology, showing a consistent pattern of high rates in the Wan Chai (HK4 & 5) area of Hong Kong Island and the Yau Ma Tei/Mong Kok areas (KL4 & 5) of Kowloon, often considered the most residential of "red light" districts. Other districts along the north and the west shoreline of Hong Kong Island and to the north of Kowloon also show a tendency to reappear with elevated rates. In the New Territories, however, no district shows recurrent high rates.

Leukaemia

The global geography of mortality follows broad patterns: high rates for affluent areas including Canada, northwestern Europe including France and some Scandinavian countries, New Zealand and Israel; and low rates in poorer countries in Latin America, southern and eastern Europe, North Africa and Asia.[25, 43] Ionizing radiation is the cause most widely known, and lay people are aware of the risks from sources including military tests, nuclear power station disasters such as at Chernobyl, more controversially the neighbourhood effects from nuclear power stations, and medical procedures.[82–90] Background radon and the electromagnetic fields from power lines have been implicated.[90–96] A leukaemogenic interaction of different viruses within mixing populations in new towns has been suggested,[97] as has a risk to the foetus from viral infections of the mother.[98–101] Chemical risk factors include benzene (convincingly) and insecticides and herbicides (less clearly); high rates have been found amongst workforces in the electricity, printing, rubber and petrochemical industries; the last has been implicated in "neighbourhood leukaemia".[26, 54, 102–3] Genetic influences may underlie the tendency for familial aggregation and also the increased risk among people with Down's syndrome.[104]

In Hong Kong, leukaemia provides only 2.5–3% of mortality from total cancer, male and female rates are stable, and the sex ratio shows only a slight male dominance. Although the high levels of natural radiation in parts of the Territory may be a potential risk, the inconsistency in the spatial patterns seems to discount that view. Such risks may exist, however, but may be obscured by other effects, such as by chemicals at work or in polluted neighbourhoods, viral mixing inevitable in overcrowded, immigrant-heavy populations of Hong Kong, or the epidemiological jumbling from incessant residential migration between districts (the jumbling effect being compounded by the statistical instability inherent in the small numbers of deaths). Nevertheless, further attention seems merited for Kowloon City/Wong Tai Sin (KL20) with its high rates for females in the first two periods and for males in the first period; and Cheung Sha Wan southern (KL15) in the second and third period. Other districts with recurring high rates include Wan Chai southern (HK5), Shau Kei Wan (HK16), Tsim Sha Tsui (KL1), Mid-level/Peak/Tai Hang (HK6) in females only, Shek Kip Mei (KL14), Kwun Tong/Jordan Valley (KL24) and Tsuen Wan (NT2).

Ischaemic Heart Disease (IHD)

Like lung cancer, IHD is now accepted as commonplace in modern life. It was rare in the West earlier this century and is still uncommon in under-developed countries, but is increasing in developing countries as their affluence increases.[45, 105–7] Like lung cancer, therefore, IHD is inflicting a slow but gigantic epidemic on developed societies, particularly on the younger age-groups of males. The wide differences in mortality between and within countries strongly implicate environmental causes, a view supported by migration studies: IHD for migrants from low-risk countries (such as Japan) to high-risk countries begins to rise after the migrants have adopted the lifestyles of their host countries. The recognized risk factors, in order of importance, include Western-style diets rich in animal fats and low in fruit and vegetable fibre, tobacco, hypertension, diabetes mellitus, and probably physical inactivity and stress; populations drinking "soft" water also tend to have high rates.[45, 108–16] The low mortality in southern Europe has led to the recognition of the protective value of the "Mediterranean diet" rich in fish (for unsaturated oils), red wine, olive oil and vegetables and fruit (for fibre and anti-oxidant vitamins).[114, 116]

Despite Hong Kong's growing wealth, with the adoption of affluent Western diets weakening the hold of healthy traditional foods, rates during recent decades have stayed relatively constant. However, the evolving map patterns, although complex, appear to reinforce the epidemiological warnings from elsewhere. Thus, the first two periods show a near-total absence of high rates in the poorer New Territories; two of these exceptions are females in non-affluent districts of Yuen Long (NT9 & 10) in 1984–88, and these districts reappear in the final period for both sexes, joined by males in districts in Tsuen Wan and Islands. High rates are found persistently in a few districts in Kowloon, but these can be wealthier districts such as Tsim Sha Tsui (KL1) and Kowloon Tong (KL17), or poorer districts such as Cheung Sha Wan (KL15) and Kowloon City/Wong Tai Sin (KL23). On Hong Kong Island, similarly, the many high-mortality districts during the first period comprise the strong band of affluent districts including the Peak and Mid-levels (HK6–9) among males, but not females; but this pattern weakens visibly in the middle period and almost vanishes in the last period; the eastern district of Chai Wan South (HK17) and the poor area of southern Wanchai (HK5) follow a similar evolution; however, the poor area of Aberdeen (HK20) shows high mortality for females throughout the three periods. Thus, the strong gradient by social class in the West today (where an unhealthy diet and tobacco cause the high rates amongst the poor) does not fit Hong Kong precisely, where the maps may illustrate a more complex pattern of the epidemiological transition often described: low rates in poor groups practising the traditional lifestyles of the New Territories and also in affluent Pokfulam (HK18), high rates not only in affluent groups in Kowloon and Hong Kong Island but also in poor areas there.

Cerebrovascular Disease (CVA) and Hypertension (HBP)

(Hypertension is included here because it is a main risk factor for CVA, and so mortality can often be attributed to either cause of death.)

CVA, or "stroke", includes intracerebral and subarachnoid haemorrhage and brain infarction from embolism, thrombosis or atheroma, causing typically a sudden focal deficit in the function of the central nervous system. The exact pathological mechanism is often unclear, and this condition is often misdiagnosed, so that study findings require cautious interpretation. Globally, high rates are found notoriously in Japan, but it is also an important cause of death in the West. Risk factors, in approximate descending order of importance, include hypertension, hyperlipidaemia, diabetes mellitus, obesity, rheumatic heart disease and atrial fibrillation, tobacco, alcohol, "soft" drinking water, salty diet, oral contraceptives and a cold climate.[22, 117–18] CVA has an important economic dimension through the costs of hospitalization and rehabilitation of survivors.

In Hong Kong, the maps for CVA show affluent areas spared but poorer areas repeatedly suffering high rates. On Hong Kong Island, these include Aberdeen (HK20), Shau Kei Wan (HK16) and southern Wanchai (HK5); of these, however, only Aberdeen persists with high mortality in the final period. In Kowloon, a persistent "hot spot" is present in southern Cheung Sha Wan (KL15). Remarkably, the poor Kowloon City/Wong Tai Sin (KL23), which in the last two periods shows high rates in both sexes, adjoins the affluent northern Ho Man Tin (KL6) which is similarly afflicted. In the New Territories, high mortality is found repeatedly in Tsing Yi Island (NT7), western Tsuen Wan (NT3), Yuen Long districts (NT9–11) and Cheung Chau Island (NT18).

For hypertension, the maps show equally striking patterns. Hong Kong Island has remarkably few districts with high mortality. Kowloon has high rates persistently in Yau Ma Tei (KL5) and in and near Kowloon City/Wong Tai Sin (KL23) and Kowloon Tong (KL17) where CVA rates are also high. In the New Territories, unexpectedly, high rates develop and persist during the middle and last periods across the central, horizontal band of districts, of which those on the west also have high CVA rates. These patterns, which are in sharp contrast with those of IHD, may result from such factors such as tobacco, hereditary and dietary factors.

Non-malignant Respiratory Diseases: Chronic Obstructive Airways Disease (COAD), Pneumonia, Tuberculosis (TB)

COAD encompasses a spectrum of respiratory disorders with overlapping features: chronic bronchitis, asthma and emphysema. High rates are common in industrialized countries. For bronchitis and emphysema, risk factors include tobacco, general urban and industrial air pollution, and some occupational factors including toxic fumes and respirable dusts in quarries, foundries and similar workplaces.[119–20] For asthma, a genetic component is often present, but environmental and occupational allergens such as pollens, fungi, house mites and chemicals are important factors.[121–25] Poorer people suffer more from COAD because they tend to smoke more and live in neighbourhoods with more air pollution.[126–27] The disease remains a major cause of occupational morbidity and inefficiency in many countries.[119] Mortality from chronic bronchitis has declined in Western countries since the 1960s as a result of the cleaning of air in towns and within industries and the effects of health education on smoking. For asthma, by contrast, reports from many countries suggest that asthma is a growing problem for reasons which are not yet clear.[128–33] Pneumonia (included here because it is a common outcome in the damaged lungs of sufferers from bronchitis) historically was caused by "traditional" bacteria which have now been controlled by antibiotics and by the improved immune status from better nutrition. However, influenza continues to reap its epidemic harvests, particularly amongst the young, the old and those with damaged lungs; and newer pathogens such as mycoplasma and legionella have been recognized.[134–35] A further scenario is where the immune defence has been weakened, whether by medication, through infection with human immunodeficiency virus (HIV) and the acquired immune deficiency syndrome (AIDS) or as a result of chronic exposure to environmental chemicals. Tuberculosis, long expected to become of historical interest as "Captain of the Men of Death" because of modern medication and improved natural resistance, is showing an alarming resurgence as a result of HIV infection and AIDS, increasing drug resistance and heavy migration from countries where it has yet to be properly controlled.[136–37]

In Hong Kong, respiratory disease is the commonest cause of morbidity, with attendant costs on industrial productivity, general welfare and medical spending. The maps show noteworthy patterns of mortality. For COAD, low rates are present in most of the affluent areas such as in Mid-levels (HK6–9) and also in northern Ho Man Tin (KL6). Remarkably, the poor district of Aberdeen (HK20) with its notorious record for other diseases has high rates only in males in the last period. With the exception of Wan Chai southern (HK5) and the Eastern Districts (HK16 & 17), high rates affect Hong Kong Island only rarely and sporadically. They are found more frequently in the northern districts of Kowloon (KL14, 15 & 23). But the most dramatic pattern is in the New Territories, where the red stain of high mortality can be seen to spread from its relatively isolated districts in the first period to embrace a very large number of districts in the final period, particularly for males. The contiguity of many districts with high rates may reflect the transmission of underlying infective agents; and the persistence of high rates for both males and females in many districts perhaps results from exacerbating factors such as air pollution from traffic, domestic sources or local industries. Dietary deficiencies may also be an underlying factor.

For pneumonia, many districts show high rates strikingly consistent between sexes or persistent between periods. On Hong Kong Island, Aberdeen (HK20) and Shau Kei Wan (HK16) are notable examples. In Kowloon, the high rates in southern Kowloon City/Wong Tai Sin (KL23) and southern Cheung Sha Wan (KL15) are disturbingly persistent; and the emergence of high mortality during the final period in many districts of north-central and northwest Kowloon, including the affluent western Kowloon Tong (KL17), deserves close monitoring. In the New Territories, a striking pattern similar to COAD also emerges, with the development in the final period of high rates in the many districts lying along the west-east axis. Many of the districts with high mortality from pneumonia also show high mortality for COAD or adjoin such districts. These patterns may illustrate the vulnerability of the damaged lungs of COAD to pneumonia; the role of underlying immune deficiencies from nutritional or other causes should also be considered.

For TB, the map patterns show expected features: affluent areas with low rates, a lack of high rates on Hong Kong Island, apart from southern Wanchai (HK5), persistent "hot spots" in crowded central and western Kowloon, most notably Shek Kip Mei (KL14), its persistence in Sheung Shui/Fanling/Tai Po (NT15) and Sai Kung (NT17) in the New Territories, and a slight decline in the number of significantly high-rate districts with time. However, concern must arise from the persistence of high rates in the northern districts of Kowloon through to the final period, and from the unexpected appearance of high rates in the affluent western Kowloon Tong (KL17), where the social ecology might have been expected to inhibit its emergence.

Comparison of the SMR Ranks between Quinquennia

The stability of the ranking of the diseases in the districts was examined by correlation analysis and compared between the periods and between the sexes. Hong Kong Island shows the greatest stability of ranking, and this stability persists throughout the whole period. Kowloon shows substantially less stability during the comparison of the earlier quinquennia, but the stability has increased to match that of Hong Kong Island in the comparison of the middle and the last quinquennia. The New Territories, however, starts with very low stability and shows only a slight gain.

Differences in the stability are seen between the sexes, with more statistically significant associations appearing between males in the different periods than between females. The associations are stronger, by sex, in Hong Kong Island than in the New Territories.

For Hong Kong as a whole (Appendix 4.1), the correlation coefficients between the disease ranks in the first (1979–83) and last (1989–93) quinquennia shows a high degree of statistical significance for males (12 of the 15 diseases) and to a lesser extent for females (6 of the 17 diseases). These values are intermediate between those in the comparisons of 1979–83 versus 1984–88 and 1984–88 versus 1989–93. In the latter of these two comparisons, significant female correlations increases substantially from 6 to 11. Negative correlations are few: only male leukaemia in the earliest comparison; and male leukaemia and female ischaemic heart disease and gastric cancer in the wider comparison of 1979–83 versus 1989–93. Hence, even with the inherent heterogeneity of Hong Kong taken as a whole, the patterns show a remarkable degree of statistical significance.

If the three regions are analyzed individually, the ranks of more diseases are statistically significantly correlated in the later comparison of 1984–88 versus 1989–93 (34) than in the comparison of the earlier periods (28)(Appendices 4.2–4.4); in the later period, 34 are significant, of which 62% are significant at $p \leq 0.01$; in the earlier period, 28 are significant with only 57% at $p \leq 0.01$.

An analysis of the rank correlations by the three regions (i.e. Hong Kong Island, Kowloon and the New Territories) shows marked differences. In these regions the numbers of statistically significant correlations in, respectively, the earlier (1979–83, 1984–88) and later (1984–88, 1989–93) periods are: 14 & 12; 7 & 13; and 7 & 9; these figures suggest a pattern of increasing demographic or epidemiological stability as time progresses in Kowloon particularly and to a much lesser extent in the New Territories. Of the ten male diseases in Hong Kong Island with statistically significant correlation coefficients (r_s) in the earlier comparison, eight are also significant in the later comparison; for females, the replicability is less. A lower replicability is also seen for correlation coefficients of the male diseases in the other two regions; but for the females there, replicability is absent.

The three regions have the same order of communities, i.e. 21, 25 and 19. Hence, the differences between their proportions of r_s with statistical significance and also of positive correlations can be attributed to differences in the changes of their demographic and environmental variables over the three periods. Accordingly, the high replicability found for the r_s on Hong Kong Island during the three quinquennia may reflect the relatively high stability of its demography and environment; similarly, the increasing proportions of significant r_s with time in the other two regions, particularly Kowloon, may reflect the increasing stability of these variables there during the second half of the period 1984–93.

Statistical differences appear between the sexes. Statistical significance is achieved far more frequently for the male correlations (19) than for the females (9) during the earlier comparison and in the later comparison (20 & 14 respectively). In both comparisons, both Hong Kong Island and Kowloon maintain the differences in r_s between the sexes with time, whereas the difference in the New Territories, which was small in the earlier comparison, reverses in the later comparison. The reason for these differences is unclear; perhaps, in Hong Kong Island and Kowloon the traditional occupational or other socio-economic factors which produce the disparities are weaker in the more mobile societies in the New Territories.

The socio-economic index (the F-Score) is correlated negatively with most diseases (Appendix 5). There are only three exceptions: colorectal cancer, breast cancer and ischaemic heart disease. However, the positive associations with both colorectal cancer and ischaemic heart disease in both males and females, which were highly significant in the first period, show substantial declines over the three periods; in the last period, they are non-significant — barely positive for the males and negative for the females. For breast cancer the association is positive throughout, but significant only in the middle period. For the negative associations, on the other hand, significant correlations are maintained or increased throughout the periods for all causes, male all cancer, NPC, liver cancer, male lung cancer, male COAD, TB, male pneumonia and male CVA; weaker negative correlations are shown by oesophageal cancer, female lung cancer, gastric cancer, cervical cancer, leukaemia, female COAD, female CVA and male HBP. The associations for both female CVA and HBP, although initially weak, show steady increases during the period.

Public Health Implications

Overview

The data, when reviewed over the three quinquennia, provide a sharp picture of the districts in Hong Kong where mortality rates from a range of diseases are consistently high, and of the districts where they are consistently low. Looking first at the locations with high mortality: when the numbers of all diseases in the top 20% of SMR ranks for each sex in all periods are combined, an enormous range is found. The highest numbers (Appendix 2) appear in Kowloon City/southern Wong Tai Sin and southern Cheung Sha Wan (KL23 & 15) with 52 each, followed by part of Yuen Long (NT9) with 37, Cheung Chau (NT18) with 35, Shau Kei Wan and Aberdeen (HK16 & 20) each with 33, southern Wan Chai (HK5) with 32, and Sham Shui Po (KL16) with 28. If the data are re-examined by excluding those diseases whose SMRs are not statistically significant, the "hot spots" remain essentially the same.

What about the "healthy" districts, i.e. those with low mortality rates ? By finding the districts with the largest number of diseases in the bottom 20% of SMR ranks (Appendix 3), for both sexes and all periods, the following districts emerged as "healthy": Pok Fu Lam (HK18) with 47, Quarry Bay (HK14) with 40, Mid-level and Mid-level/Peak (HK8 & 9) with 36 and 33 respectively, Cheung Sha Wan (KL12) with 32, and Mid-level/Peak/Tai Hang (HK6) and eastern North Point (HK13) with 28 each. After excluding diseases without statistically significant SMRs, only two districts, Cheung Sha Wan and eastern North Point are removed from the above list.

These findings, therefore, can be used as a ready starting point for public health surveillance in Hong Kong. The data provide validated signposts to the locations where preventive medicine, through successful investigations, diagnoses and interventions, can bring most benefit to the public's health.

Individual Diseases

Despite the encouragingly downward trends for both incidence and mortality from NPC, it is disturbing that the causal origins and mechanisms still remain obscure despite several valuable studies of this disease; the "hot spots" districts, particularly Aberdeen, are ripe for epidemiological investigation of lifestyle factors which undoubtedly underlie this disease. For bronchogenic cancer, the persistence of the patterns and their correlations with other diseases provide a strong incentive for investigating systematically the lifestyles and environments of the affected communities in the search for carcinogenic agents. If tobacco is found to be the main culprit, these map patterns also provide baselines for evaluating the effects of health education (and perhaps higher taxation) on tobacco consumption. The strange immunity of the poor districts in the New Territories certainly warrants further study. For oesophageal and gastric cancers, the striking and persistent geographical patterns demonstrate a pressing need for public health practitioners to investigate and eliminate the causal factors of these painful and totally preventable cancers within the high risk communities. Colorectal cancer, with its increasing frequency in Hong Kong and its geographical patterns at least partly explicable through known risk factors, is an apt target for vigorous preventive medicine. For liver cancer, although the systematic immunization programme with the vaccine against HBV can be expected to lower the incidence in future, public health doctors should continue to seek other aetiological factors and to eliminate them. Breast cancer, despite its current "low profile" in Hong Kong as a whole, shows map patterns (including the unexplained "hot spots" near Kai Tak Airport) which challenge health education here because of its known links with an affluent lifestyle with unwise dietary habits; there exists ample scope for primary prevention, guiding people towards healthier diets, and perhaps for secondary prevention through screening services for high-risk individuals in high-rate areas — perhaps by means of mobile clinics moving from one such area to another. Although the rates for cervical cancer in Hong Kong are declining, studies in other countries are a warning that the youngest age-groups here may start to show increasing rates during the coming years; given the strong links between this cancer and behavioural factors, it is almost entirely preventable, in Hong Kong as elsewhere, through a combination of effective health education and screening services. The map patterns for IHD, CVA and hypertension, if confirmed by further studies, also suggest targetting health education at specified communities, to identify and remedy the dietary factors or other components of lifestyle responsible for those patterns, for they are largely preventable. The high rate districts of respiratory disease on Hong Kong Island and in Kowloon also merit detailed investigations and targeting by preventive medicine. And although TB is still on the decline, careful surveillance will be needed in future to block its resurgence, profiting by the immune deficiencies from AIDS or chemical pollution. In the many activities against these diseases, public health has a leading role to play. These maps suggest the most appropriate places to start.

References

1. Howe GE. *Man, Environment & Disease in Britain: A Medical Geography Through the Ages.* David & Charles, Newton Abbot, Devon 1972.
2. Needham J. *Clerks and Craftsmen in China and the West: Lectures and Addresses on the History of Science and Technology.* Cambridge University Press, Cambridge 1970.
3. Needham J. *The Grand Titration: Science and Society in East and West.* Allen and Unwin, London 1969.
4. Lloyd OL, Yu TS. Disease mapping: a valuable technique for environmental medicine. *J Hong Kong Med Ass* 1994; 46(1):3–15.
5. Underwood EA (ed). *Science, Medicine and History.* Vol 2. Oxford University Press, London 1953.
6. Howe GM. History of disease mapping. In: *An Atlas of Mortality in Scotland.* Lloyd OL, Williams FLR, Berry WG, Florey C (eds). Croom Helm, Beckenham, Kent 1987.
7. Owen I (ed). Reports of the collective Investigation Committee of the British Medical Association: Geographical distribution of the rickets, acute and subacute rheumatism, chorea, cancer and urinary calculus in the British Islands. *BMJ* 1889; 1464:113–16.
8. Howe GM. *National Atlas of Disease Mortality in the United Kingdom.* 2 vols. Nelson, London 1963–70.
9. Becker N, Frentzel-Beyme R, Wagner G. *Atlas of Cancer Mortality in the Federal Republic of Germany.* Springer Verlag, Berlin 1984.
10. Gardner MJ, Winter PD, Taylor CP, Acheson ED. *Atlas of Cancer Mortality in England and Wales 1969–78.* John Wiley, Chichester 1983.
11. McGlashan ND. Some developments in disease atlas mapping in the 1970s and 1980s. *Norsk Geogr Tidsskr* 1990; 44:211–19.
12. Lloyd OL, Williams FLR, Berry WG, Florey C (eds). *An Atlas of Mortality in Scotland.* Croom Helm, Beckenham, Kent 1987.
13. Lloyd OL. Respiratory cancer clustering associated with localized industrial air pollution. *Lancet* 1978; 8059:318–20.
14. Lloyd OL, Barclay R, Lloyd MM and Armadale Group Practice. Lung cancer and other health problems in a Scottish industrial town: a review. *Ambio* 1985; 14:322–28.
15. Gailey FAY, Lloyd OL. Spatial and temporal patterns of airborne metal pollution: the value of low technology sampling to an environmental epidemiology study. *SCI Total Environ* 1993; 133:201–19.
16. National Cancer Control Office of the Ministry of Health. *Atlas of Cancer Mortality in the People's Republic of China.* China Map Press, Shanghai 1979.

17. Chen KP, Wu HY, Yeh CC, Cheng YU. *Color Atlas of Cancer Mortality by Administrative and Other Classified Districts in Taiwan area: 1968–76.* National Science Council, Taipei 1979.
18. Chen J, Campbell TC, Li J, Peto R. *Diet, Life-style and Mortality in China: A Study of the Characteristics of 65 Chinese Counties.* Oxford University Press, Oxford 1991.
19. Lloyd OL, Wong SL, Wong TW, Yu TS. Mortality mapping in Hong Kong, 1979–83 and 1984–88. Feasibility study and the patterns of cancers. *Asia Pac J Public Health* 1995; 8(2):66–73.
20. Yu TS, Wong SL, Wong TW, Lloyd OL. Mortality mapping in Hong Kong 1979–83 and 1984–88: non-malignant disease patterns and their associations with cancers and socio-economic factors. *Asia Pac J Public Health* 1995; 8(2):74–80.
21. Muir CS, Boyle P, Smans M. The plans for a European cancer atlas: discussion. In: *Maps and Cancer.* Southampton MRC Environmental Epidemiology Unit, Southampton 1983.
22. Wong SL, Donnan SPB. Influence of socioeconomic status on cardiovascular diseases in Hong Kong. *J Epidemiol Comm Hlth* 1992; 46:148–50.
23. Bailar JC. Significance factors for the ratio of a Poisson variable to its expectation. *Biometrics* 1964; 9:639–49.
24. Illsley R. Mortality trends in UK. *Lancet* 1995; 346:313–14.
25. Alderson M. *International Mortality Statistics.* MacMillan, London 1981.
26. Alderson M. *Occupational Cancer.* Butterworths, London 1985.
27. Kleinbaum DG, Kupper LL. *Applied Regression Analysis and Other Multivariable Methods.* Duxbury Press, North Scituate, Massachusetts 1978.
28. West PB, McIver SM. Spatial variations in mortality: a contribution from medical sociology. In: *An Atlas of Mortality in Scotland.* Lloyd OL, Williams FLR, Berry WG, Florey C (eds). Croom Helm, Beckenham, Kent 1987.
29. English D. Geographical epidemiology and ecological studies. In: *Geographical and Environmental Epidemiology: Methods for Small Area Studies.* Elliot P, Cuzick J, English D, Stern R (eds). Oxford University Press, Hong Kong 1992.
30. Huang DP. Epidemiology and aetiology. In: *Nasopharyngeal Carcinoma.* Van Hasselt CA, Gibb AG (eds). The Chinese University Press, Hong Kong 1991.
31. Ho JHC. Chemical risk factors for nasopharyngeal carcinoma (NPC) — a review. In: *Changing Cancer Patterns and Topics in Cancer Epidemiology.* Kurihara M, Aoki K, Miller RW, Muir CS (eds). Gann Monograph on Cancer Research 33. Plenum Press, New York 1987; 157–64.
32. Prasad U, Rampal L. Descriptive epidemiology of nasopharyngeal carcinoma in Peninsular Malaysia. *Cancer Causes Control* 1992; 3:179.
33. Day NE. The geographic pathology of cancer of the oesophagus. In: The Geography of Disease. Doll R (ed). *Brit Med Bull* 1984; 40:329–34.
34. Fraumeni JF Jr. Etiologic clues from cancer mapping in the United States. In: *Changing Cancer Patterns and Topics in Cancer Epidemiology.* Kurihara M, Aoki K, Miller RW, Muir CS (eds). Gann Monograph on Cancer Research 33. Plenum Press, New York 1987; 171–79.

35. Wang YP, Han XY, Su W, Wang YL, Zhu YW, Sasaba T, Nakachi K, Hoshiyama Y, Tagashira Y. Esophageal cancer in Shanxi province, People's Republic of China: a case-control study in high and moderate risk areas. *Cancer Causes Control* 1992; 3:107–13.
36. Parrish KM, Higuchi S, Lucas LJ. Increased alcohol-related oesophageal cancer mortality rates in Japanese men. *Int J Epidemiol* 1993; 22:600–5.
37. Rose EF. A comparative analysis of 2 areas of differing oesophageal cancer incidence in the Transkei. *Medecine/Biologie/Environnement* 1979; July/December: 30–40.
38. Launoy G, Faivre J, Pienkowski P, Milan C, Gignoux M, Pottier D. Changing pattern of oesophageal cancer incidence in France. *Int J Epidemiol* 1994; 23:246–51.
39. Crisp WJ, Hayes N, Raimes SA, Griffin SM. Is there an epidemic of cancer? *BMJ* 1994; 308:1372.
40. Li JY, Liu BQ, Li GY, Chen ZJ, Sun XD, Rong SD. *Atlas of Cancer Mortality in the People's Republic of China:* an aid for cancer control and research. *Int J Epidemiol* 1981; 10:127–33.
41. Li JY. *Investigation of Geographic Patterns of Cancer Mortality in China.* In: NCI Monograph 62, Third Symposium on Epidemiology and Cancer Registries in the Pacific Basin. US Dept of Health, Education and Welfare, Bethesda 1982; 17–42.
42. Li JY. *Epidemiology of Esophageal Cancer in China.* In: NCI Monograph 62, Third Symposium on Epidemiology and Cancer Registries in the Pacific Basin. US Dept of Health, Education and Welfare, Bethesda 1982; 113–22.
43. Schottenfield D, Fraumeni JF Jr. *Cancer Epidemiology and Prevention.* WB Saunders, Philadelphia 1982.
44. Coggon D, Acheson ED. The geography of cancer of the stomach. In: The Geography of Disease. Doll R (ed). *Brit Med Bull* 1984; 40:335–41.
45. Muir CS, Malhotra A. Changing patterns of cancer incidence in five Continents. In: *Changing Cancer Patterns and Topics in Cancer Epidemiology.* Kurihara M, Aoki K, Miller RW, Muir CS (eds). Gann Monograph on Cancer Research 33. Plenum Press, New York 1987; 3–23.
46. Aird I, Bentall HH, Fraser Roberts JA. A relationship between cancer of the stomach and ABO blood group. *BMJ* 1953; I:799–801.
47. Nazario CM, Szklo M, Diamond E, Roman-Franco A, Climent C, Suarez E, Conde JG. Salt and gastric cancer: a case-control study in Puerto Rico. *Int J Epidemiol* 1993; 22:790–97.
48. Memik F. Differences in the distribution of gastrointestinal cancer in Turkey; the possible causative environmental factors in etiology. *Medecine/Biologie/Environnement* 1989; October/December:15–23.
49. Ramon JM, Serra-Majem L, Cerdo C, Oromi J. Nutrient intake and gastric cancer risk: a case-control study in Spain. *Int J Epidemiol* 1993; 22:983–88.
50. Lee JK, Park BJ, Yoo KY, Ahn YO. Dietary factors and stomach cancer: a case-control study in Korea. *Int J Epidemiol* 1995; 24:33–41.
51. Forman D, Newell DG, Fullerton F, Yarnell JWG, Stacey AR, Wald N, Sitas F. Association between infection with

helicobacter pylori and risk of gastric cancer: evidence from a prospective investigation. *BMJ* 1991; 302:1302–5.
52. Jankowski J. Helicobacter pylori infection and gastric cancer. *BMJ* 1991; 302:1534.
53. Wynder EL, Hyams L, Shigematsu T. Correlations of international cancer death rates. *Cancer* 1967; 20:113–26.
54. Logan WPD. *Cancer Mortality by Occupation and Social Class 1851–1971.* IARC Scientific Publications 36. IARC, Lyon 1982.
55. Finlay IG, Pickford IR. *Colorectal Carcinoma.* In: Current Medicine 4. Royal College of Physicians of Edinburgh. Churchill Livingstone, London 1994; 51–64.
56. Cook-Mozaffari P, van Rensburg S. Cancer of the liver. In: The Geography of Disease. Doll R (ed). *Brit Med Bull* 1984; 40:342–45.
57. Lam KC, Tong MJ. *Analytical Epidemiology of Primary Liver Carcinoma in the Pacific Basin.* In: NCI Monograph 62, Third Symposium on Epidemiology and Cancer Registries in the Pacific Basin. US Dept of Health, Education and Welfare, Bethesda 1982; 123–28.
58. Beasley RP, Hwang LY, Lin CC, Chien CS. Hepatocellular carcinoma and hepatitis B virus — a prospective study of 22,707 men in Taiwan. *Lancet* 1981; 2:1129–33.
59. Adler I. *Primary Malignant Growths of the Lung and Bronchi.* Longmans Green, New York 1912.
60. Kurihara M. Trends in lung cancer mortality in 24 countries. In: *Changing Cancer Patterns and Topics in Cancer Epidemiology.* Kurihara M, Aoki K, Miller RW, Muir CS (eds). Gann Monograph on Cancer Research 33. Plenum Press, New York 1987; 45–54.
61. Hirayama T. Passive smoking and cancer: an epidemiological review. In: *Changing Cancer Patterns and Topics in Cancer Epidemiology.* Kurihara M, Aoki K, Miller RW, Muir CS (eds). Gann Monograph on Cancer Research 33. Plenum Press, New York 1987; 127–135.
62. Liu Q, Sasco AJ, Riboli E, Hu MX. Indoor air pollution and lung cancer in Guangzhou, People's Republic of China. *Am J Epidemiol* 1993; 137:145–54.
63. Brownson RC, Alavanja MCR, Hock ET, Loy TS. Passive smoking and lung cancer in nonsmoking women. *Am J Publ Hlth* 1992; 82:1525–30.
64. Heath CW. Passive smoking. *Lancet* 1993; 341:526.
65. Peto R. Smoking and death: the past 40 years and the next 40. *BMJ* 1994; 309:937–39.
66. Lloyd OL, Gailey FAY. Techniques of low technology sampling of air pollution by metals. *Br J Ind Med* 1987; 44:494–504.
67. Ho JHC, Chan CL, Lau WH, Au LGKH, Koo LC. *Cancer in Hong Kong: Some Epidemiological Observations.* In: NCI Monograph 62, Third Symposium on Epidemiology and Cancer Registries in the Pacific Basin. US Dept of Health, Education and Welfare, Bethesda 1982; 47–55.
68. Pike MC, Ross RK. Breast cancer. In: The Geography of Disease. Doll R (ed). *Brit Med Bull* 1984; 40:351–54.
69. Henderson BE, Ross RK, Bernstein L. Exogenous hormones and the risk of cancer. In: *Changing Cancer Patterns and Topics in Cancer Epidemiology.* Kurihara M, Aoki K, Miller RW, Muir CS (eds). Gann Monograph on Cancer Research 33. Plenum Press, New York 1987; 137–47.
70. Bruzzi P. Epidemiological approach to breast cancer etiology.

In: *Epidemiology and Quantitation of Environmental Risk in Humans from Radiation and Other Agents.* Castellani A (ed). NATO Advanced Science Institute Series. Plenum Press, New York 1985.

71. McPherson K, Steel CM, Dixon JM. Breast cancer — epidemiology, risk factors, and genetics. *BMJ* 1994; 309: 1003–6.
72. Eidson M, Becker TM, Wiggins CL, Key CR, Samet MJ. Breast cancer among Hispanics, American Indians and non-Hispanic Whites in New Mexico. *Int J Epidemiol* 1994; 23:231–37.
73. Ekbom A, Trichopoulos D, Adami HO, Hsieh CC, Lan SJ. Evidence of prenatal influences on breast cancer risk. *Lancet* 1992; 340:1015–18.
74. UK National Case Control Study Group. Breast feeding and risk of breast cancer in young women. *BMJ* 1993; 307:17–20.
75. Milne R, Vessey M. The pill and mortality — an overview. *J Publ Hlth Med* 1992; 14:9–16.
76. Ferraroni M, Gerber M, Decarli A, Richardson S, Marubini E, Paulet PCD, Paulet ACD, Pujol J. HDL cholesterol and breast cancer: a joint study in northern Italy and southern France. *Int J Epidemiol* 1993; 22:772–80.
77. Bennicke K, Conrad C, Sabroe S, Sorensen HT. Cigarette smoking and breast cancer. *BMJ* 1995; 310:1431–33.
78. Parazzini F, La Vecchia C, Negri E, Franceschi S, Tozzi L. Family history of breast, ovarian and endometrial cancer and risk of breast cancer. *Int J Epidemiol* 1993; 22: 614–18.
79. Lee HP, Cuello C, Singh K. *Review of the Epidemiology of Cervical Cancer in the Pacific Basin.* In: NCI Monograph 62, Third Symposium on Epidemiology and Cancer Registries in the Pacific Basin. US Dept of Health, Education and Welfare, Bethesda 1982; 197–99.
80. Vet HCWde, Knipschild PG, Sturmans F. The role of sexual factors in the aetiology of cervical dysplasia. *Int J Epidemiol* 1993; 22:798–803.
81. Murphy MFG, Goldblatt PO, Mant D. Marital stability and cancer of uterine cervix: changing patterns in post-War Britain. *Int J Epidemiol* 1993; 22:385–92.
82. Darby SC, Kendall GM, Fell TP, O'Hagan JA, Murihead CR, Ennis JR, Ball AM, Dennis JA, Doll RA. A summary of mortality and incidence of cancer in men from the United Kingdom who participated in the United Kingdom's atmospheric nuclear weapon tests and experimental programmes. *BMJ* 1988; 296:332–38.
83. Anssi A, Hakama M, Arvela H, Hakulinen T, Rahola T, Suomela M, Soderman B, Rytomaa T. Fallout from chernobyl and incidence of childhood leukaemia in Finland, 1976–92. *BMJ* 1994; 309:151–54.
84. Roman E, Beral V, Carpenter L, Watson A, Barton C, Ryder H, Aston DL. Childhood leukaemia in the West Berkshire and Basingstoke and North Hampshire District health authorities in relation to nuclear establishments in the vicinity. *BMJ* 1987; 294:597–602.
85. Darby SC, Doll R. Fallout, Radiation doses near Dounreay, and childhood leukaemia. *BMJ* 1987; 294:603–7.
86. McLaughlin JR, King WD, Anderson TW, Clarke EA, Ashmore JP. Paternal radiation exposure and leukaemia in

offspring; the Ontario case-control study. *BMJ* 1993; 307:959–66.

87. Gardner MJ. Childhood cancer and nuclear installations. *Publ Hlth Lond* 1991; 105:277–85.

88. Bithell JF, Dutton SJ, Draper GJ, Neary NM. Distribution of childhood leukaemias and non-Hodgkin's lymphomas near nuclear installations in England and Wales. *BMJ* 1994; 309:501–5.

89. MacMahon B. Leukaemia clusters around nuclear facilities in Britain. *Cancer Causes Control* 1992; 3:283–88.

90. Godlee F. Environmental radiation: a cause for concern? *BMJ* 1992; 304:299–304.

91. Battista G, Belli S, Carboncini F, Comba P, Levante G, Sartorelli P, Strambi F, Valentini F, Axelson O. Mortality among pyrite miners with low-level exposure to radon daughters. *Scand J Work Environ Hlth* 1988; 14:280–85.

92. Court Brown WM, Spiers FS, Doll R, Duffy BJ, McHugh MJ. Geographical variation in leukaemia mortality in relation to background radiation and other factors. *BMJ* 1960; 5188:1753–59.

93. Axelson O, Edling C, Kling H. Lung cancer and residency: a case-referent study on the possible impact of exposure to radon and its daughters in dwellings. *Scand J Work Environ Hlth* 1979; 5:10–15.

94. Chaffey CM, Bowie C. Radon and health — an update. *J Publ Hlth Med* 1994; 16:465–70.

95. Viel JF. Radon exposure and leukaemia in adulthood. *Int J Epidemiol* 1993; 22:627–31.

96. Hawkins LH. Does electromagnetic radiation cause cancer? *Occup Med* 1992; 42:98–100.

97. Kinlen LJ, Clarke K, Hudson C. Evidence from population mixing in British new towns 1946–85 of an infective basis for childhood leukaemia. *Lancet* 1990; 336:577–82.

98. Kinlen LJ, John SM. Wartime evacuation and mortality from childhood leukaemia in England and Wales in 1945–9. *BMJ* 1994; 309:1197–202.

99. Kinlen LJ, O'Brien F, Clarke K, Balkwill A, Matthews F. Rural population mixing and childhood leukaemia: effects of the North Sea oil industry in Scotland, including the area near Dounreay Nuclear Site. *BMJ* 1993; 306:743–48.

100. Alexander FE, Mckinney PM, Cartwright RA. Migration patterns of children with leukaemia and non-Hodgkin's lymphoma in three areas of Northern England. *J Publ Hlth Med* 1993; 15:9–15.

101. Nerurkar LS, Wong-Staal F, Gallo RC. Human retroviruses, leukaemia and AIDS. In: *Leukaemia.* Henderson ES, Lister TA (eds). Saunders, Philadelphia 1990.

102. Rosner F, Grunwald HW. Chemicals and leukaemia. In: *Leukaemia.* Henderson ES, Lister TA (eds). Saunders, Philadelphia 1990.

103. Knox EG. Leukaemia clusers in childhood: geographical analysis in Britain. *J Epidemiol Commun Hlth* 1994; 369–76.

104. Linet MS, Devesa SS. Descriptive epidemiology of the leukaemias. In: *Leukaemia.* Henderson ES, Lister TA (eds). Saunders, Philadelphia 1990.

105. Yu TS, Wong SL, Lloyd OL, Wong TW. Ischaemic heart

disease: trends in mortality in Hong Kong, 1970–1989. *J Epidemiol Comm Hlth* 1995; 49:16–21.
106. Family Heart Study Group. British family heart study: its design and method, and prevalence of cardiovascular risk factors. *Br J General Practice* 1994; 44:62–67.
107. Li LN, Tuomilehto J et al. Electrocardiographic abnormalities and associated factors in Chinese living in Beijing and in Mauritius. *BMJ* 1992; 304:1596–601.
108. Puska P, Tuomilehto J, Salonen J et al. Changes in coronary risk factors during comprehensive five-year community programme to control cardiovascular diseases (North Karelia project). *BMJ* 1979; 2:1173–78.
109. Beaglehole R. Cardiovascular disease in developing countries. *BMJ* 1991; 305:1170–71.
110. Porrini M, Simonetti P, Testolin G, Roggi C, Laddomada MS, Tenconi MT. Relation between diet composition and coronary heart disease risk factors. *J Epidemiol Comm Hlth* 1991; 45:148–51.
111. VanSaase JLCM, Noteboom WMP, Vandenbroucke JP. Longevity of men capable of prolonged vigorous physical exercise: a 32–year follow up of 2259 participants in the Dutch eleven cities ice skating tour. *BMJ* 1990; 301:1409–11.
112. Faculty of Public Health Medicine, the Royal College of Physicians of the United Kingdom. *Epidemiology of Coronary Heart Disease Risk Factors: an Update.* Guidelines for Health Promotion 38, 1994.
113. Hong Y, Bots ML, Pan X, Wang J, Jing J, Hofman A, Chen H. Physical activity and cardiovascular risk factors in rural Shanghai, China. *Int J Epidemiol* 1994; 23:1154–58.
114. Burr ML, Gilbert JF, Holliday RM, Elwood PC, Fehily AM, Rogers S, Sweetnam PM, Deadman NM. Effects of changes in fat, fish and fibre intakes on death and myocardial reinfarction: diet and reinfarction trial (DART). *Lancet* 1989; 8666:757–61.
115. Helmert U, Herman B, Shea S. Moderate and vigorous leisure-time physical activity and cardiovascular disease risk factors in West Germany 1984–91. *Int J Epidemiol* 1994; 23:285–92.
116. Ornish D, Brown SE et al. Can lifestyle changes reverse coronary heart disease? *Lancet* 1990; 336:129–33.
117. Shaper AG, Phillips AN, Pocock SJ, Walker M, Macfarlane PW. Risk factors for stroke in middle aged British men. *BMJ* 1991; 302:1111–15.
118. Barker DJP, Osmond C. Death rates from stroke in England and Wales predicted from past maternal mortality. *BMJ* 1987; 295:83–86.
119. Hunter D. *Diseases of Occupations.* Hodder & Stoughton, London 1975.
120. Florey C. Bronchitis, emphysema, asthma. In: *An Atlas of Mortality in Scotland.* Lloyd OL, William FLR, Berry WG, Florey C (eds). Croom Helm, Beckenham, Kent 1987.
121. Tattersfield AE. *Asthma — Where Now?* In: Current Medicine 4. Royal College of Physicians of Edinburgh. Churchill Livingstone, Edinburgh 1994.
122. Cullinan P, Taylor AJN. Asthma in children: environmental factors. *BMJ* 1994; 308:1585–86.
123. Seaton A, Godden DJ, Brown K. Increase in asthma: a more

toxic environment or a more susceptible population? *Thorax* 1994; 49:171–74.

124. Temple JMF, Sykes AM. Asthma and open cast mining. *BMJ* 1992; 305:396–97.

125. Picado C. Barcelona's asthma epidemics: clinical aspects and intriguing findings. *Thorax* 1992; 47:197–200.

126. Bobak M, Leon DA. Air pollution and infant mortality in the Czech Republic, 1986–8. *Lancet* 1992; 340:1010–14.

127. Williams FLR, Lloyd OL, Berry WG. Mortality from non-malignant respiratory diseases in Scotland between 1959 and 1983. *Ambio* 1987; 16:206–10.

128. Ninan TK, Russell G. Respiratory symptoms and atopy in Aberdeen school children: evidence from two surveys 25 years apart. *BMJ* 1992; 304:873–75.

129. Robertson CF, Heycock E, Biship J, Nolan T, Olinsky A, Phelan PD. Prevalence of asthma in Melbourne school children: changes over 26 years. *BMJ* 1991; 302:1116–18.

130. Burney PG, Chinn S, Rona RJ. Has the prevalence of asthma increased in children? Evidence from the national study of health and growth 1973–86. *BMJ* 1990; 300:1306–10.

131. Phelan PD. Asthma in children: epidemiology. *BMJ* 1994; 308:1584–85.

132. Peat JK, vdBerg RH, Green WF, Mellis CM, Leeder SR, Woolcock AJ. Changing prevalence of asthma in Australian children. *BMJ* 1994; 308:1591–96.

133. Laor A, Cohen L, Danon YL. Effects of time, sex, ethnic origin, and area of residence on prevalence of asthma in Israeli adolescents. *BMJ* 1993; 307:841–44.

134. Reid D. Acute respiratory infection: influenza and pneumonia. In: *An Atlas of Mortality in Scotland.* Lloyd OL, Williams FLR, Berry WG, Florey C (eds). Croom Helm, Beckenham, Kent 1987.

135. Webster RG. While awaiting the next pandemic of influenza A. *BMJ* 1994; 309:1179–80.

136. Spence DPS, Hotchkiss J, Williams CSD, Davies PDO. Tuberculosis and poverty. *BMJ* 1993; 307:759–61.

137. Godlee F. Tuberculosis — 'a global emergency'. *BMJ* 1993; 306:1147.

General

a. Kaln HA, Sempos CT. *Statistical Methods in Epidemiology.* Oxford University Press, New York 1989.

b. Trowell HC, Burkitt DP (eds). *Western Diseases: Their Emergence and Prevention.* Edward Arnold, London 1981.

c. Miller DL, Farmer RDT (eds). *Epidemiology of Diseases.* Blackwell, London 1981.

d. International Agency for Research on Cancer. *Cancer Incidence in Five Continents.* IARC Scientific Publications, vol. 6, no. 1120. IARC, Lyon 1992.

e. Kurihara M, Aoki K, Tominaga S (eds). *Cancer Mortality Statistics in the World: Commemorative Publication for Professor Mitsuo Segi.* University of Nagoya Press, Nagoya 1984.

f. Hill AB. *Principles of Medical Statistics.* Oxford University Press, New York 1971.

g. Boice JD, Fraumeni JF (eds). *Radiation Carcinogenesis. Epidemiology and Biological Significance.* Raven Press, London 1984.

General Maps

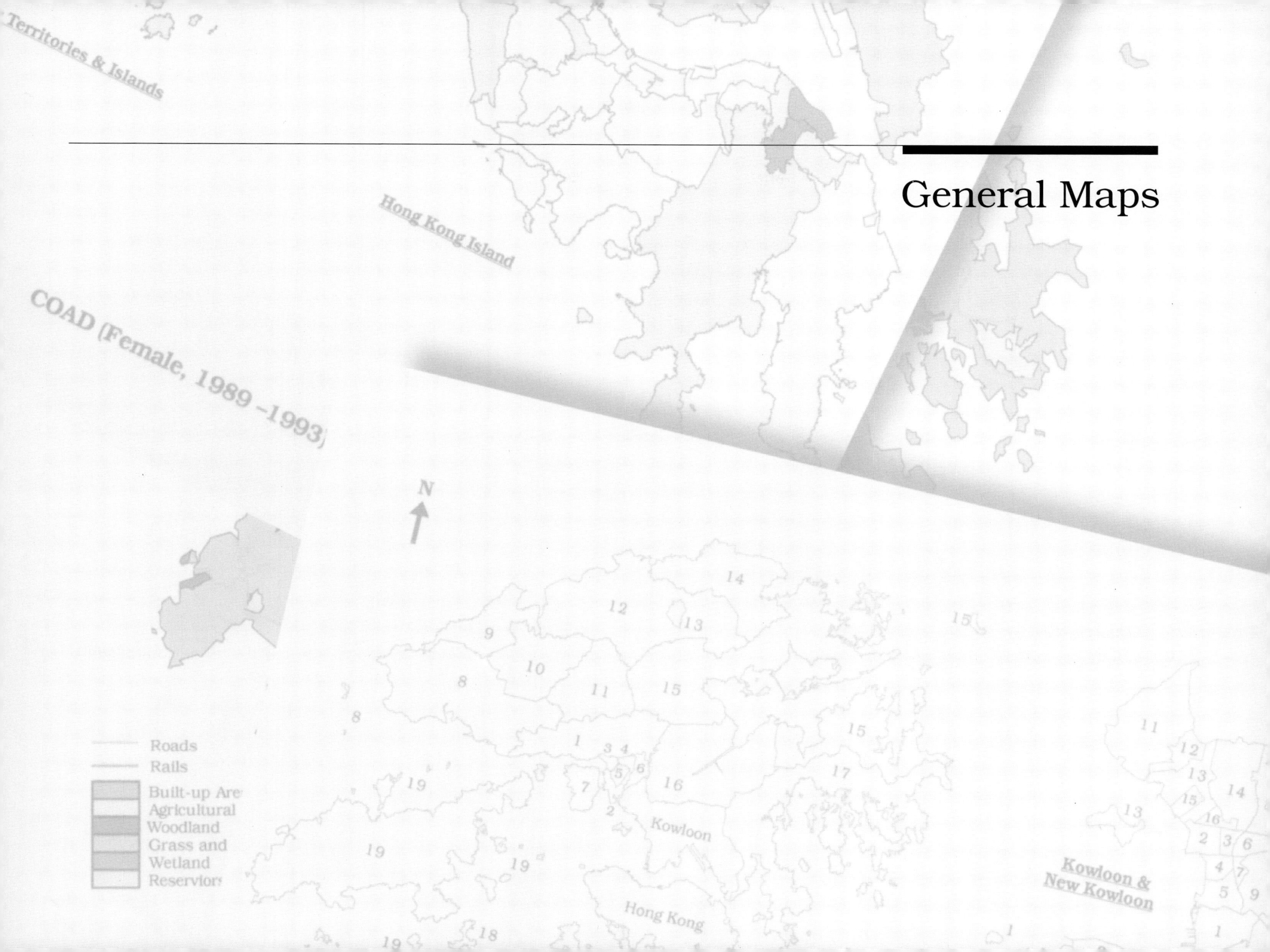

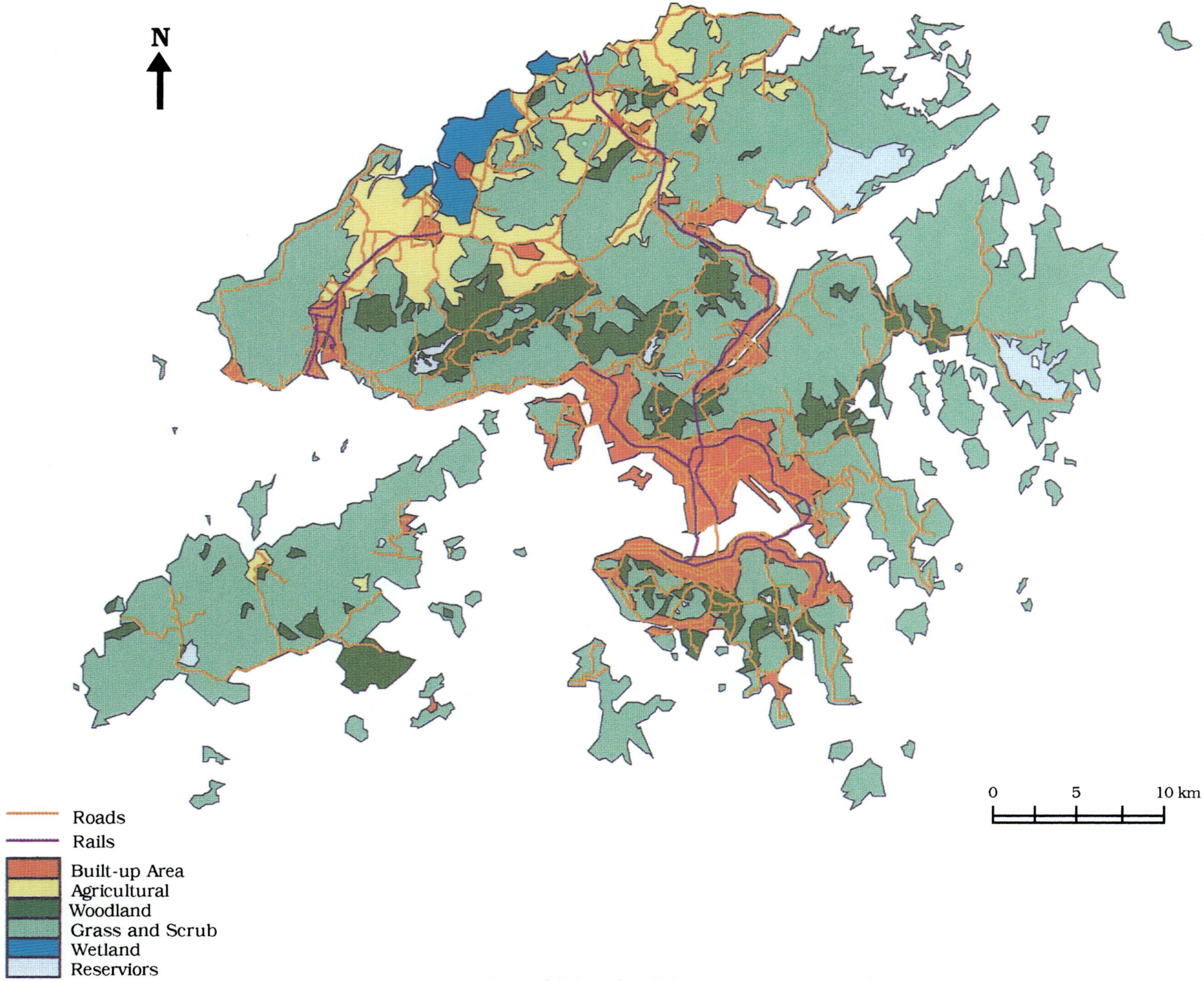

Land Use in Hong Kong in 1984

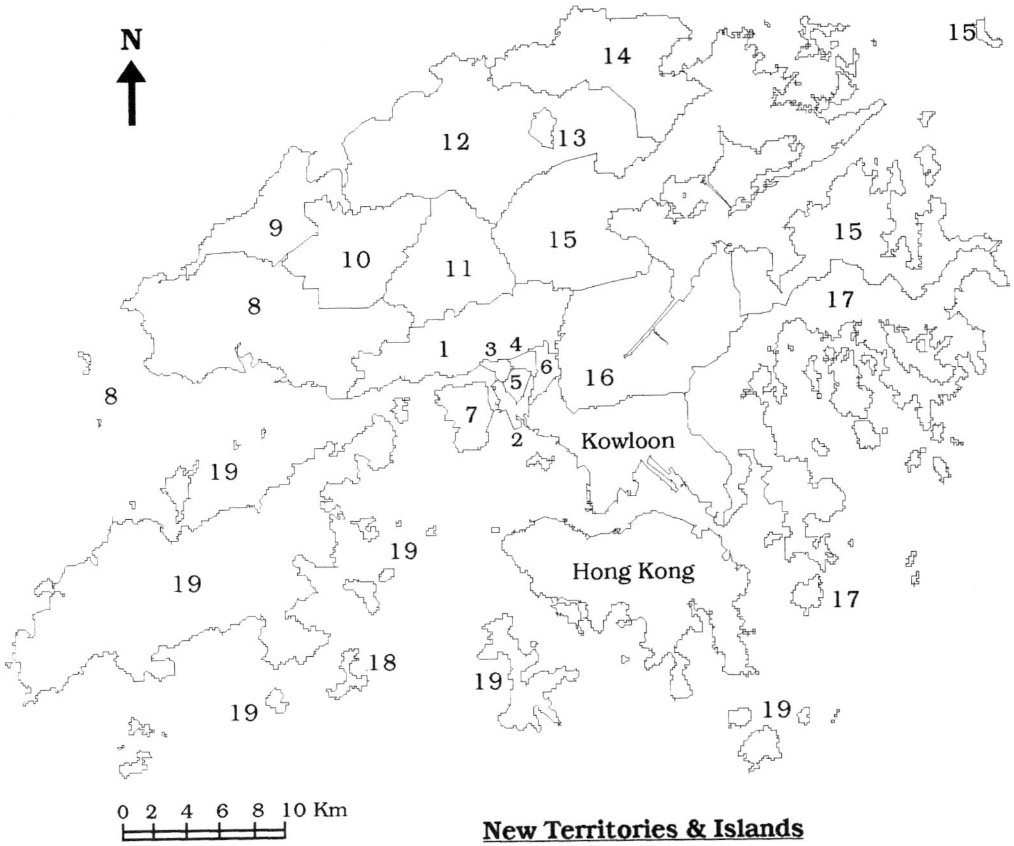

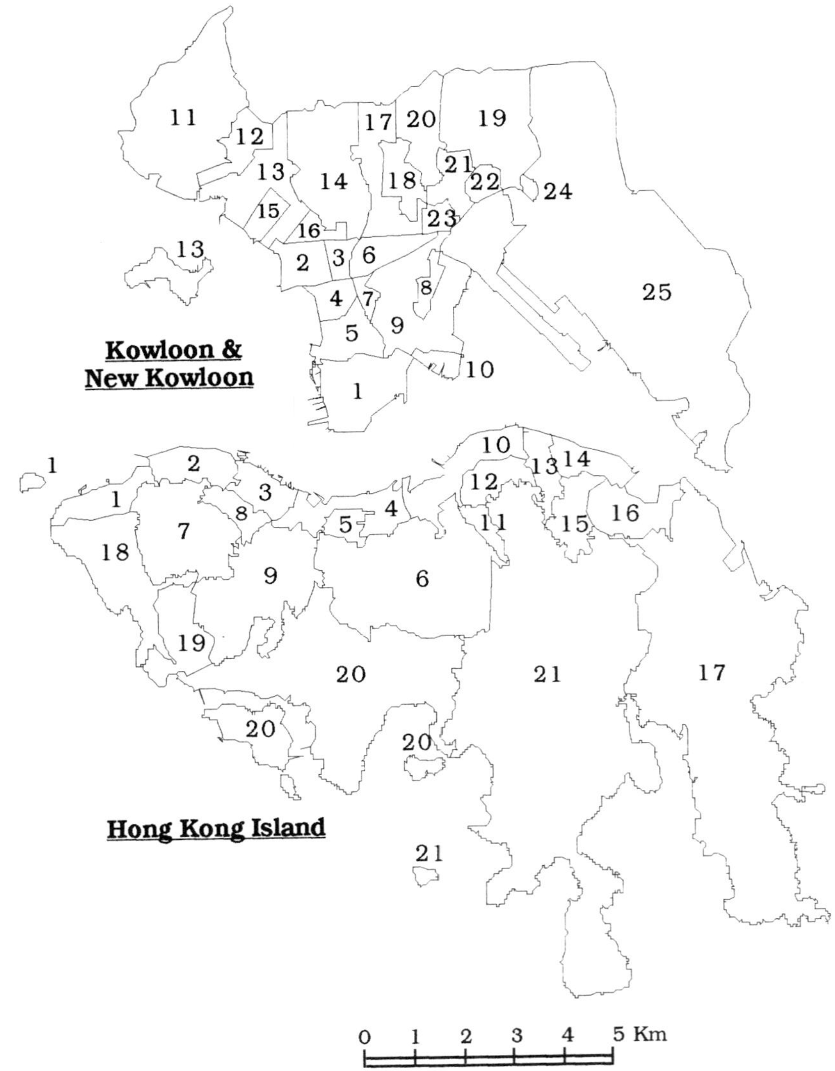

65 communities:

21 communities in Hong Kong Island
25 communities in Kowloon & New Kowloon
19 communities in New Territories

Location of 65 Communities

(See Appendix 1 for the names of the communities)

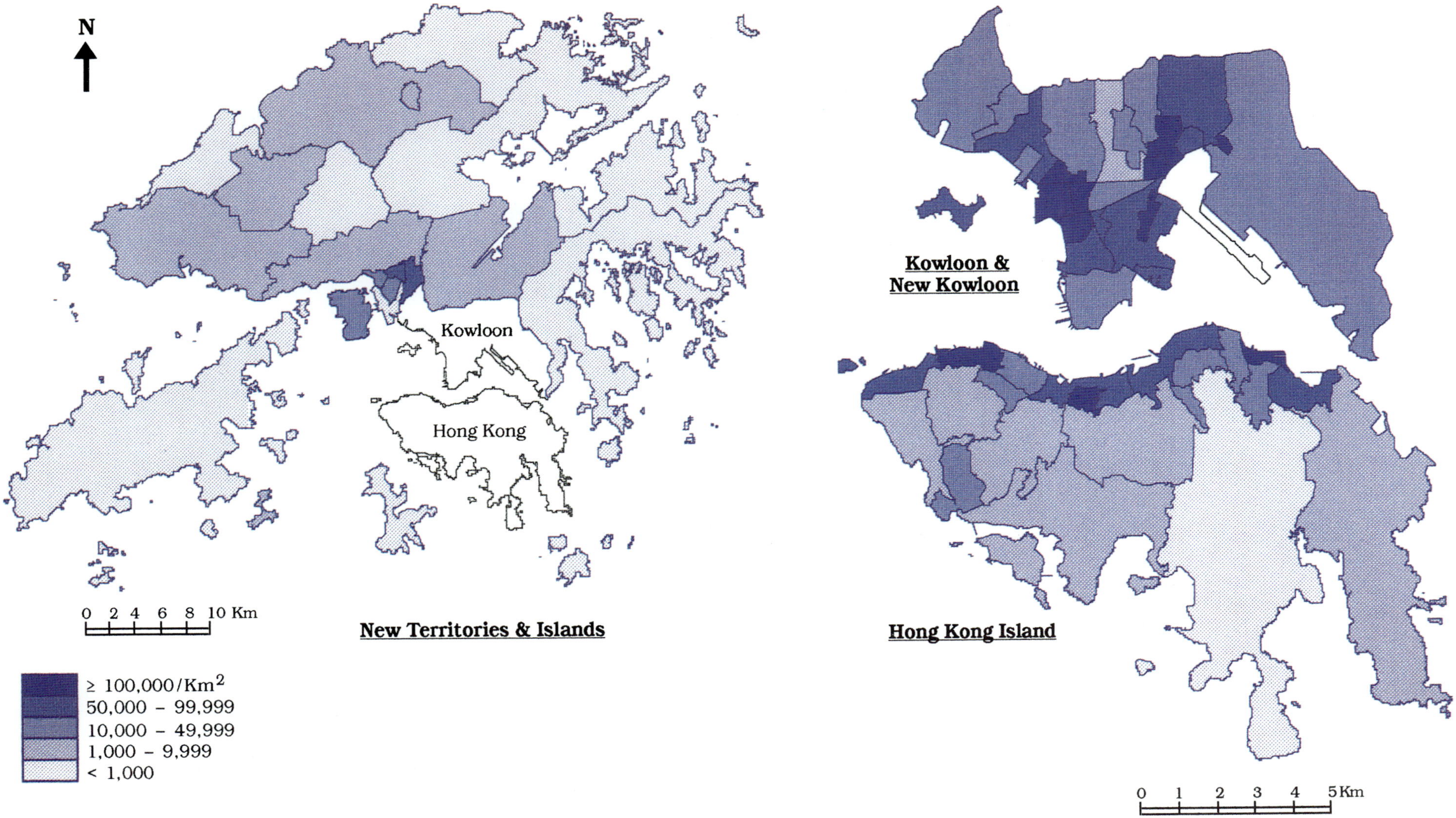

Population Density in 1981

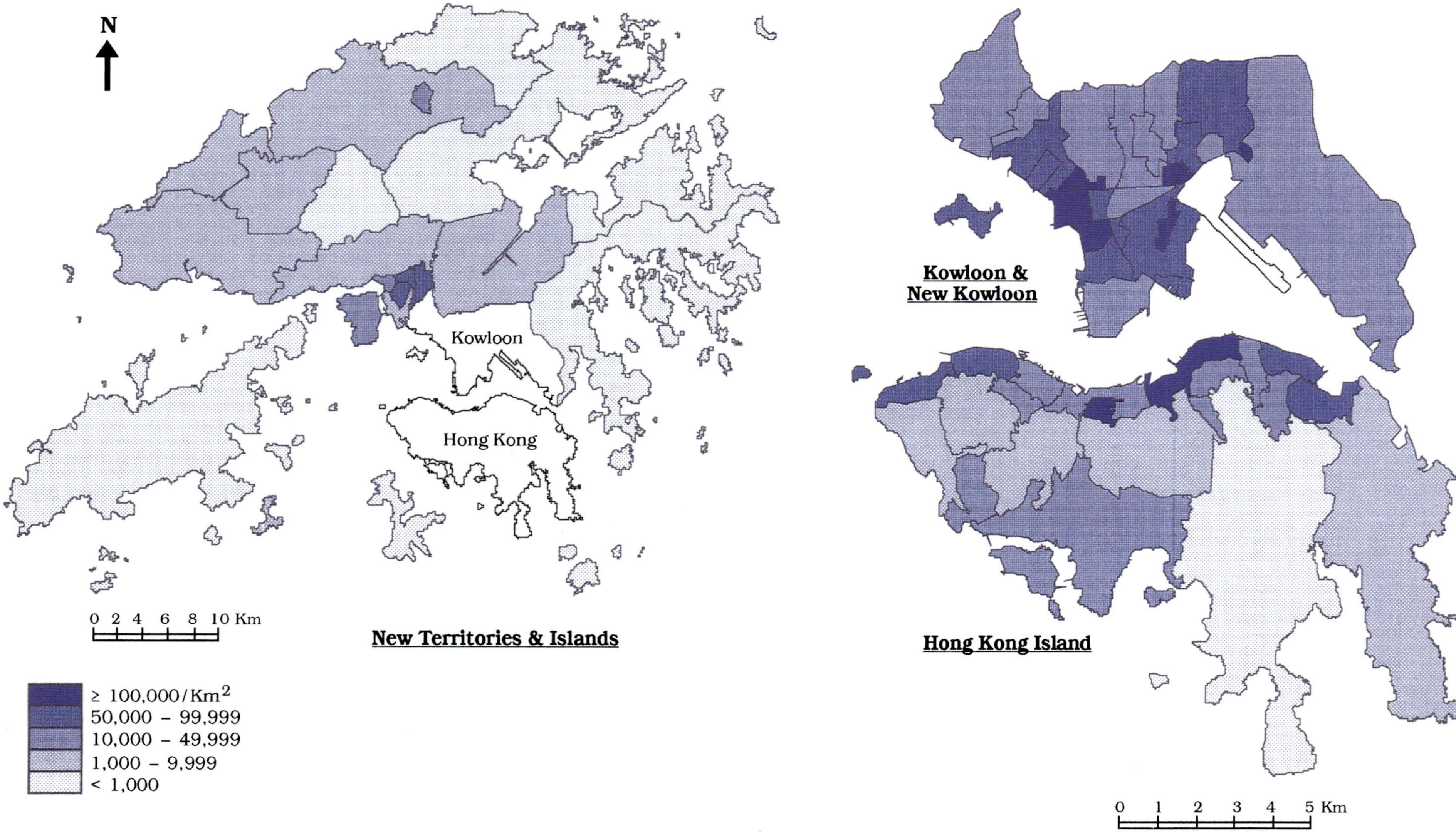

Population Density in 1986

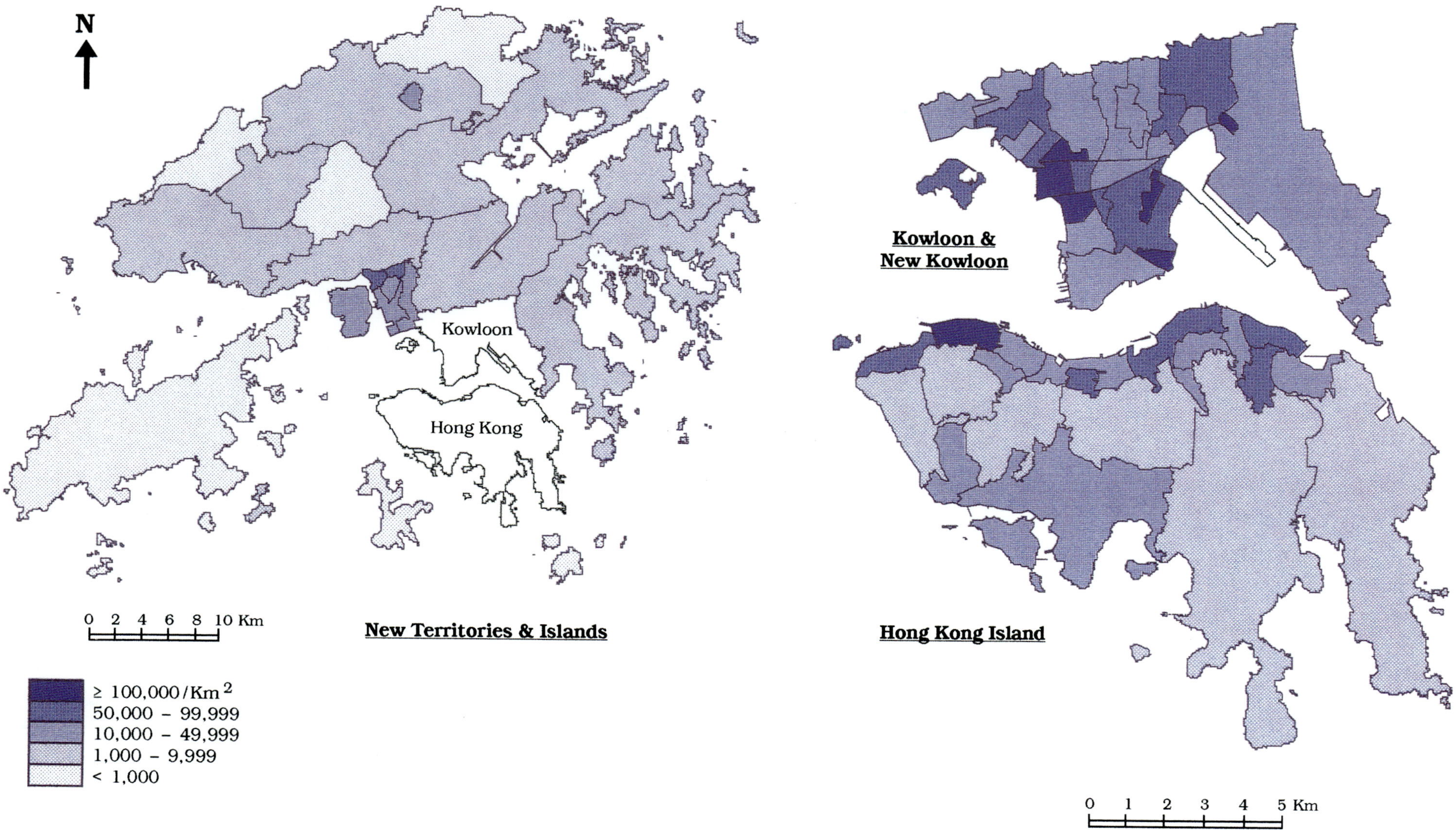

Population Density in 1991

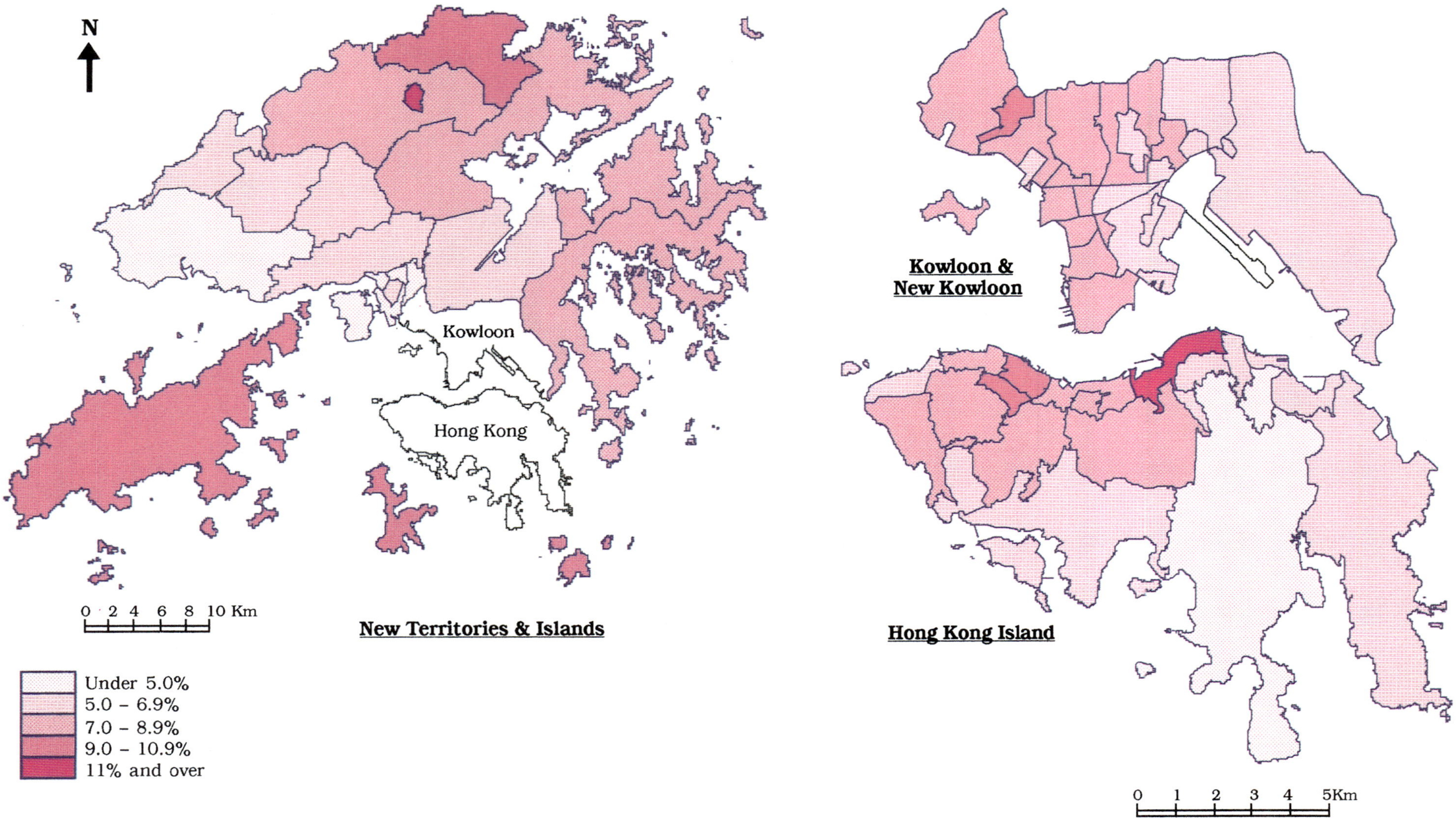

Percentage of Population Aged 65 and over in 1981

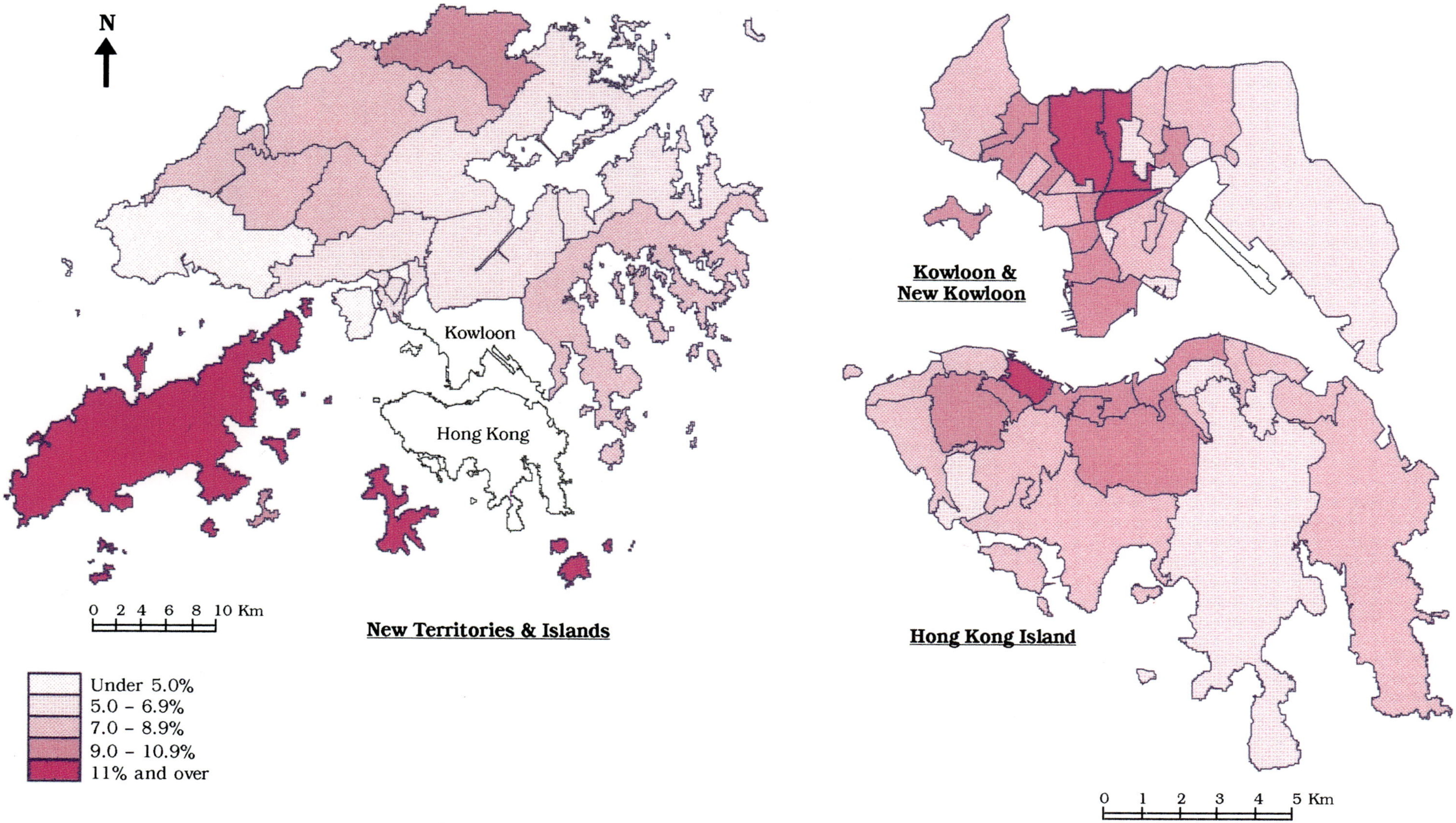

Percentage of Population Aged 65 and over in 1986

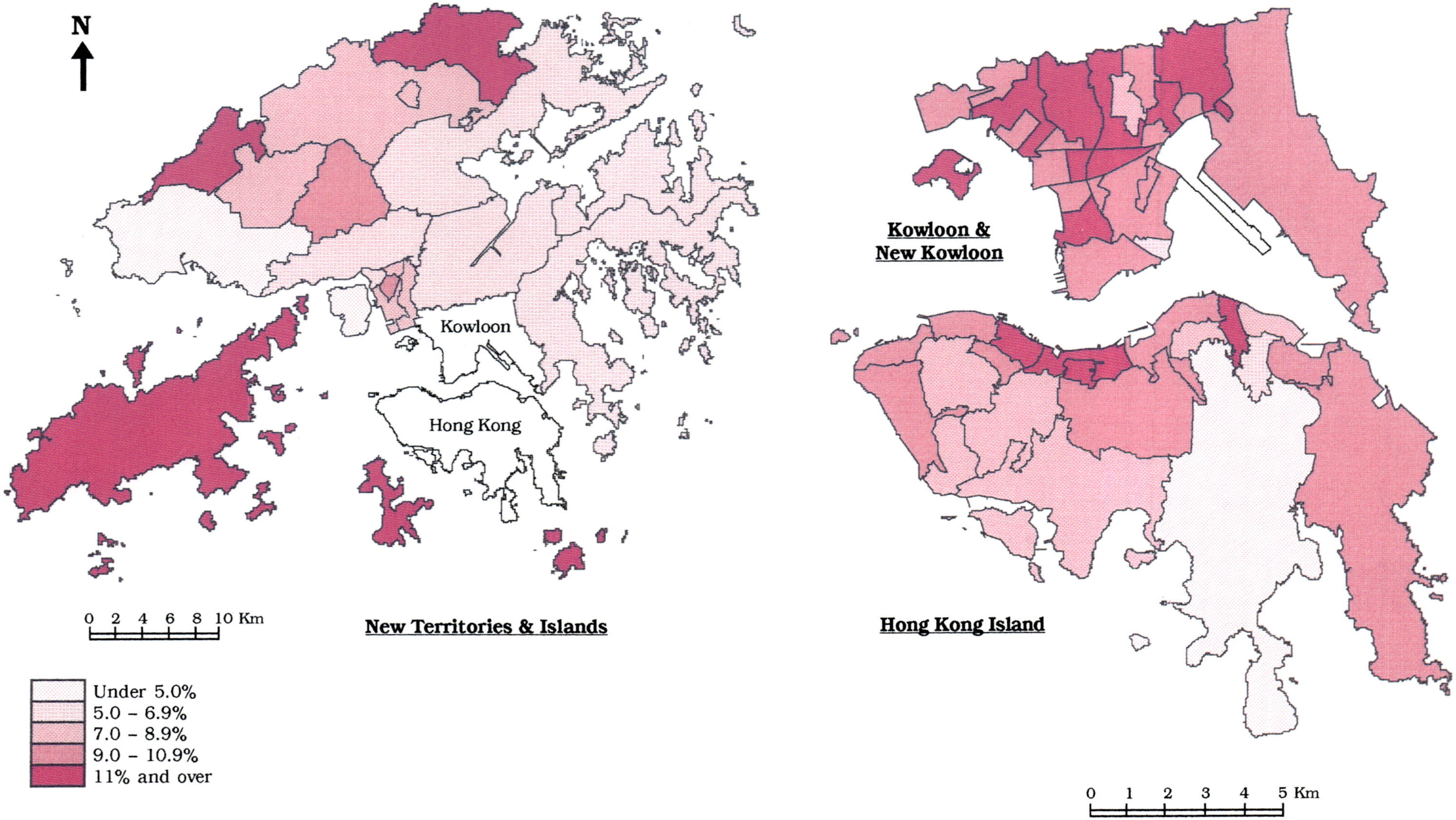

Percentage of Population Aged 65 and over in 1991

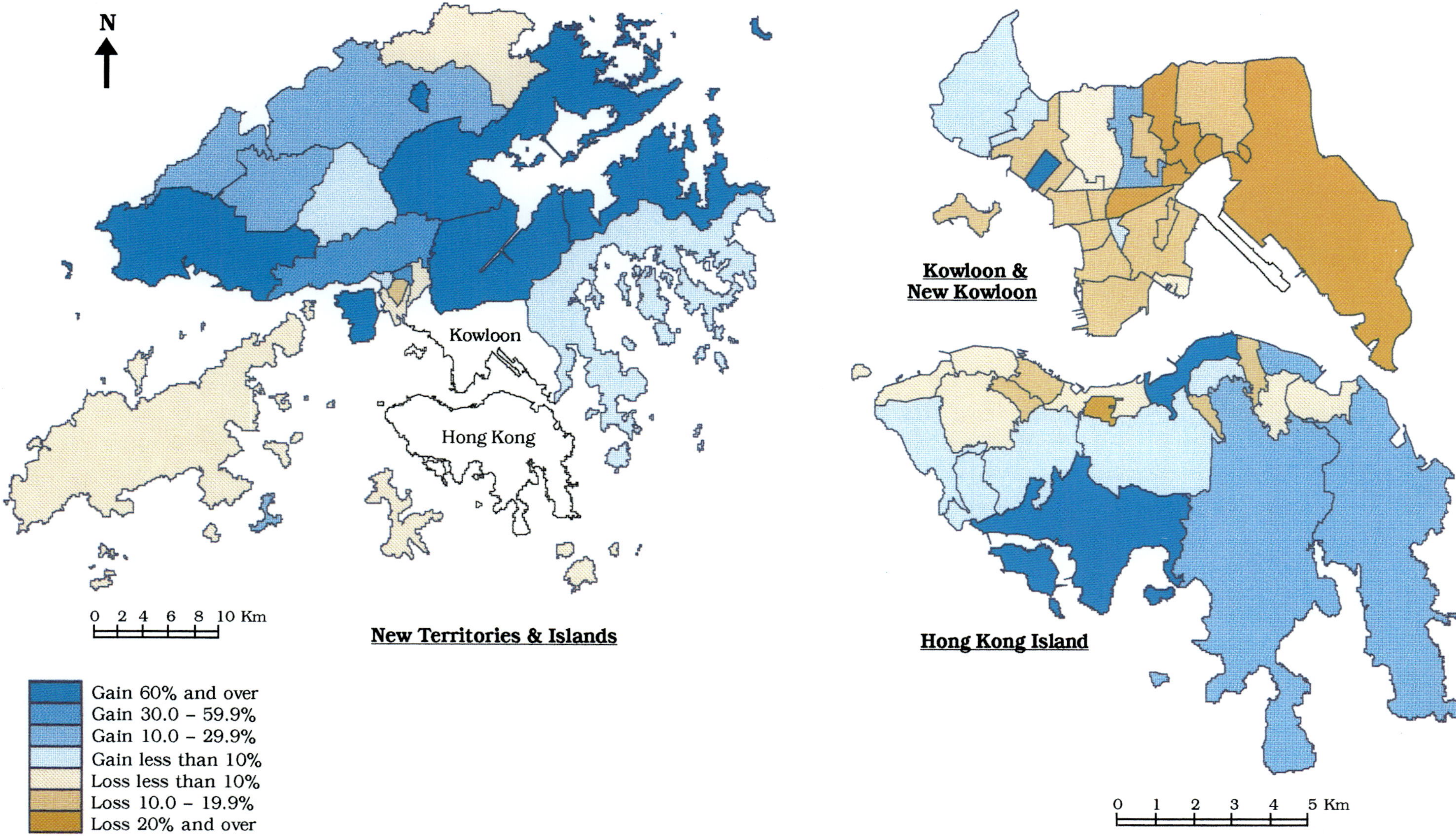

Change in Total Population: 1981 -1986

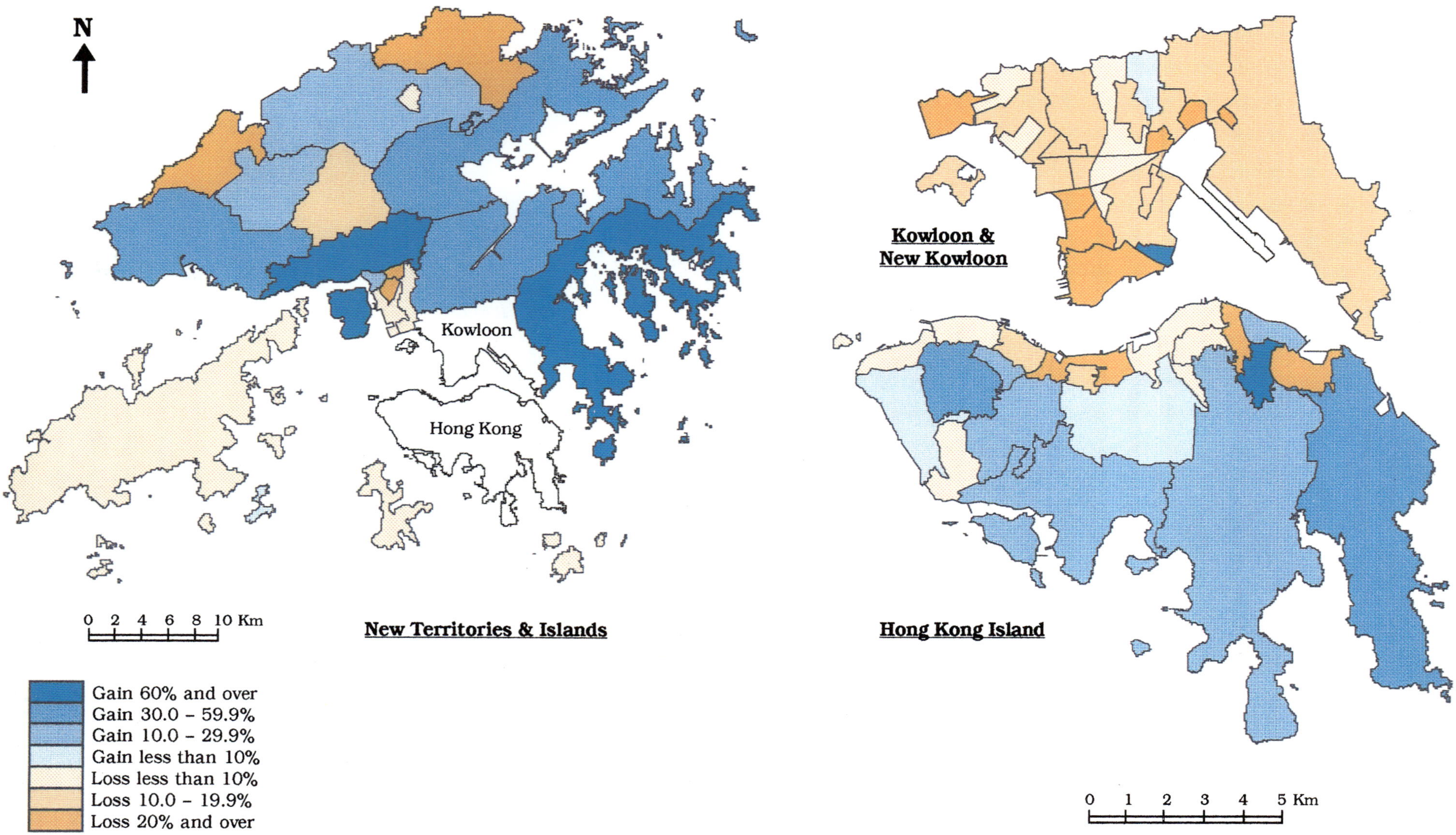

Change in Total Population: 1986 -1991

Maps, Tables and Graphs of the Disease Mortalities in Hong Kong, 1979–83, 1984–88 and 1989–93

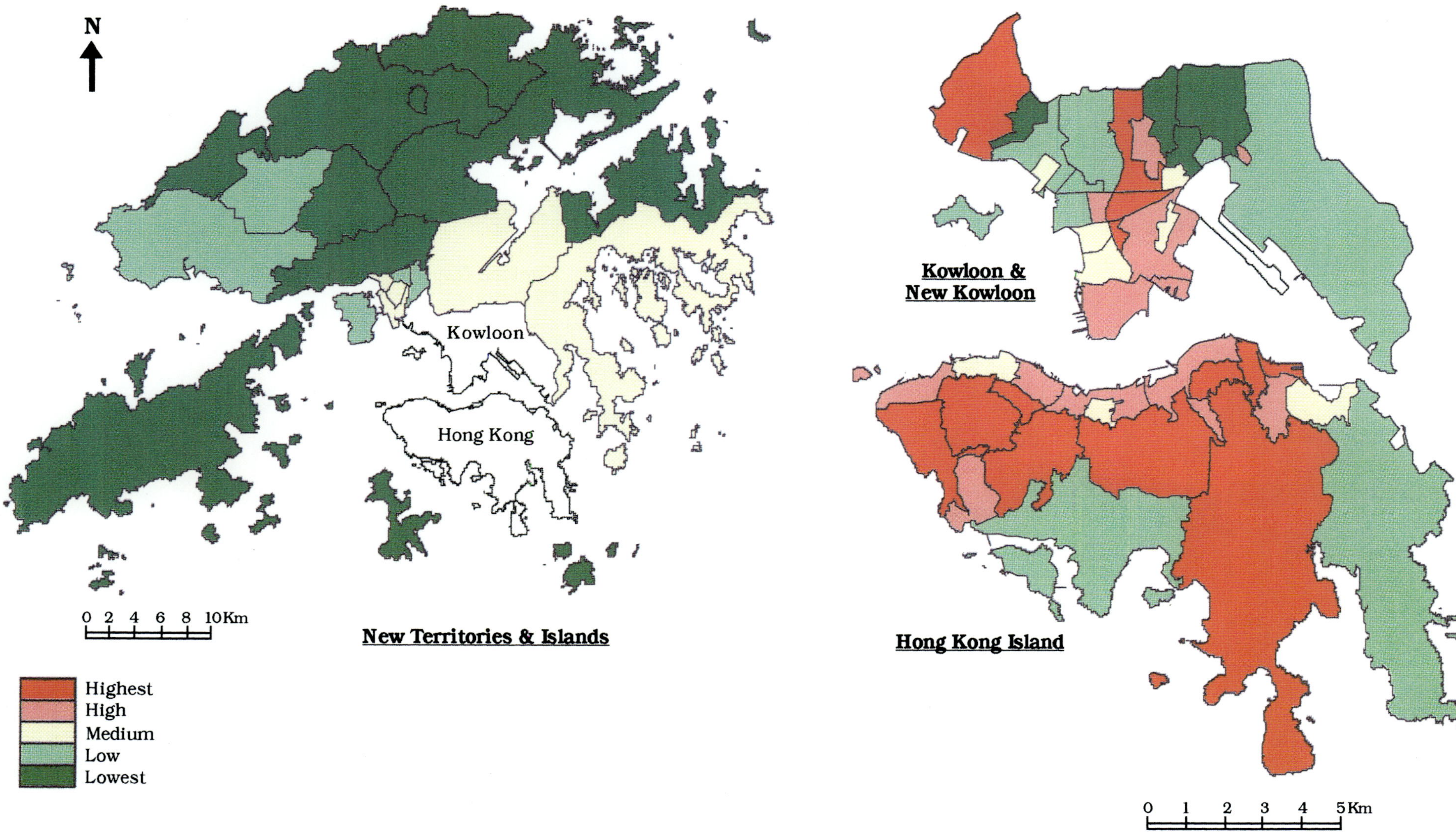

F-Score (in quintiles), 1981

(A composite score indicating socio-economic status)

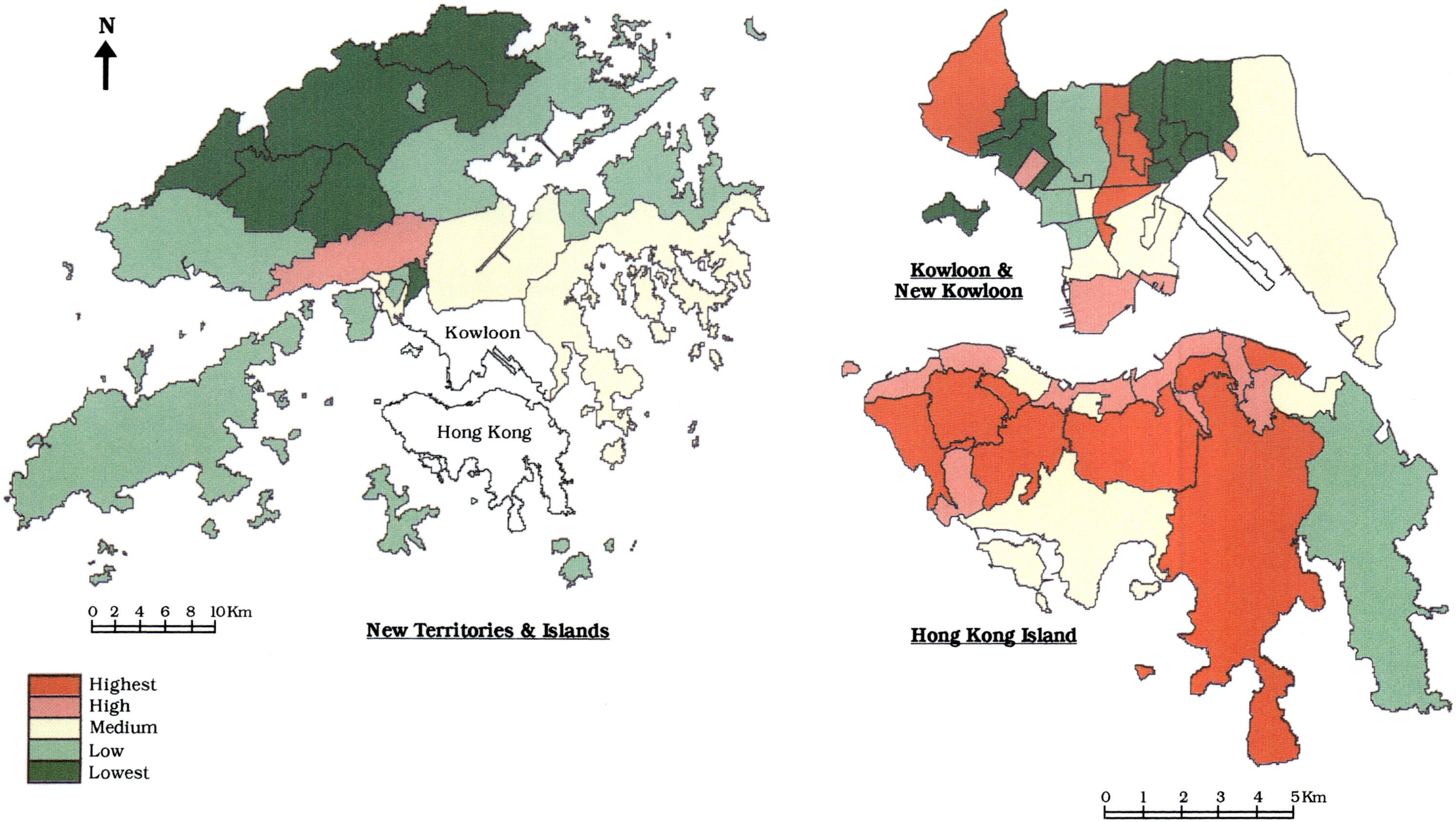

F-Score (in quintiles), 1986
(A composite score indicating socio-economic status)

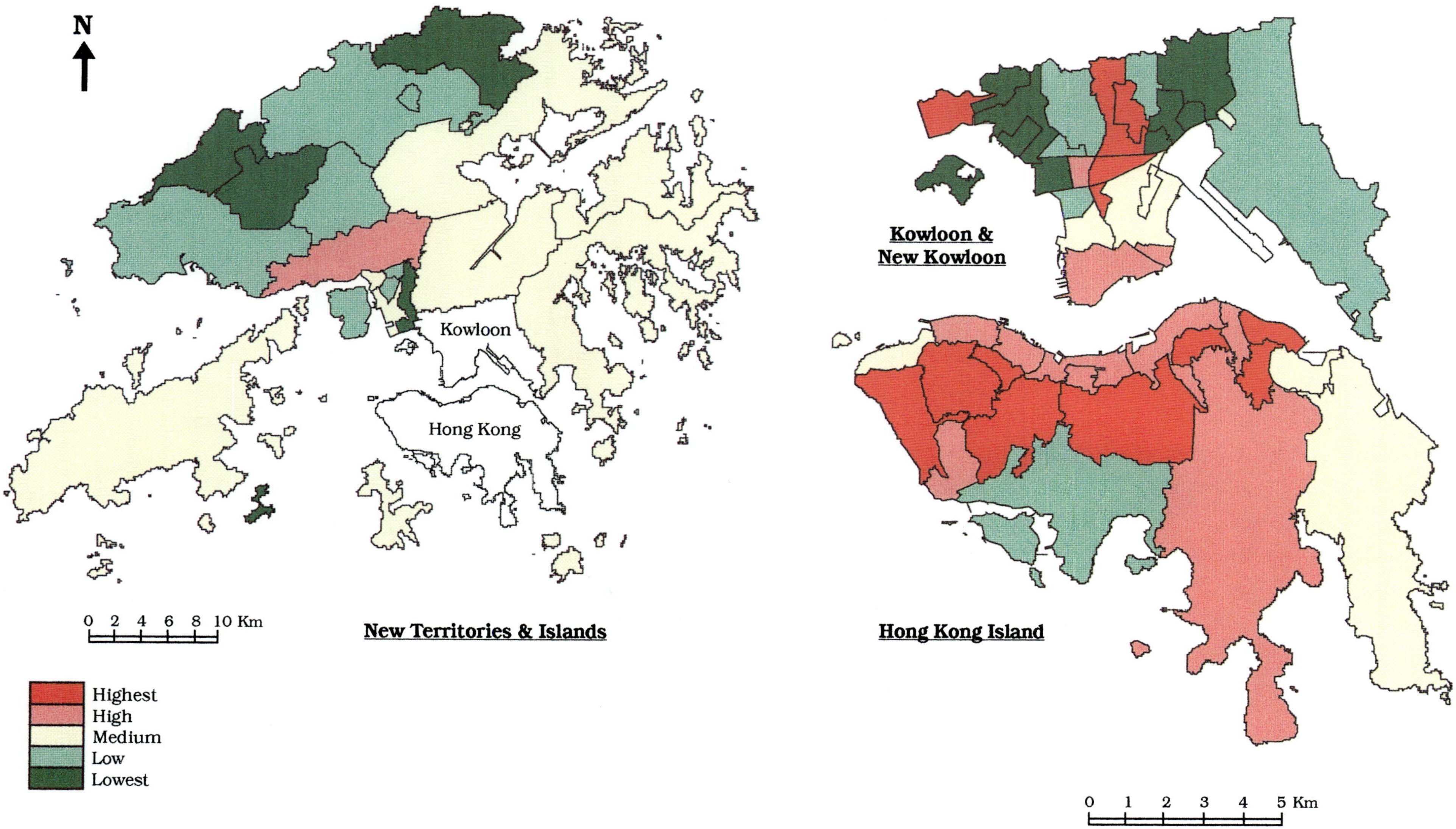

F-Score (in quintiles), 1991

(A composite score indicating socio-economic status)

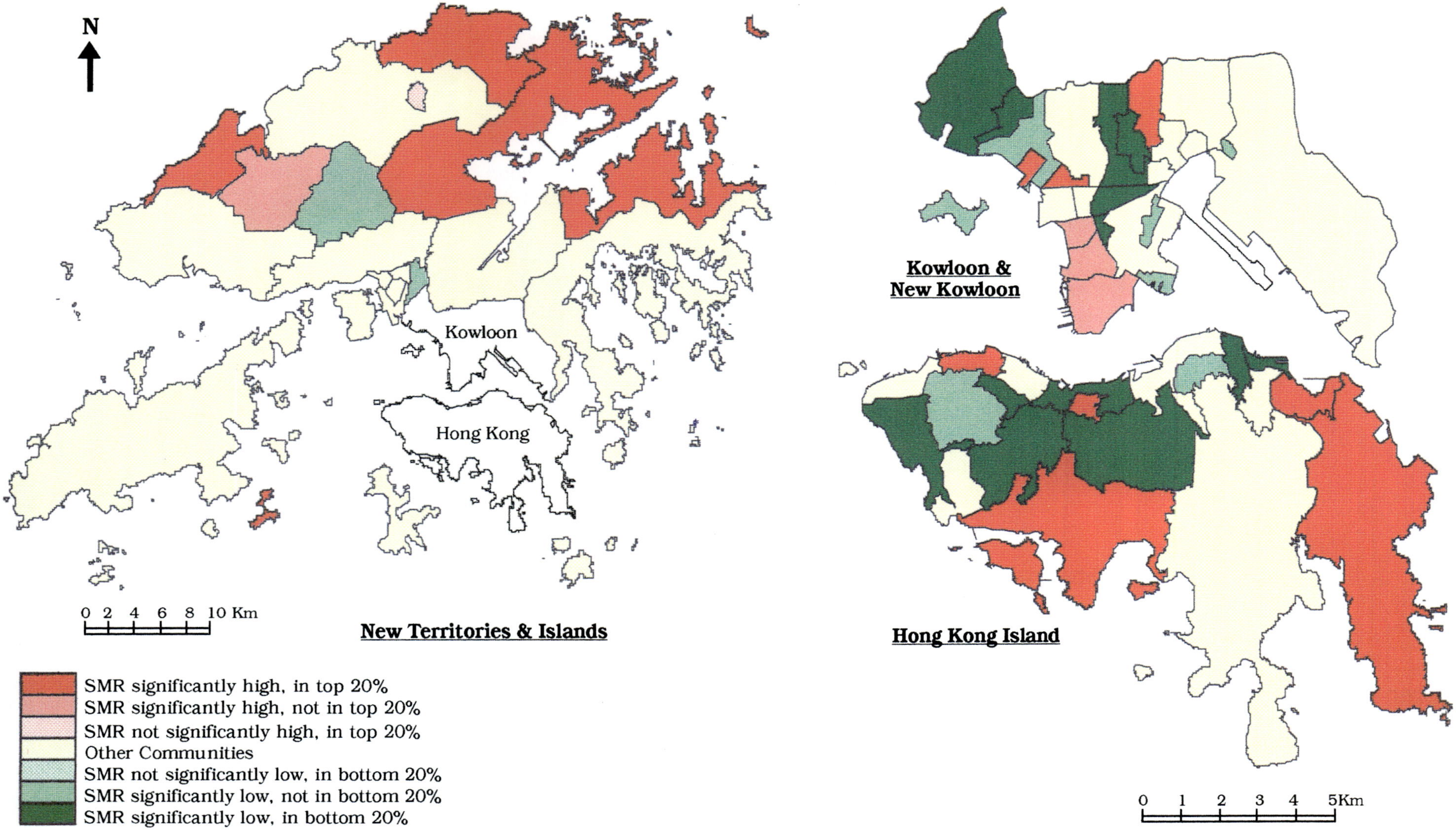

All Causes (Male, 1979 –1983)

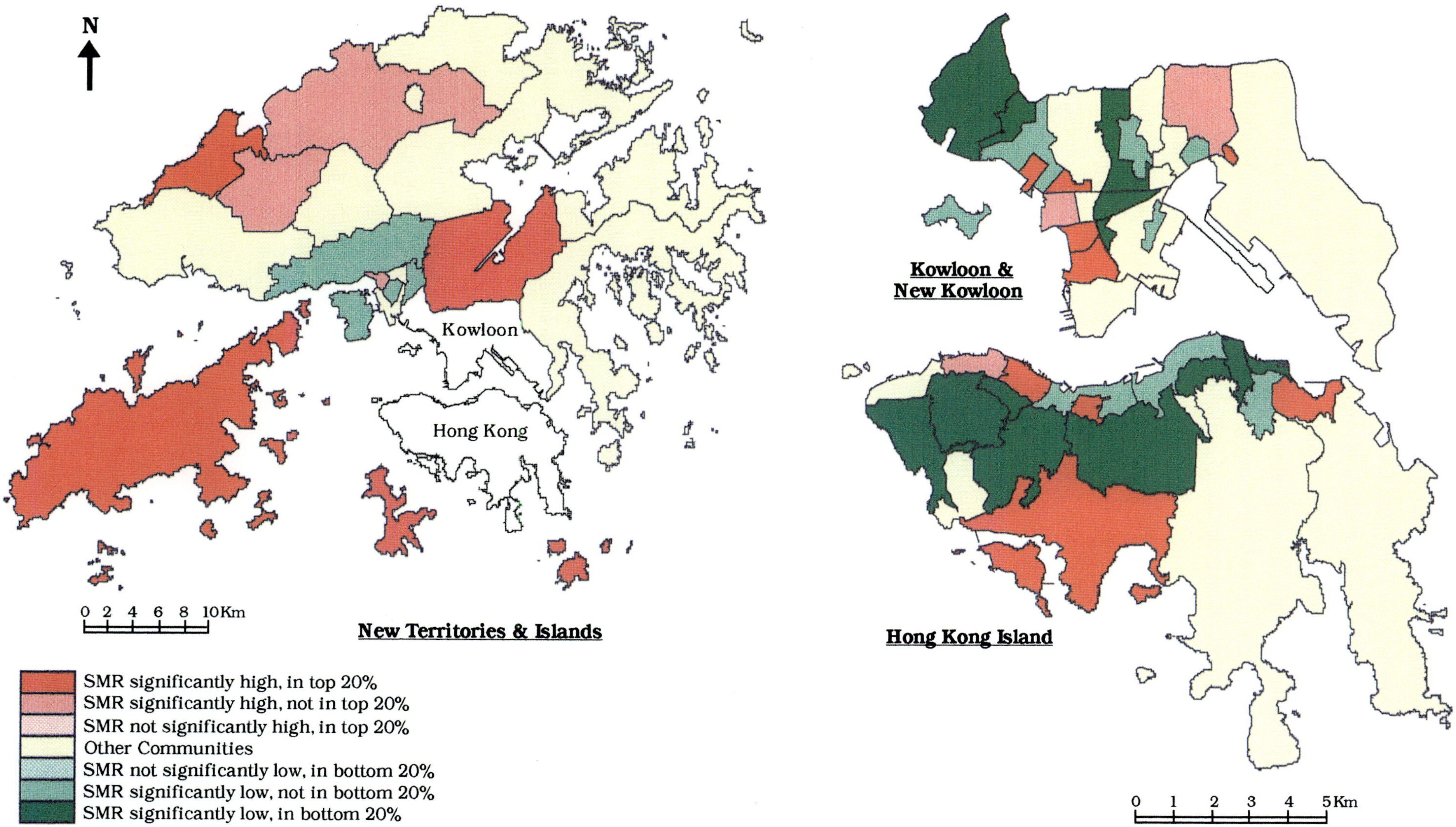

All Causes (Female, 1979 – 1983)

Number of Deaths, Standardised Mortality Ratio (SMR) and 95% Confidence Interval of All Causes by 65 Communities in 1979–1983

Community	Male			Female		
	Number of deaths	SMR	95% C.I.	Number of deaths	SMR	95% C.I.
HK1	1133	96.2	90.6 - 101.8	938	100.1	93.7 - 106.5
HK2	2011	108.3	103.6 - 113.0	1490	109.6	104.1 - 115.2
HK3	723	100.0	92.7 - 107.3	559	112.2	102.9 - 121.4
HK4	879	77.6	72.5 - 82.7	753	86.9	80.7 - 93.1
HK5	1307	120.0	113.5 - 126.5	1037	126.3	118.6 - 133.9
HK6	680	75.5	69.9 - 81.2	688	72.5	67.1 - 78.0
HK7	153	83.4	70.2 - 96.7	153	78.9	66.4 - 91.4
HK8	284	80.0	70.7 - 89.2	309	79.2	70.4 - 88.0
HK9	92	57.2	45.5 - 68.9	82	48.0	37.6 - 58.4
HK10	2409	96.2	92.4 - 100.1	2131	91.3	87.5 - 95.2
HK11	216	97.3	84.3 - 110.3	142	86.7	72.4 - 100.9
HK12	160	84.4	71.3 - 97.5	149	67.6	56.8 - 78.5
HK13	198	67.6	58.2 - 77.0	204	78.7	67.9 - 89.5
HK14	569	77.7	71.3 - 84.1	495	78.4	71.5 - 85.3
HK15	282	93.2	82.3 - 104.1	217	80.5	69.8 - 91.3
HK16	1549	114.7	109.0 - 120.4	1163	112.4	105.9 - 118.8
HK17	1587	108.2	102.8 - 113.5	1128	98.8	93.0 - 104.5
HK18	128	60.6	50.1 - 71.1	129	65.1	53.9 - 76.3
HK19	731	103.0	95.5 - 110.4	645	107.2	99.0 - 115.5
HK20	1776	113.2	107.9 - 118.4	1406	115.3	109.3 - 121.4
HK21	175	87.6	74.6 - 100.6	126	87.6	72.3 - 102.9
KL1	1054	108.1	101.6 - 114.6	758	102.3	95.0 - 109.6
KL2	2078	102.5	98.1 - 107.0	1670	105.5	100.4 - 110.5
KL3	600	102.1	94.0 - 110.3	516	100.8	92.1 - 109.5
KL4	1744	106.5	101.5 - 111.5	1430	115.9	109.9 - 121.9
KL5	1464	107.2	101.7 - 112.7	1164	115.8	109.1 - 122.4
KL6	260	77.2	67.8 - 86.6	234	60.8	53.0 - 68.6
KL7	190	75.0	64.3 - 85.6	211	79.4	68.7 - 90.1
KL8	777	88.8	82.6 - 95.1	690	92.5	85.6 - 99.4
KL9	3149	96.7	93.3 - 100.0	2774	99.7	96.0 - 103.4
KL10	291	87.1	77.1 - 97.1	280	93.2	82.3 - 104.1
KL11	715	80.2	74.3 - 86.0	617	76.1	70.1 - 82.1
KL12	187	70.0	59.9 - 80.0	156	78.4	66.1 - 90.8
KL13	2937	89.5	86.2 - 92.7	2395	94.2	90.4 - 97.9
KL14	2023	103.9	99.4 - 108.4	1432	102.2	96.9 - 107.5
KL15	235	148.6	129.6 - 167.6	210	165.4	143.0 - 187.8
KL16	958	122.1	114.4 - 129.9	757	117.8	109.5 - 126.2
KL17	183	82.3	70.4 - 94.2	196	72.7	62.5 - 82.9
KL18	116	75.9	62.1 - 89.8	116	82.7	67.7 - 97.8
KL19	2933	101.4	97.7 - 105.1	2644	107.2	103.1 - 111.3
KL20	1091	109.3	102.8 - 115.8	829	101.7	94.7 - 108.6
KL21	1628	101.2	96.3 - 106.1	1299	98.6	93.3 - 104.0
KL22	265	94.4	83.0 - 105.7	172	85.8	72.9 - 98.6
KL23	825	94.0	87.6 - 100.4	641	95.9	88.5 - 103.3
KL24	468	90.6	82.4 - 98.8	454	112.1	101.8 - 122.5
KL25	8107	100.1	97.9 - 102.2	6355	98.2	95.8 - 100.7
NT1	398	92.9	83.8 - 102.0	316	87.4	77.8 - 97.1
NT2	593	96.5	88.7 - 104.2	429	91.9	83.2 - 100.6
NT3	1254	104.2	98.5 - 110.0	896	111.6	104.3 - 118.9
NT4	650	97.9	90.4 - 105.4	543	96.2	88.1 - 104.3
NT5	2349	102.0	97.9 - 106.2	1715	94.4	89.9 - 98.8
NT6	1013	89.5	84.0 - 95.0	804	86.1	80.1 - 92.0
NT7	410	100.4	90.7 - 110.1	279	88.9	78.5 - 99.3
NT8	1329	100.4	95.0 - 105.8	1019	102.5	96.2 - 108.8
NT9	511	131.0	119.7 - 142.4	331	114.2	101.9 - 126.6
NT10	1750	108.1	103.0 - 113.1	1327	111.0	105.1 - 117.0
NT11	301	88.6	78.6 - 98.6	252	105.7	92.7 - 118.8
NT12	1586	104.0	98.9 - 109.1	1251	107.5	101.5 - 113.4
NT13	310	108.7	96.6 - 120.8	254	110.2	96.6 - 123.7
NT14	298	113.0	100.2 - 125.9	258	108.6	95.3 - 121.8
NT15	1263	118.3	111.8 - 124.8	922	102.7	96.1 - 109.4
NT16	1381	103.7	98.2 - 109.1	1319	116.5	110.2 - 122.8
NT17	649	103.6	95.6 - 111.5	554	107.9	98.9 - 116.9
NT18	400	131.6	118.7 - 144.4	372	140.0	125.8 - 154.3
NT19	541	104.5	95.7 - 113.3	510	114.7	104.7 - 124.7

ALL CAUSES

Sex-Age specific mortality rate (1/100,000) of all causes in Hong Kong (1979–1983)

	Male		Female	
Age	No. of deaths	Mortality rate	No. of deaths	Mortality rate
0–4	2087	197.92	1650	166.75
5–9	746	70.32	545	55.27
10–14	471	41.15	387	36.18
15–19	744	52.09	413	30.98
20–24	1056	68.95	593	42.58
25–29	1104	83.61	589	50.64
30–34	1182	107.16	612	66.77
35–39	1147	158.87	526	94.60
40–44	1992	283.07	861	155.65
45–49	3372	467.45	1557	257.27
50–54	5355	779.46	2380	390.26
55–59	7130	1253.46	3522	658.57
60–64	9057	1982.10	4817	1055.96
65+	32866	4820.69	36844	3649.91
TOTAL	68309	518.10	55296	454.17

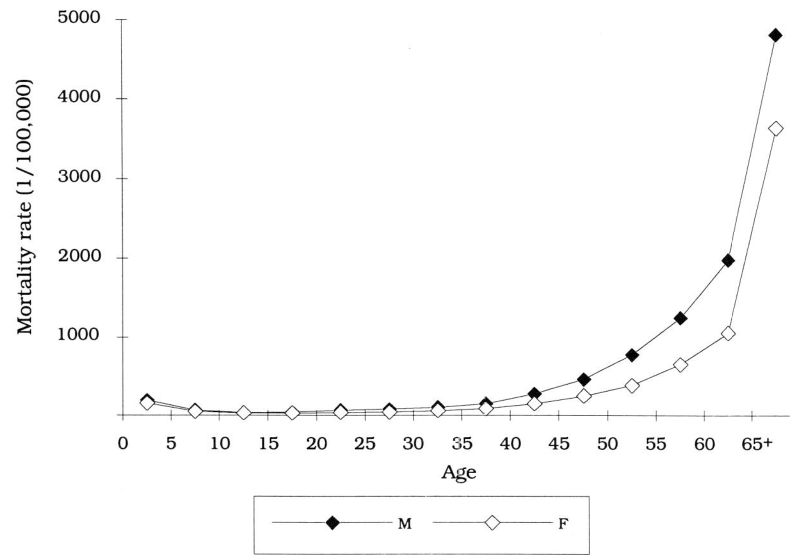

Number of communities on map by category based on standardized mortality ratio (SMR) during 1979–1983

Category	Number of communities Male	Female
SMR significantly high, in top 20%	12	13
SMR significantly high , not in top 20%	4	6
SMR not significantly high, in top 20%	1	0
SMR not significantly low, in bottom 20%	0	0
SMR significantly low, not in bottom 20%	8	11
SMR significantly low, in bottom 20%	13	13
other communities	27	22

Values of the standardized mortality ratio (SMR) which divide the 65 communities into quintile

Percentile	Male	Female
20th	82.28	79.38
40th	94.36	93.21
60th	102.02	102.30
80th	108.08	111.59
Lowest SMR	57.23	47.99
Highest SMR	148.61	165.41
No. of communities with zero death	0	0

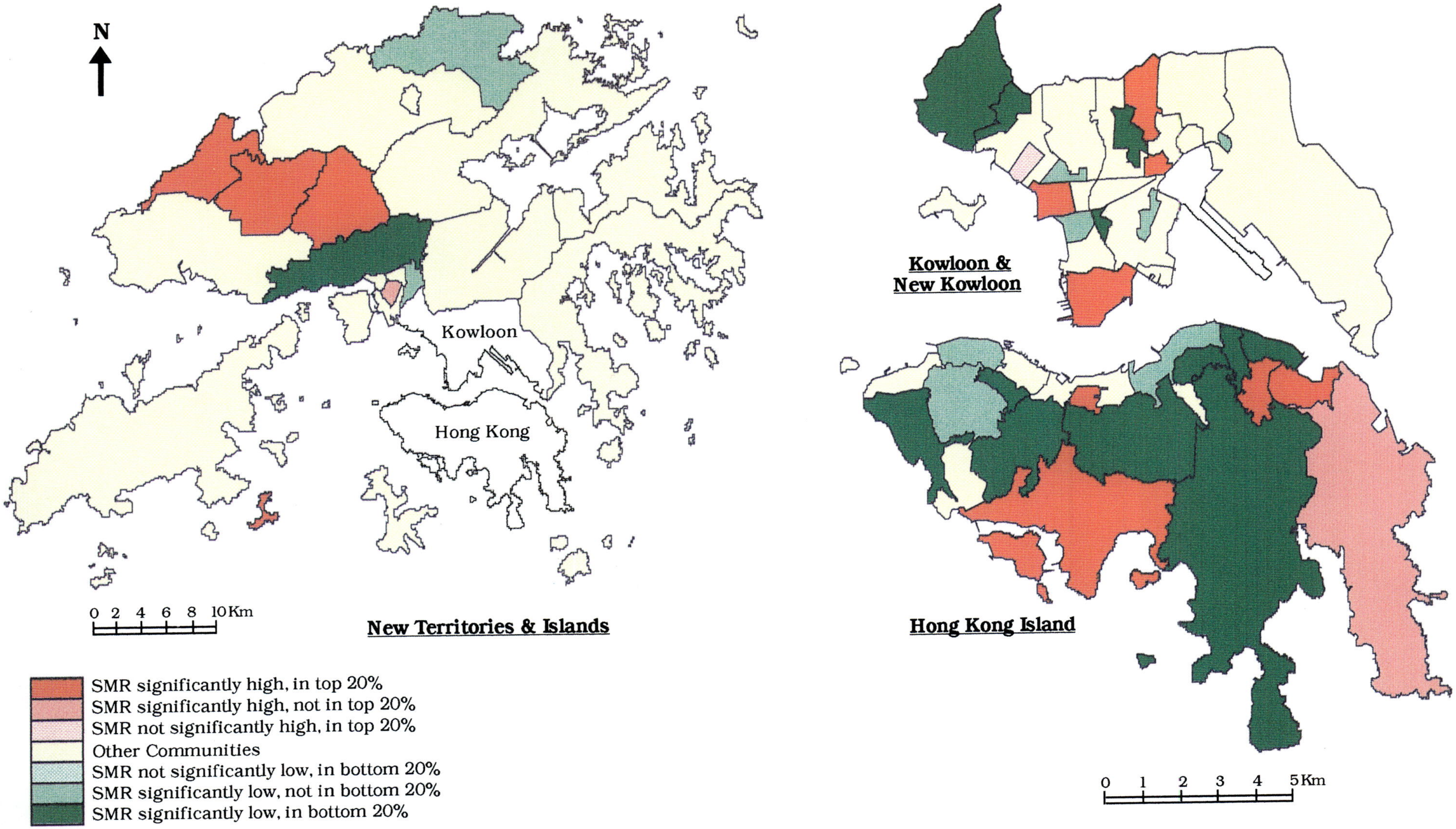

All Causes (Male, 1984 – 1988)

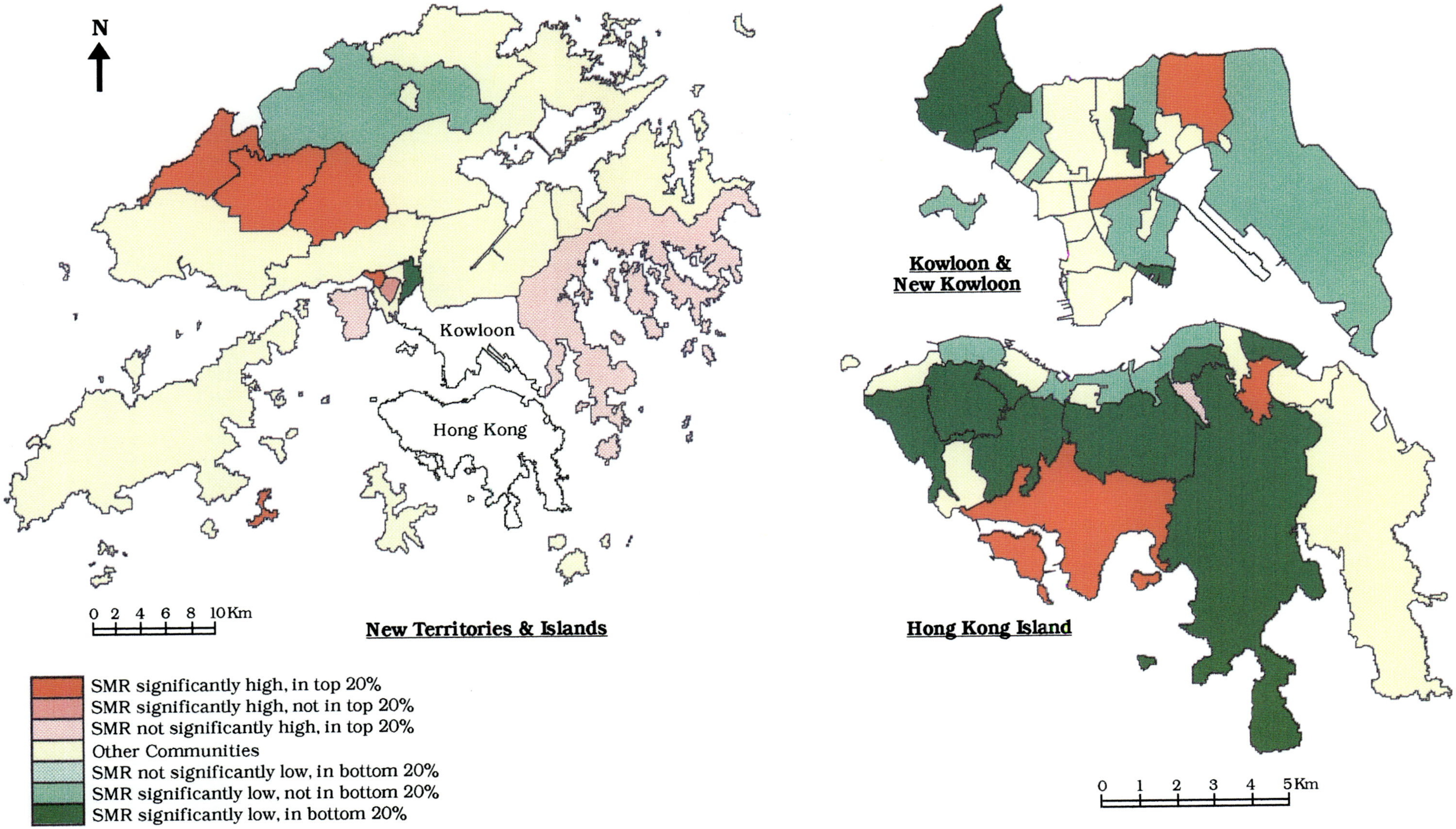

All Causes (Female, 1984 - 1988)

Number of Deaths, Standardised Mortality Ratio (SMR) and 95% Confidence Interval of All Causes by 65 Communities in 1984–1988

Community	Male			Female		
	Number of deaths	SMR	95% C.I.	Number of deaths	SMR	95% C.I.
HK1	1115	97.1	91.4 - 102.8	881	98.4	91.9 - 104.9
HK2	1520	93.6	88.9 - 98.3	1175	92.9	87.6 - 98.2
HK3	566	94.3	86.5 - 102.1	393	94.4	85.1 - 103.8
HK4	917	95.0	88.9 - 101.2	700	92.5	85.7 - 99.4
HK5	992	115.9	108.7 - 123.1	711	100.4	93.1 - 107.8
HK6	719	81.7	75.7 - 87.7	740	84.2	78.1 - 90.2
HK7	153	85.5	71.9 - 99.0	139	79.0	65.9 - 92.2
HK8	194	59.4	51.0 - 67.7	238	75.6	66.0 - 85.2
HK9	67	47.2	35.9 - 58.5	77	49.2	38.2 - 60.2
HK10	2317	94.6	90.7 - 98.4	2158	93.9	89.9 - 97.8
HK11	213	98.1	84.9 - 111.2	160	108.2	91.5 - 125.0
HK12	147	72.3	60.6 - 84.0	147	77.3	64.8 - 89.8
HK13	240	81.7	71.3 - 92.0	218	99.5	86.3 - 112.7
HK14	593	64.9	59.7 - 70.2	619	74.1	68.2 - 79.9
HK15	387	132.8	119.5 - 146.0	346	125.0	111.8 - 138.1
HK16	1389	110.5	104.6 - 116.3	1045	105.3	98.9 - 111.7
HK17	1815	108.7	103.7 - 113.7	1342	101.5	96.0 - 106.9
HK18	86	46.0	36.3 - 55.8	84	46.4	36.4 - 56.3
HK19	795	100.3	93.3 - 107.3	663	100.5	92.8 - 108.1
HK20	2100	120.9	115.7 - 126.1	1698	122.9	117.1 - 128.8
HK21	152	70.1	59.0 - 81.2	119	64.8	53.1 - 76.4
KL1	960	110.0	103.0 - 117.0	683	104.2	96.4 - 112.0
KL2	1887	112.7	107.6 - 117.7	1343	103.0	97.5 - 108.5
KL3	498	97.1	88.5 - 105.6	476	105.7	96.2 - 115.2
KL4	1406	90.2	85.5 - 95.0	1075	97.4	91.5 - 103.2
KL5	1204	104.7	98.8 - 110.6	876	102.9	96.1 - 109.8
KL6	292	90.1	79.8 - 100.4	380	115.2	103.6 - 126.7
KL7	181	76.3	65.2 - 87.4	213	105.0	90.9 - 119.1
KL8	705	87.9	81.4 - 94.3	587	92.7	85.2 - 100.2
KL9	3019	95.5	92.1 - 98.9	2444	95.0	91.2 - 98.8
KL10	309	97.5	86.6 - 108.3	233	84.6	73.8 - 95.5
KL11	767	82.6	76.8 - 88.5	651	83.3	76.9 - 89.7
KL12	199	78.4	67.5 - 89.3	115	61.8	50.5 - 73.1
KL13	2794	98.9	95.3 - 102.6	2086	95.9	91.7 - 100.0
KL14	2129	103.0	98.6 - 107.4	1523	98.4	93.4 - 103.3
KL15	377	109.4	98.4 - 120.5	303	101.3	89.9 - 112.7
KL16	638	89.1	82.2 - 96.0	521	99.0	90.5 - 107.5
KL17	292	91.0	80.6 - 101.5	416	97.4	88.0 - 106.8
KL18	105	77.5	62.7 - 92.4	87	78.5	62.0 - 95.0
KL19	3025	103.6	99.9 - 107.3	2559	109.5	105.2 - 113.7
KL20	822	115.4	107.5 - 123.3	546	90.2	82.7 - 97.8
KL21	1288	105.1	99.4 - 110.9	963	105.7	99.0 - 112.4
KL22	237	93.2	81.4 - 105.1	175	91.5	77.9 - 105.1
KL23	957	149.1	139.6 - 158.5	740	153.3	142.3 - 164.4
KL24	527	90.6	82.8 - 98.3	410	101.7	91.9 - 111.6
KL25	9007	96.3	94.3 - 98.3	6856	94.5	92.3 - 96.8
NT1	458	84.2	76.5 - 91.9	432	97.4	88.2 - 106.6
NT2	627	95.8	88.3 - 103.3	502	102.5	93.5 - 111.5
NT3	1238	105.4	99.6 - 111.3	853	110.7	103.3 - 118.2
NT4	965	96.8	90.7 - 102.9	763	95.5	88.7 - 102.3
NT5	2261	108.2	103.7 - 112.7	1635	106.1	101.0 - 111.3
NT6	1133	91.7	86.4 - 97.0	818	90.0	83.8 - 96.2
NT7	669	104.7	96.8 - 112.6	478	107.6	97.9 - 117.2
NT8	2284	99.4	95.4 - 103.5	1954	103.1	98.6 - 107.7
NT9	538	138.8	127.1 - 150.5	430	133.6	120.9 - 146.2
NT10	2221	121.3	116.3 - 126.4	1934	141.8	135.5 - 148.1
NT11	369	112.9	101.4 - 124.5	356	127.2	114.0 - 140.4
NT12	1637	101.3	96.4 - 106.2	1211	91.0	85.9 - 96.1
NT13	411	96.5	87.2 - 105.9	295	101.5	89.9 - 113.0
NT14	229	87.6	76.2 - 98.9	218	101.0	87.6 - 114.4
NT15	1577	103.7	98.6 - 108.8	1414	105.1	99.6 - 110.6
NT16	3297	98.9	95.6 - 102.3	2992	97.2	93.7 - 100.7
NT17	678	106.2	98.2 - 114.1	545	108.1	99.0 - 117.1
NT18	415	131.5	118.8 - 144.1	399	147.6	133.1 - 162.0
NT19	492	102.8	93.8 - 111.9	411	106.6	96.3 - 116.9

ALL CAUSES

Sex-Age specific mortality rate (1/100,000) of all causes in Hong Kong (1984–1988)

	Male		Female	
Age	No. of deaths	Mortality rate	No. of deaths	Mortality rate
0–4	1427	133.36	1152	115.87
5–9	517	47.11	443	43.55
10–14	360	31.59	272	26.07
15–19	523	43.66	303	27.50
20–24	800	55.36	470	33.86
25–29	1039	66.20	613	41.46
30–34	1195	88.30	670	54.15
35–39	1444	130.17	730	75.26
40–44	1648	224.83	658	109.74
45–49	2709	384.80	1122	192.29
50–54	4980	679.49	2056	325.57
55–59	7095	1068.20	3187	524.61
60–64	9267	1715.79	4734	884.36
65+	40091	4440.25	41730	3381.14
TOTAL	73095	512.61	58140	433.17

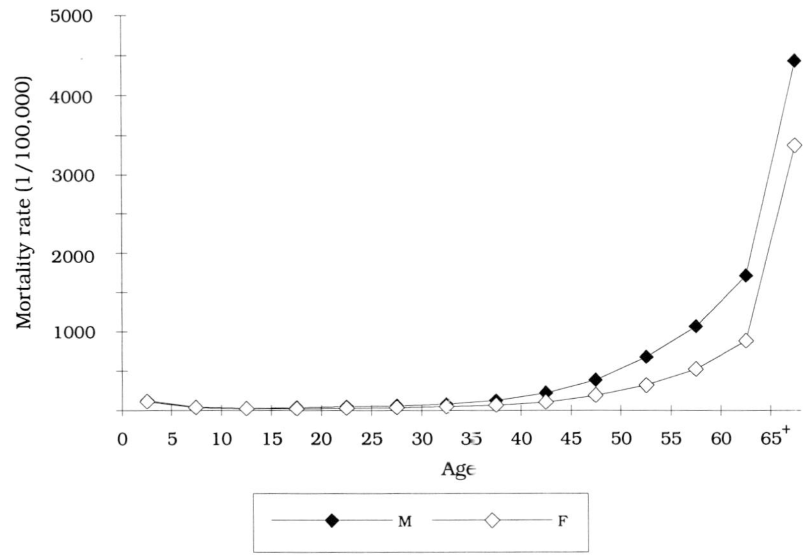

Number of communities on map by category based on standardized mortality ratio (SMR) during 1984–1988

Category	Number of communities Male	Female
SMR significantly high, in top 20%	12	10
SMR significantly high , not in top 20%	2	1
SMR not significantly high, in top 20%	1	3
SMR not significantly low, in bottom 20%	0	0
SMR significantly low, not in bottom 20%	9	8
SMR significantly low, in bottom 20%	13	13
other communities	28	30

Values of the standardized mortality ratio (SMR) which divide the 65 communities into quintile

Percentile	Male	Female
20th	84.19	90.00
40th	94.55	97.17
60th	99.45	101.47
80th	108.68	106.59
Lowest SMR	46.05	46.35
Highest SMR	149.08	153.34
No. of communities with zero death	0	0

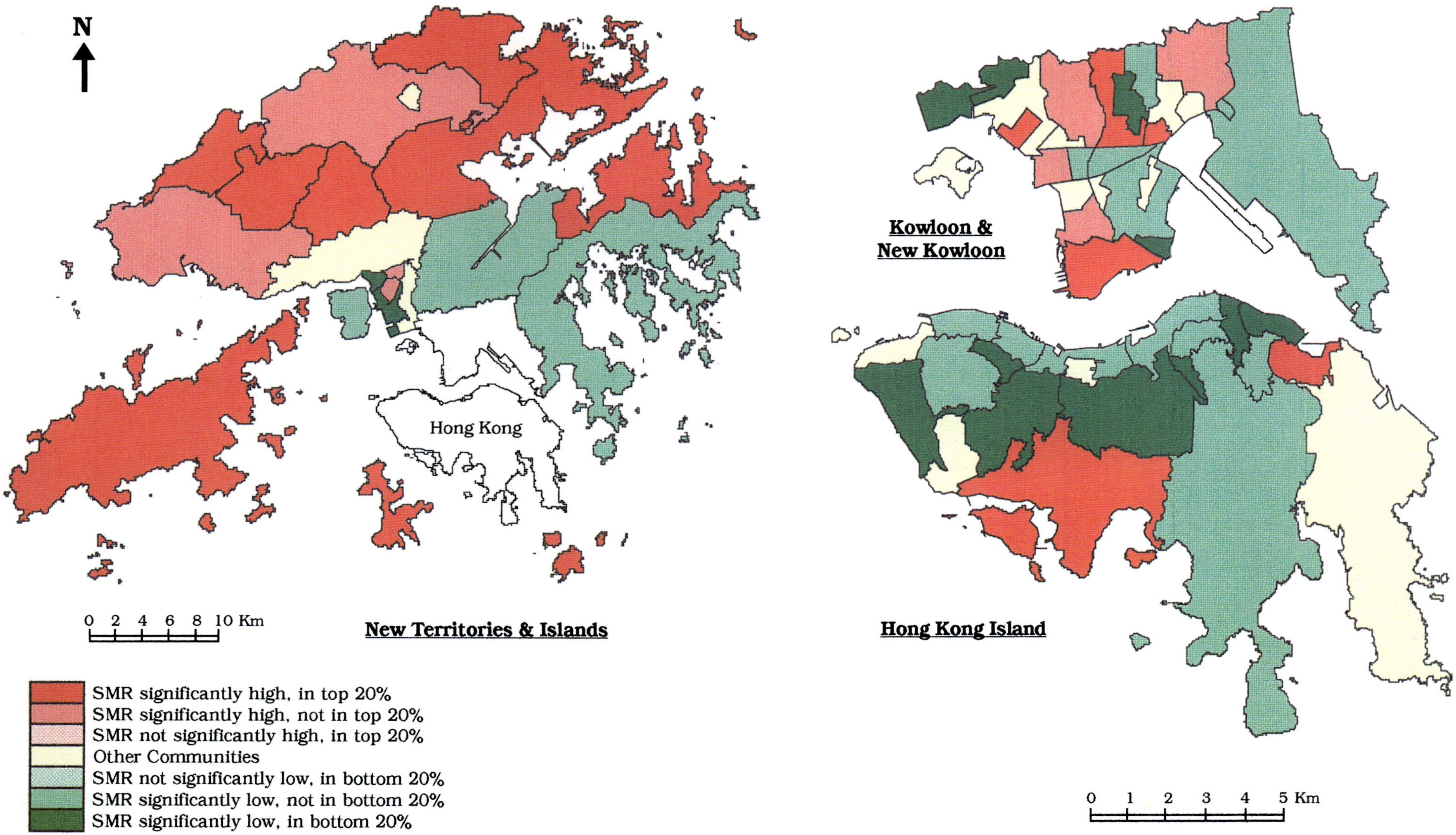

All Causes (Male, 1989 -1993)

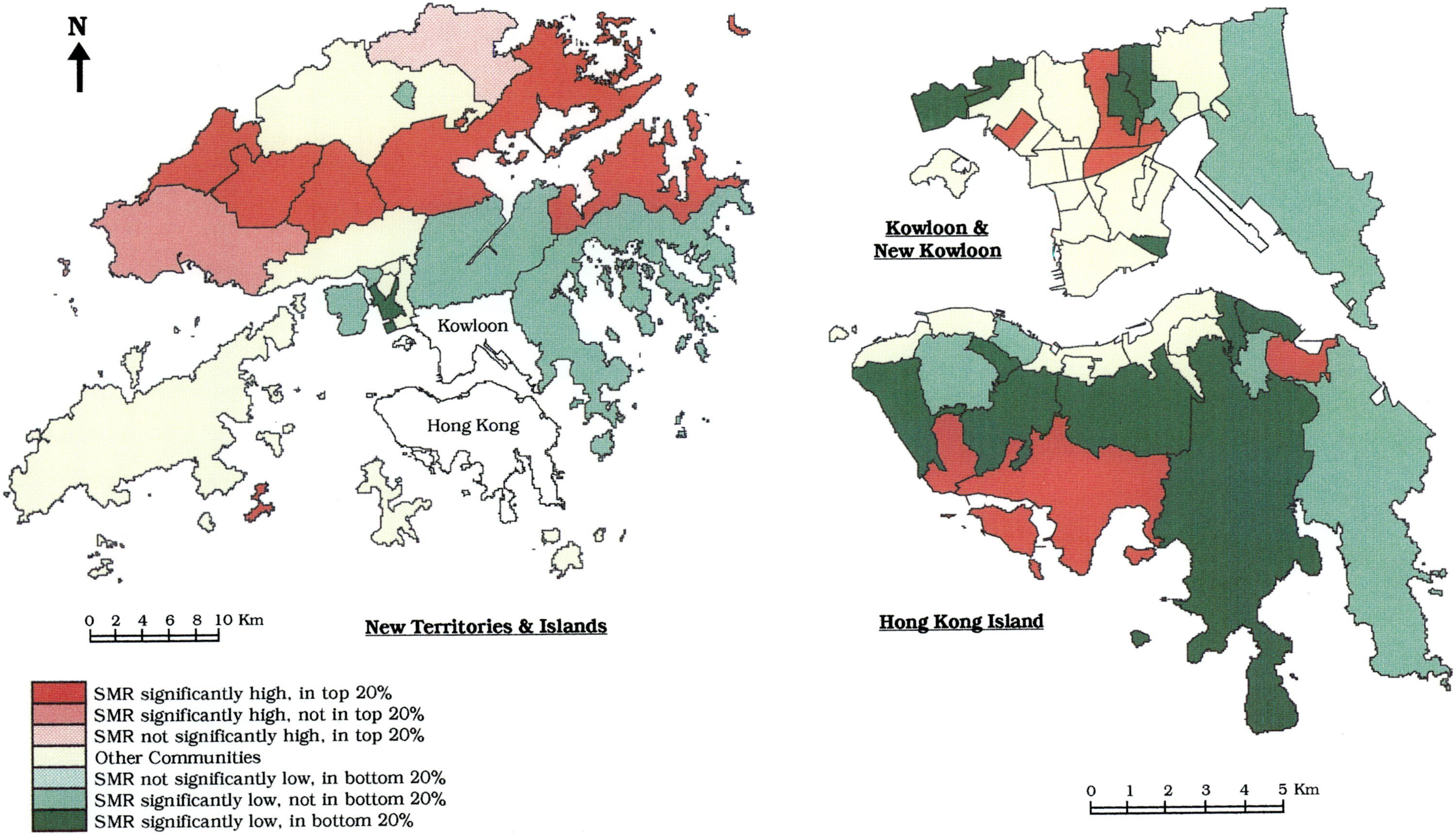

All Causes (Female, 1989 -1993)

Number of Deaths, Standardised Mortality Ratio (SMR) and 95% Confidence Interval
of All Causes by 65 Communities in 1989–1993

Community	Male			Female		
	Number of deaths	SMR	95% C.I.	Number of deaths	SMR	95% C.I.
HK1	1144	95.5	89.9 - 101.0	896	97.3	90.9 - 103.7
HK2	1497	92.8	88.1 - 97.5	1087	97.4	91.7 - 103.2
HK3	506	91.8	83.8 - 99.8	321	87.8	78.2 - 97.4
HK4	825	91.9	85.6 - 98.2	631	97.2	89.6 - 104.7
HK5	909	106.0	99.2 - 112.9	644	105.4	97.2 - 113.5
HK6	742	75.8	70.4 - 81.3	777	85.0	79.0 - 91.0
HK7	187	85.9	73.6 - 98.3	186	85.5	73.2 - 97.8
HK8	240	68.8	60.1 - 77.5	209	71.2	61.5 - 80.8
HK9	101	65.1	52.4 - 77.8	103	73.6	59.4 - 87.8
HK10	2564	93.3	89.7 - 96.9	2369	96.4	92.6 - 100.3
HK11	206	82.1	70.9 - 93.3	170	100.4	85.3 - 115.4
HK12	190	85.2	73.1 - 97.3	188	95.0	81.4 - 108.6
HK13	197	66.6	57.3 - 75.9	184	83.6	71.5 - 95.7
HK14	701	64.2	59.4 - 68.9	667	76.7	70.9 - 82.6
HK15	554	85.4	78.3 - 92.6	465	88.8	80.7 - 96.8
HK16	1248	111.8	105.6 - 118.0	1027	121.0	113.6 - 128.4
HK17	2449	103.5	99.4 - 107.6	1722	94.0	89.6 - 98.5
HK18	115	44.7	36.5 - 52.8	139	52.9	44.1 - 61.8
HK19	967	102.6	96.1 - 109.1	783	112.5	104.6 - 120.3
HK20	2441	114.6	110.0 - 119.1	1938	114.5	109.4 - 119.6
HK21	181	84.1	71.8 - 96.3	111	76.4	62.2 - 90.6
KL1	789	110.5	102.8 - 118.2	560	106.0	97.2 - 114.8
KL2	1735	105.1	100.2 - 110.1	1198	100.5	94.8 - 106.2
KL3	438	90.2	81.8 - 98.7	392	98.2	88.5 - 108.0
KL4	1389	100.5	95.2 - 105.8	921	101.0	94.5 - 107.6
KL5	1087	108.0	101.5 - 114.4	766	107.2	99.6 - 114.8
KL6	326	85.0	75.8 - 94.2	461	111.6	101.4 - 121.8
KL7	239	89.3	78.0 - 100.7	262	98.7	86.7 - 110.6
KL8	807	96.9	90.2 - 103.6	589	95.5	87.8 - 103.2
KL9	3072	92.2	89.0 - 95.5	2443	96.9	93.1 - 100.7
KL10	456	79.1	71.9 - 86.4	395	77.6	70.0 - 85.3
KL11	561	73.1	67.1 - 79.2	475	74.3	67.6 - 81.0
KL12	181	73.7	63.0 - 84.5	136	71.5	59.5 - 83.6
KL13	2970	97.0	93.5 - 100.5	2131	97.9	93.7 - 102.0
KL14	2112	104.8	100.4 - 109.3	1505	95.9	91.1 - 100.8
KL15	518	136.9	125.1 - 148.7	369	122.0	109.6 - 134.5
KL16	732	106.2	98.5 - 113.8	506	103.1	94.2 - 112.1
KL17	456	147.6	134.1 - 161.2	674	182.7	168.9 - 196.5
KL18	86	60.7	47.9 - 73.5	79	58.3	45.4 - 71.2
KL19	3428	106.7	103.2 - 110.3	2662	98.7	94.9 - 102.4
KL20	607	82.7	76.1 - 89.3	453	81.8	74.3 - 89.3
KL21	1205	104.0	98.1 - 109.9	845	90.3	84.2 - 96.3
KL22	233	98.2	85.6 - 110.8	185	103.7	88.8 - 118.7
KL23	881	180.2	168.3 - 192.0	722	195.9	181.6 - 210.2
KL24	547	85.8	78.6 - 92.9	432	103.1	93.4 - 112.8
KL25	9328	95.9	93.9 - 97.8	6945	91.3	89.2 - 93.5
NT1	768	95.3	88.6 - 102.1	615	93.2	85.9 - 100.6
NT2	611	76.0	70.0 - 82.0	522	80.8	73.9 - 87.8
NT3	1210	82.0	77.4 - 86.7	875	90.8	84.8 - 96.8
NT4	1069	106.7	100.3 - 113.1	821	102.9	95.8 - 109.9
NT5	2311	109.0	104.5 - 113.4	1579	101.1	96.1 - 106.1
NT6	1421	101.1	95.8 - 106.3	1018	95.1	89.3 - 101.0
NT7	1321	93.8	88.7 - 98.8	930	92.3	86.4 - 98.3
NT8	3602	107.2	103.7 - 110.7	2803	107.7	103.7 - 111.6
NT9	698	165.1	152.9 - 177.4	555	152.8	140.1 - 165.5
NT10	2906	137.7	132.7 - 142.7	2631	164.9	158.6 - 171.2
NT11	476	121.7	110.7 - 132.6	475	144.0	131.0 - 156.9
NT12	2066	106.0	101.4 - 110.5	1570	101.2	96.2 - 106.2
NT13	395	98.5	88.8 - 108.2	310	89.4	79.5 - 99.4
NT14	285	129.4	114.3 - 144.4	219	110.7	96.1 - 125.4
NT15	2563	115.6	111.1 - 120.1	2223	117.5	112.6 - 122.3
NT16	5177	96.2	93.6 - 98.8	4423	91.7	89.0 - 94.4
NT17	1265	92.4	87.3 - 97.5	1028	89.0	83.5 - 94.4
NT18	411	111.8	101.0 - 122.6	353	116.6	104.4 - 128.7
NT19	504	111.4	101.7 - 121.2	423	110.1	99.6 - 120.6

ALL CAUSES

Sex-Age specific mortality rate (1/100,000) of all causes in Hong Kong (1989–1993)

	Male		Female	
Age	No. of deaths	Mortality rate	No. of deaths	Mortality rate
0–4	871	91.43	774	87.61
5–9	335	31.69	279	28.52
10–14	297	27.21	229	22.72
15–19	453	41.48	297	29.66
20–24	686	60.09	366	32.27
25–29	1038	71.97	523	35.36
30–34	1292	82.85	732	48.18
35–39	1666	124.43	900	71.52
40–44	2188	198.67	1038	106.78
45–49	2426	332.06	1015	169.99
50–54	3933	566.88	1624	285.21
55–59	6579	941.47	2817	462.49
60–64	9602	1555.48	4434	767.26
65+	49843	4499.68	49069	3492.70
TOTAL	81209	555.27	64097	458.07

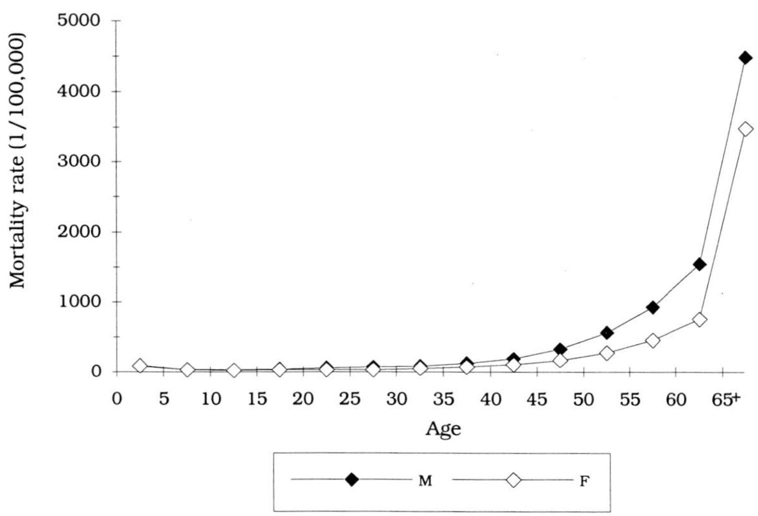

Number of communities on map by category based on standardized mortality ratio (SMR) during 1989–1993

Category	Number of communities Male	Female
SMR significantly high, in top 20%	13	12
SMR significantly high , not in top 20%	8	1
SMR not significantly high, in top 20%	0	1
SMR not significantly low, in bottom 20%	0	0
SMR significantly low, not in bottom 20%	17	11
SMR significantly low, in bottom 20%	13	13
other communities	14	28

Values of the standardized mortality ratio (SMR) which divide the 65 communities into quintile

Percentile	Male	Female
20th	82.08	85.00
40th	92.40	95.03
60th	101.06	100.36
80th	108.96	110.11
Lowest SMR	44.67	52.95
Highest SMR	180.15	195.92
No. of communities with zero cases	0	0

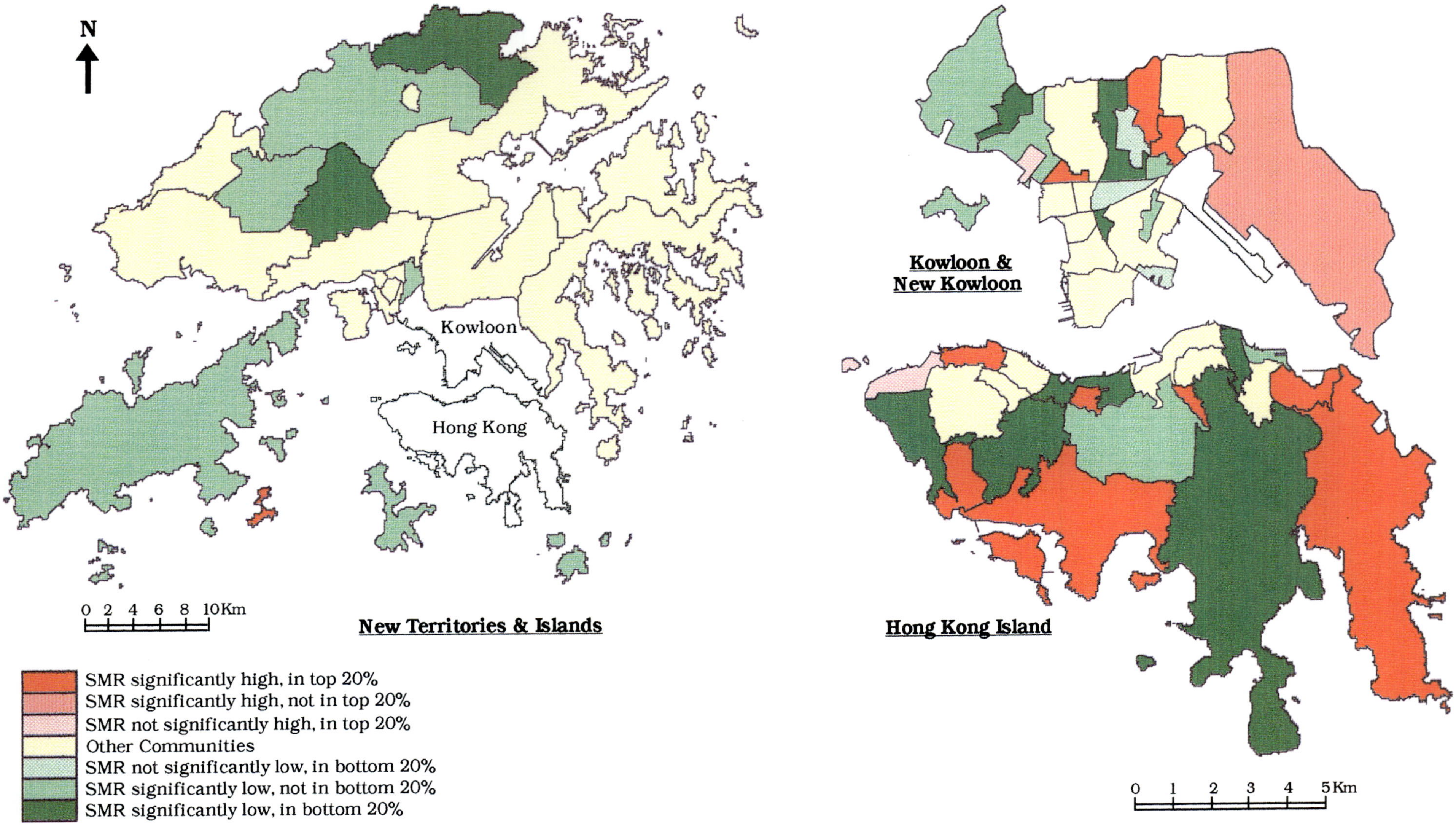

All Cancers (Male, 1979 – 1983)

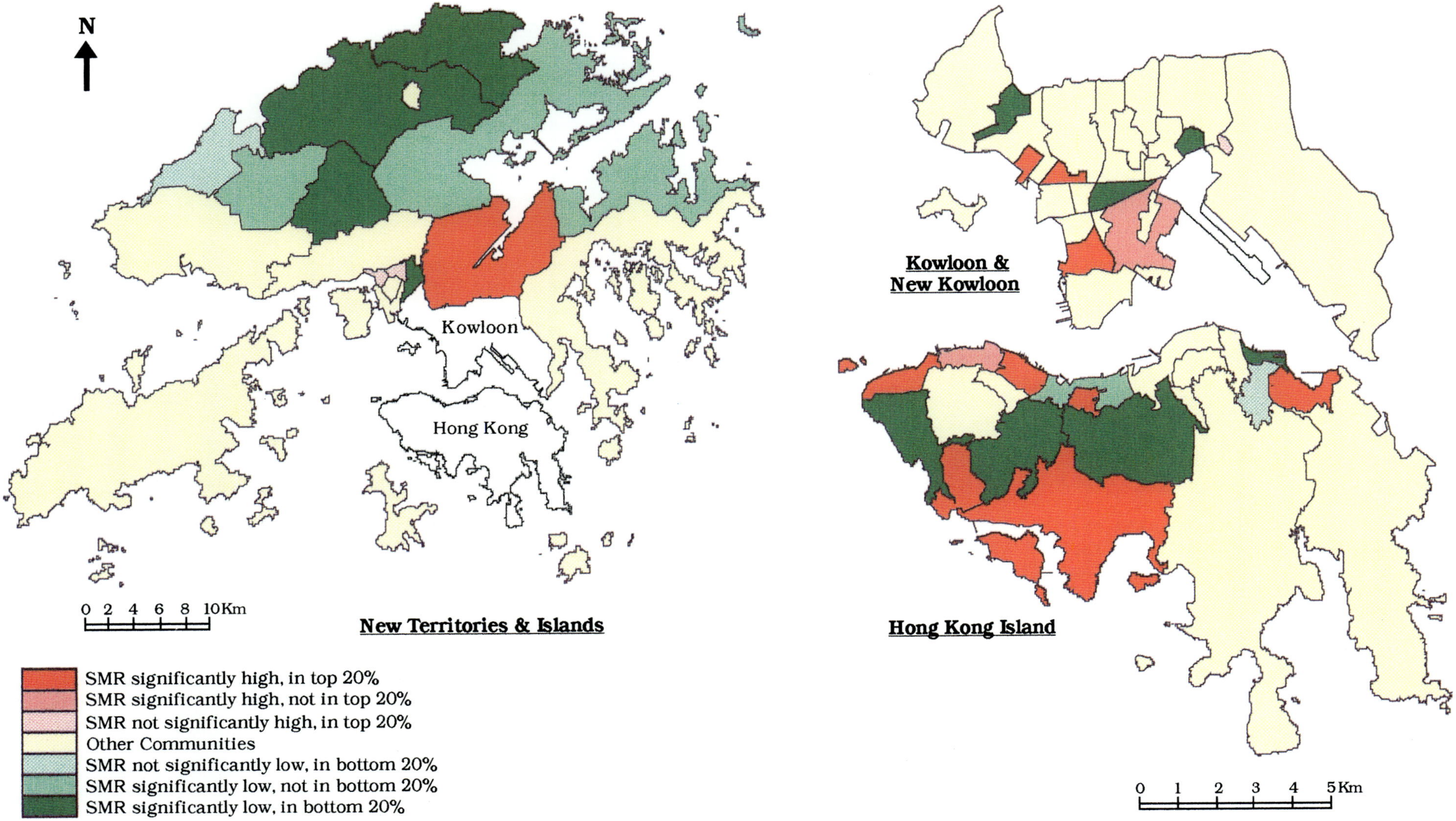

All Cancers (Female, 1979 – 1983)

Number of Deaths, Standardised Mortality Ratio (SMR) and 95% Confidence Interval of All Cancers by 65 Communities in 1979–1983

	Male			Female				Male			Female		
Community	Number of deaths	SMR	95% C.I.	Number of deaths	SMR	95% C.I.	Community	Number of deaths	SMR	95% C.I.	Number of deaths	SMR	95% C.I.
HK1	384	110.7	99.7 - 121.8	249	115.5	101.1 - 129.8	KL13	865	87.3	81.5 - 93.1	557	96.7	88.7 - 104.7
HK2	606	111.5	102.6 - 120.3	342	112.1	100.2 - 123.9	KL14	595	105.3	96.9 - 113.8	324	100.2	89.3 - 111.1
HK3	220	103.2	89.6 - 116.9	136	123.4	102.6 - 144.1	KL15	57	119.6	88.5 - 150.6	51	183.8	133.4 - 234.3
HK4	253	74.9	65.7 - 84.2	164	82.9	70.2 - 95.6	KL16	301	129.1	114.5 - 143.7	188	133.1	114.1 - 152.1
HK5	434	134.4	121.8 - 147.1	272	147.9	130.3 - 165.5	KL17	47	70.0	50.0 - 90.0	54	86.8	63.7 - 110.0
HK6	234	87.2	76.0 - 98.4	179	81.4	69.5 - 93.3	KL18	38	83.9	57.2 - 110.6	29	90.4	57.5 - 123.3
HK7	46	85.5	60.8 - 110.2	39	85.7	58.8 - 112.6	KL19	856	99.0	92.3 - 105.6	576	102.1	93.8 - 110.5
HK8	92	87.6	69.7 - 105.5	87	96.8	76.5 - 117.2	KL20	345	116.4	104.2 - 128.7	187	99.8	85.5 - 114.1
HK9	18	36.4	21.5 - 57.5	20	47.8	29.1 - 73.8	KL21	529	111.3	101.8 - 120.8	297	98.4	87.2 - 109.6
HK10	730	98.4	91.3 - 105.6	546	100.7	92.2 - 109.1	KL22	71	84.6	64.9 - 104.3	27	59.9	37.3 - 82.5
HK11	93	135.3	107.8 - 162.8	37	91.3	61.9 - 120.7	KL23	227	88.0	76.5 - 99.4	146	96.0	80.5 - 111.6
HK12	48	83.9	60.2 - 107.7	43	83.2	58.3 - 108.0	KL24	163	106.4	90.1 - 122.7	116	115.9	94.8 - 137.0
HK13	62	69.2	52.0 - 86.4	53	87.1	63.6 - 110.5	KL25	2531	104.4	100.3 - 108.5	1447	97.2	92.2 - 102.2
HK14	186	87.1	74.6 - 99.6	115	78.3	64.0 - 92.6	NT1	104	84.5	68.2 - 100.7	68	87.1	66.4 - 107.8
HK15	84	94.5	74.3 - 114.7	52	81.0	58.9 - 103.0	NT2	188	104.0	89.1 - 118.8	108	101.2	82.1 - 120.3
HK16	454	113.6	103.1 - 124.0	287	120.5	106.6 - 134.5	NT3	344	94.5	84.5 - 104.5	217	114.9	99.6 - 130.2
HK17	487	113.9	103.8 - 124.0	254	97.2	85.3 - 109.2	NT4	195	96.8	83.2 - 110.4	148	115.2	96.6 - 133.8
HK18	40	64.9	44.8 - 85.1	33	73.7	48.5 - 98.8	NT5	730	106.1	98.4 - 113.8	426	102.2	92.5 - 111.9
HK19	247	116.5	102.0 - 131.0	167	118.1	100.2 - 136.0	NT6	306	89.3	79.3 - 99.3	162	75.2	63.6 - 86.8
HK20	561	123.1	113.0 - 133.3	319	114.9	102.3 - 127.5	NT7	125	106.5	87.8 - 125.2	70	99.8	76.4 - 123.2
HK21	45	73.5	52.1 - 95.0	31	88.3	57.2 - 119.3	NT8	348	93.5	83.6 - 103.3	201	94.4	81.4 - 107.5
KL1	272	93.1	82.0 - 104.2	185	107.6	92.1 - 123.2	NT9	103	91.5	73.8 - 109.2	51	79.7	57.8 - 101.6
KL2	583	96.0	88.2 - 103.7	346	98.8	88.4 - 109.2	NT10	415	88.9	80.3 - 97.4	230	86.7	75.5 - 97.9
KL3	170	97.4	82.8 - 112.1	116	101.9	83.4 - 120.5	NT11	62	63.8	47.9 - 79.7	37	70.5	47.8 - 93.3
KL4	499	101.6	92.7 - 110.5	309	112.4	99.8 - 124.9	NT12	394	89.2	80.4 - 98.1	181	71.0	60.7 - 81.4
KL5	414	101.8	92.0 - 111.6	271	120.6	106.2 - 134.9	NT13	71	85.9	65.9 - 105.9	46	91.0	64.7 - 117.3
KL6	83	83.6	65.6 - 101.6	56	64.3	47.4 - 81.1	NT14	60	79.2	59.2 - 99.2	33	64.1	42.2 - 85.9
KL7	56	74.9	55.3 - 94.6	58	95.6	71.0 - 120.2	NT15	325	106.8	95.2 - 118.5	163	83.4	70.6 - 96.2
KL8	234	87.8	76.5 - 99.0	169	99.1	84.2 - 114.1	NT16	416	108.1	97.7 - 118.5	288	114.7	101.5 - 128.0
KL9	996	101.6	95.3 - 107.9	711	110.2	102.1 - 118.3	NT17	188	105.6	90.5 - 120.7	105	93.5	75.6 - 111.4
KL10	81	83.1	65.0 - 101.2	60	86.6	64.7 - 108.5	NT18	111	129.6	105.5 - 153.7	58	100.4	74.6 - 126.3
KL11	221	85.0	73.8 - 96.3	170	92.5	78.6 - 106.4	NT19	127	84.8	70.1 - 99.6	80	84.7	66.1 - 103.2
KL12	62	77.2	58.0 - 96.4	31	73.1	47.4 - 98.8							

ALL CANCERS

Sex-Age specific mortality rate (1/100,000) of all cancers in Hong Kong (1979–1983)

	Male		Female	
	No. of	Mortality	No. of	Mortality
Age	deaths	rate	deaths	rate
0–4	51	4.84	36	3.64
5–9	66	6.22	37	3.75
10–14	68	5.94	55	5.14
15–19	119	8.33	55	4.13
20–24	146	9.53	100	7.18
25–29	194	14.69	130	11.18
30–34	338	30.64	194	21.17
35–39	448	62.05	226	40.65
40–44	828	117.66	402	72.68
45–49	1496	207.39	669	110.54
50–54	2290	333.33	1049	172.01
55–59	2920	513.34	1418	265.15
60–64	3312	724.82	1669	365.87
65+	7958	1167.26	6538	647.68
TOTAL	20234	153.47	12578	103.31

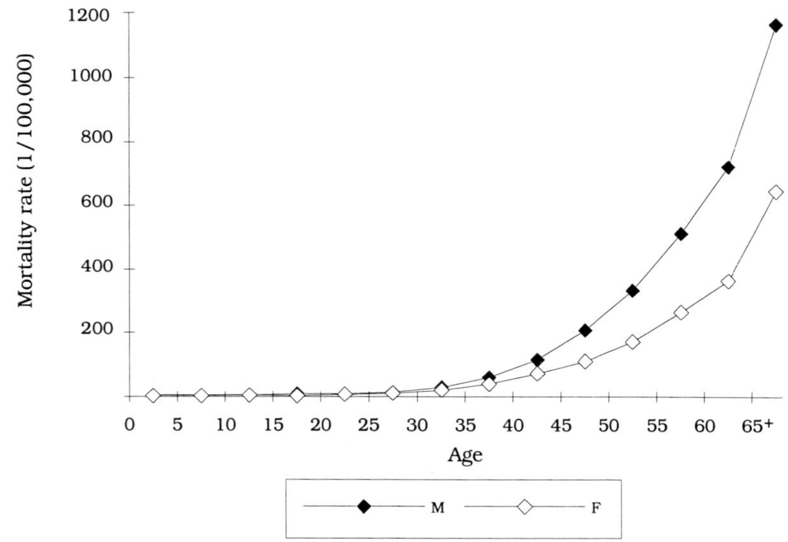

Number of communities on map by category based on standardized mortality ratio (SMR) during 1979–1983

	Number of communities	
Category	Male	Female
SMR significantly high, in top 20%	11	10
SMR significantly high , not in top 20%	1	2
SMR not significantly high, in top 20%	2	3
SMR not significantly low, in bottom 20%	3	2
SMR significantly low, not in bottom 20%	10	3
SMR significantly low, in bottom 20%	10	11
other communities	28	34

Values of the standardized mortality ratio (SMR) which divide the 65 communities into quintile

Percentile	Male	Female
20th	83.91	81.40
40th	87.97	91.02
60th	98.97	99.14
80th	108.13	112.35
Lowest SMR	36.37	47.75
Highest SMR	135.33	183.85
No. of communities with zero death	0	0

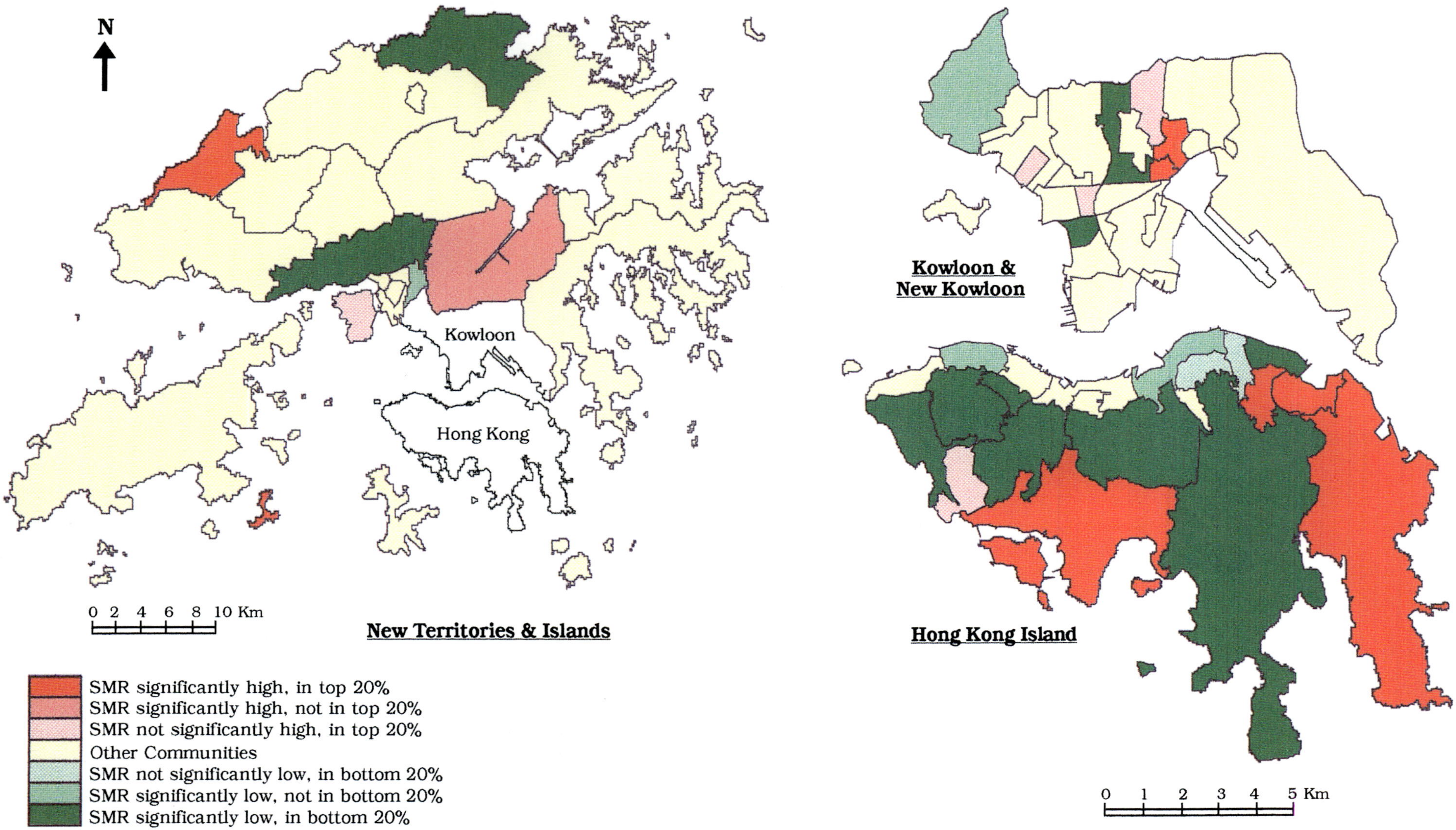

All Cancers (Male, 1984 -1988)

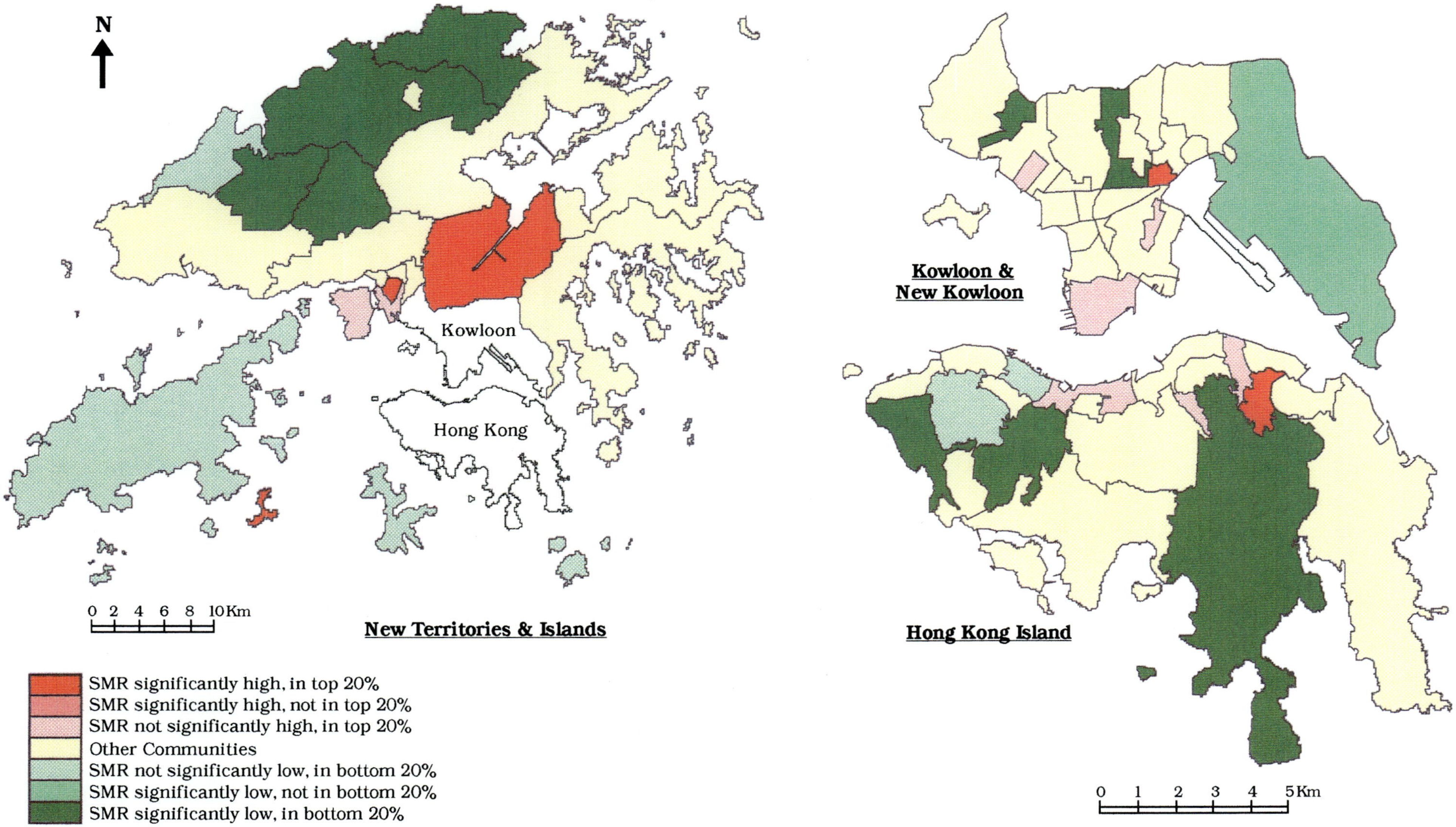

All Cancers (Female, 1984 – 1988)

Number of Deaths, Standardised Mortality Ratio (SMR) and 95% Confidence Interval of All Cancers by 65 Communities in 1984–1988

Community	Male			Female		
	Number of deaths	SMR	95% C.I.	Number of deaths	SMR	95% C.I.
HK1	402	104.8	94.5 - 115.0	246	104.2	91.1 - 117.2
HK2	480	88.7	80.8 - 96.7	346	106.3	95.1 - 117.5
HK3	183	90.4	77.3 - 103.5	90	83.5	66.2 - 100.7
HK4	301	92.9	82.4 - 103.4	219	111.7	96.9 - 126.5
HK5	295	100.9	89.4 - 112.4	195	106.4	91.4 - 121.3
HK6	226	77.0	67.0 - 87.1	207	90.2	77.9 - 102.5
HK7	44	74.7	52.6 - 96.7	41	87.5	60.7 - 114.3
HK8	53	48.5	35.4 - 61.6	77	91.4	71.0 - 111.9
HK9	15	30.4	15.0 - 45.7	28	64.4	40.6 - 88.3
HK10	725	88.3	81.8 - 94.7	624	102.7	94.6 - 110.7
HK11	79	106.3	82.8 - 129.7	56	128.6	94.9 - 162.3
HK12	55	80.1	59.0 - 101.3	50	96.9	70.0 - 123.8
HK13	82	83.2	65.2 - 101.2	65	110.0	83.3 - 136.8
HK14	219	72.5	62.9 - 82.1	212	95.4	82.6 - 108.3
HK15	134	136.0	113.0 - 159.0	99	133.3	107.0 - 159.6
HK16	512	122.0	111.4 - 132.6	284	109.3	96.6 - 122.0
HK17	641	117.0	107.9 - 126.0	352	102.0	91.3 - 112.6
HK18	35	57.0	38.1 - 75.9	21	45.3	25.9 - 64.6
HK19	302	111.9	99.3 - 124.6	195	109.0	93.7 - 124.3
HK20	731	128.0	118.8 - 137.3	384	106.8	96.1 - 117.5
HK21	38	51.9	35.4 - 68.4	26	53.1	32.7 - 73.5
KL1	285	96.8	85.6 - 108.1	194	111.4	95.7 - 127.1
KL2	605	105.7	97.2 - 114.1	365	108.0	96.9 - 119.0
KL3	185	108.8	93.2 - 124.5	106	92.6	75.0 - 110.2
KL4	443	83.8	76.0 - 91.6	277	97.9	86.4 - 109.4
KL5	403	103.9	93.8 - 114.1	240	108.8	95.0 - 122.6
KL6	98	91.3	73.2 - 109.3	80	93.9	73.3 - 114.5
KL7	73	92.8	71.5 - 114.1	49	89.3	64.3 - 114.3
KL8	275	99.7	88.0 - 111.5	184	109.4	93.6 - 125.2
KL9	1076	100.5	94.5 - 106.5	704	102.0	94.5 - 109.6
KL10	106	99.1	80.3 - 118.0	67	90.5	68.8 - 112.2
KL11	268	86.3	76.0 - 96.7	202	97.3	83.9 - 110.8
KL12	73	84.8	65.3 - 104.2	26	56.0	34.4 - 77.5
KL13	952	99.2	92.9 - 105.5	530	93.6	85.6 - 101.5
KL14	663	100.1	92.4 - 107.7	417	104.6	94.5 - 114.6
KL15	135	115.2	95.7 - 134.6	92	118.1	94.0 - 142.2
KL16	219	91.1	79.0 - 103.2	142	103.9	86.8 - 121.0
KL17	76	75.3	58.4 - 92.2	80	77.1	60.2 - 94.0
KL18	48	103.9	74.5 - 133.3	31	102.5	66.4 - 138.6
KL19	1004	103.0	96.7 - 109.4	646	104.6	96.5 - 112.7
KL20	269	113.0	99.5 - 126.5	148	93.5	78.4 - 108.5
KL21	451	112.2	101.8 - 122.5	263	109.4	96.1 - 122.6
KL22	79	90.3	70.4 - 110.2	47	94.6	67.6 - 121.7
KL23	289	134.3	118.8 - 149.8	189	148.9	127.7 - 170.1
KL24	191	95.2	81.7 - 108.7	104	91.8	74.1 - 109.4
KL25	3086	97.6	94.1 - 101.0	1782	91.5	87.2 - 95.7
NT1	141	79.0	65.9 - 92.0	117	100.7	82.4 - 118.9
NT2	199	90.4	77.8 - 102.9	151	114.1	95.9 - 132.3
NT3	391	97.9	88.2 - 107.6	226	105.8	92.0 - 119.6
NT4	371	106.2	95.4 - 117.0	217	99.9	86.6 - 113.2
NT5	762	106.3	98.7 - 113.8	472	112.4	102.2 - 122.5
NT6	378	89.8	80.7 - 98.8	227	91.7	79.8 - 103.7
NT7	244	113.4	99.2 - 127.6	135	110.8	92.1 - 129.5
NT8	740	99.9	92.7 - 107.1	488	100.6	91.7 - 109.5
NT9	163	125.9	106.6 - 145.3	67	82.0	62.3 - 101.6
NT10	589	98.5	90.6 - 106.5	298	84.6	75.0 - 94.2
NT11	96	89.2	71.4 - 107.1	55	76.6	56.4 - 96.9
NT12	527	100.2	91.6 - 108.7	242	71.9	62.8 - 80.9
NT13	145	106.4	89.1 - 123.7	78	103.2	80.3 - 126.1
NT14	67	77.3	58.8 - 95.9	38	69.9	47.6 - 92.1
NT15	525	107.1	97.9 - 116.2	341	100.0	89.4 - 110.6
NT16	1202	108.6	102.5 - 114.8	900	111.9	104.6 - 119.3
NT17	208	101.5	87.7 - 115.3	131	101.9	84.4 - 119.3
NT18	144	143.4	120.0 - 166.9	88	130.1	102.9 - 157.3
NT19	144	93.5	78.2 - 108.8	85	88.7	69.8 - 107.6

ALL CANCERS

Sex-Age specific mortality rate (1/100,000) of all cancers in Hong Kong (1984–1988)

	Male		Female	
Age	No. of deaths	Mortality rate	No. of deaths	Mortality rate
0–4	46	4.30	56	5.63
5–9	60	5.47	57	5.60
10–14	53	4.65	48	4.60
15–19	108	9.02	56	5.08
20–24	115	7.96	85	6.12
25–29	199	12.68	133	8.99
30–34	346	25.57	268	21.66
35–39	553	49.85	336	34.64
40–44	728	99.32	350	58.37
45–49	1266	179.83	602	103.17
50–54	2317	316.14	994	157.40
55–59	3255	490.06	1490	245.27
60–64	3867	715.98	1861	347.66
65+	11246	1245.54	8871	718.77
TOTAL	24159	169.42	15207	113.30

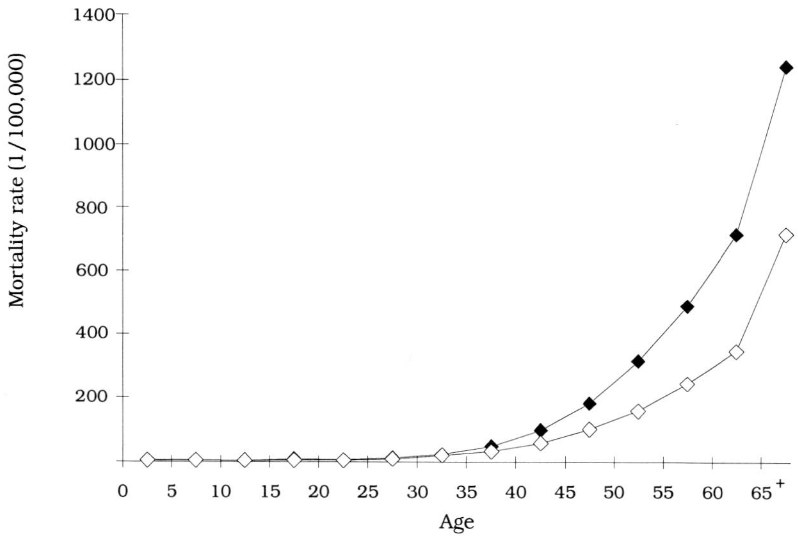

Number of communities on map by category based on standardized mortality ratio (SMR) during 1984–1988

Category	Number of communities Male	Female
SMR significantly high, in top 20%	8	5
SMR significantly high , not in top 20%	1	0
SMR not significantly high, in top 20%	5	8
SMR not significantly low, in bottom 20%	2	4
SMR significantly low, not in bottom 20%	4	1
SMR significantly low, in bottom 20%	11	9
other communities	34	38

Values of the standardized mortality ratio (SMR) which divide the 65 communities into quintile

Percentile	Male	Female
20th	83.80	88.70
40th	92.93	95.41
60th	100.47	103.23
80th	108.64	109.36
Lowest SMR	30.35	45.25
Highest SMR	143.44	148.90
No. of communities with zero death	0	0

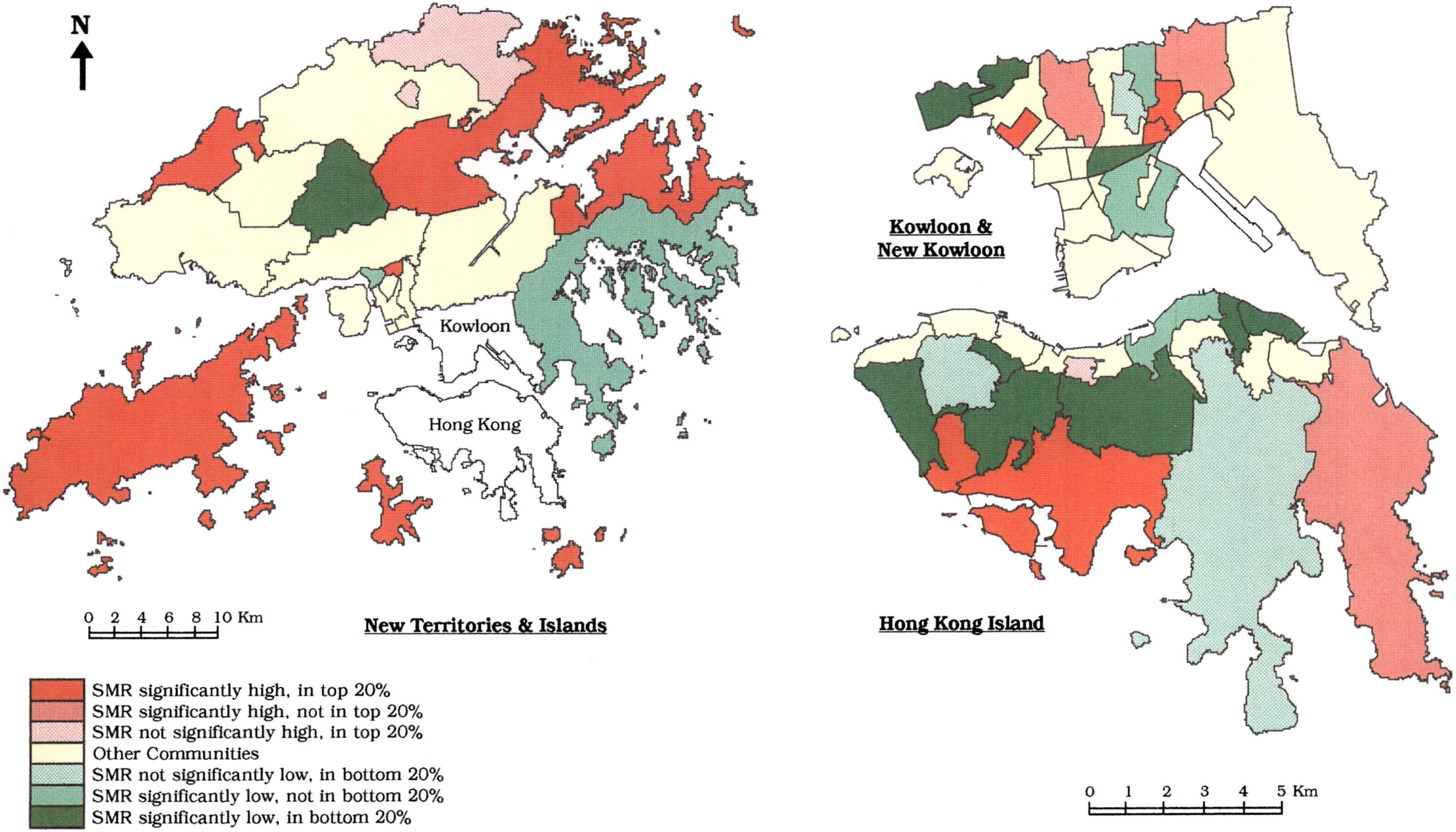

All Cancers (Male, 1989 –1993)

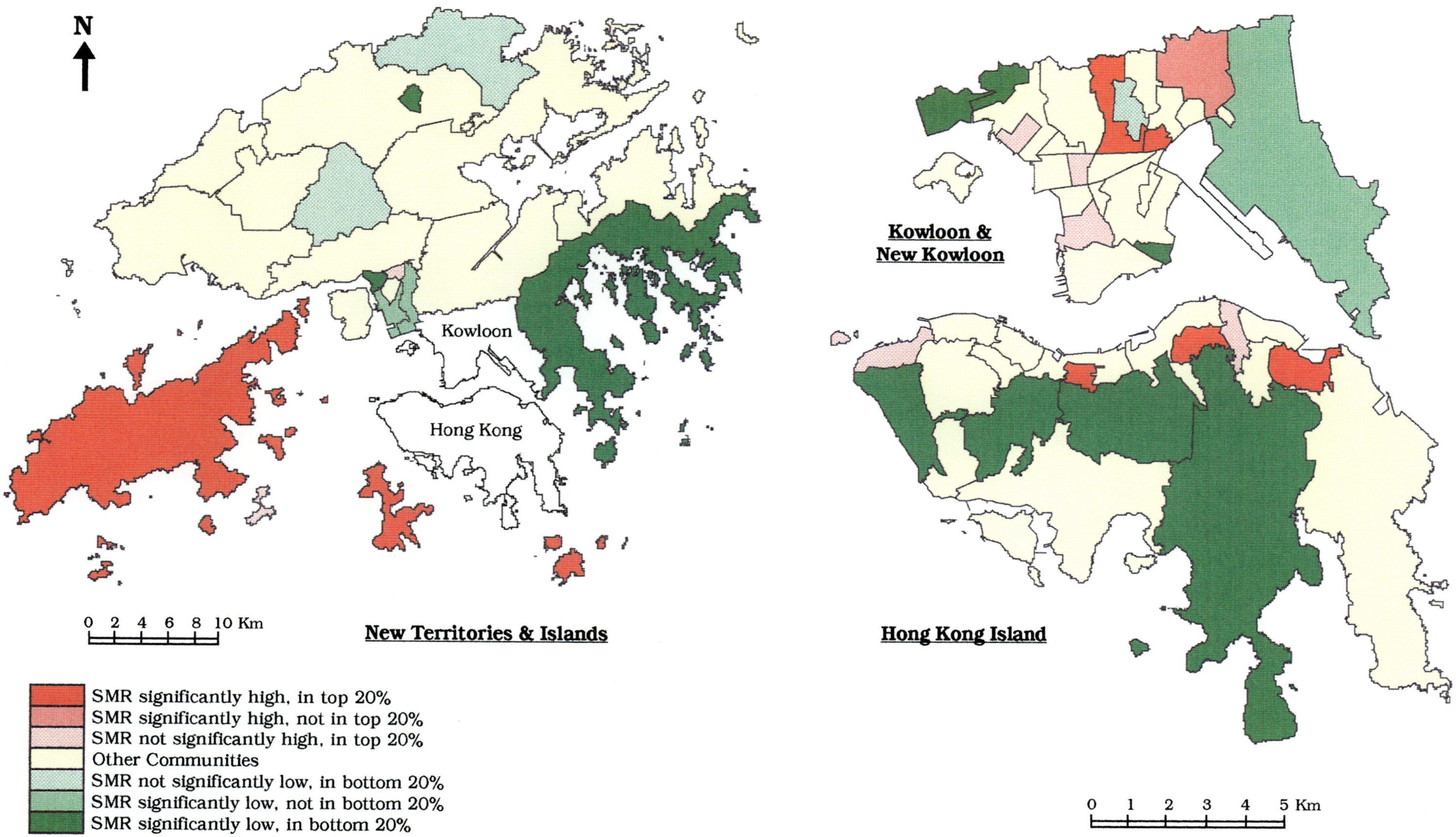

All Cancers (Female, 1989 –1993)

Number of Deaths, Standardised Mortality Ratio (SMR) and 95% Confidence Interval of All Cancers by 65 Communities in 1989–1993

Community	Male			Female		
	Number of deaths	SMR	95% C.I.	Number of deaths	SMR	95% C.I.
HK1	379	94.0	84.6 - 103.5	278	112.9	99.6 - 126.2
HK2	504	92.5	84.4 - 100.6	318	106.8	95.0 - 118.5
HK3	170	91.1	77.4 - 104.7	82	86.3	67.6 - 105.0
HK4	280	91.2	80.5 - 101.9	160	94.5	79.8 - 109.1
HK5	325	111.3	99.2 - 123.4	195	122.5	105.3 - 139.7
HK6	221	68.1	59.1 - 77.1	202	84.4	72.8 - 96.1
HK7	58	80.5	59.8 - 101.3	51	89.1	64.7 - 113.6
HK8	85	73.7	58.1 - 89.4	73	91.0	70.1 - 111.8
HK9	41	76.1	52.8 - 99.4	29	70.2	44.7 - 95.8
HK10	825	88.7	82.7 - 94.8	637	97.2	89.6 - 104.7
HK11	74	84.8	65.5 - 104.2	46	93.3	66.4 - 120.3
HK12	64	84.0	63.4 - 104.6	74	136.1	105.1 - 167.2
HK13	65	65.4	49.5 - 81.3	67	113.9	86.6 - 141.2
HK14	252	68.1	59.7 - 76.6	222	91.3	79.3 - 103.3
HK15	207	93.3	80.6 - 106.0	148	97.9	82.1 - 113.7
HK16	414	108.8	98.3 - 119.3	276	121.7	107.4 - 136.1
HK17	861	109.0	101.8 - 116.3	481	98.3	89.5 - 107.1
HK18	41	49.2	34.1 - 64.3	37	58.4	39.6 - 77.2
HK19	387	118.9	107.0 - 130.7	216	111.0	96.2 - 125.8
HK20	796	112.2	104.4 - 119.9	464	106.1	96.5 - 115.8
HK21	59	80.9	60.3 - 101.6	25	59.3	38.4 - 87.8
KL1	215	88.3	76.5 - 100.1	127	90.4	74.7 - 106.1
KL2	604	104.5	96.2 - 112.8	304	98.4	87.4 - 109.5
KL3	151	91.7	77.1 - 106.3	118	115.7	94.8 - 136.6
KL4	464	97.7	88.8 - 106.6	267	112.0	98.6 - 125.4
KL5	347	100.7	90.1 - 111.3	208	113.7	98.3 - 129.2
KL6	91	73.8	58.7 - 89.0	93	94.3	75.1 - 113.5
KL7	83	93.0	73.0 - 113.1	68	100.1	76.3 - 123.9
KL8	279	95.6	84.3 - 106.8	163	98.3	83.2 - 113.4
KL9	1078	93.8	88.2 - 99.4	708	103.6	96.0 - 111.3
KL10	173	87.2	74.2 - 100.1	111	78.2	63.7 - 92.8
KL11	206	79.6	68.7 - 90.4	141	82.2	68.6 - 95.7
KL12	58	69.1	51.3 - 86.9	30	67.3	43.2 - 91.3

Community	Male			Female		
	Number of deaths	SMR	95% C.I.	Number of deaths	SMR	95% C.I.
KL13	995	94.7	88.9 - 100.6	555	98.1	90.0 - 106.3
KL14	702	108.2	100.2 - 116.2	395	98.5	88.8 - 108.2
KL15	182	141.0	120.5 - 161.4	88	112.1	88.7 - 135.5
KL16	253	107.1	93.9 - 120.3	133	104.3	86.6 - 122.1
KL17	102	105.3	84.9 - 125.8	108	125.1	101.5 - 148.7
KL18	38	79.1	54.0 - 104.3	23	67.3	42.6 - 100.9
KL19	1148	107.1	100.9 - 113.3	750	109.1	101.3 - 116.9
KL20	218	88.2	76.5 - 99.9	134	89.0	74.0 - 104.1
KL21	430	112.1	101.5 - 122.7	241	99.5	86.9 - 112.1
KL22	76	93.6	72.6 - 114.7	51	110.6	80.2 - 140.9
KL23	271	165.3	145.6 - 185.0	153	162.1	136.4 - 187.8
KL24	206	93.3	80.5 - 106.0	118	98.9	81.1 - 116.8
KL25	3328	99.7	96.3 - 103.1	1911	94.4	90.2 - 98.7
NT1	255	93.1	81.7 - 104.6	178	99.6	84.9 - 114.2
NT2	257	93.5	82.1 - 104.9	145	85.9	72.0 - 99.9
NT3	415	81.1	73.3 - 88.9	228	84.3	73.4 - 95.2
NT4	413	116.2	105.0 - 127.4	242	112.5	98.3 - 126.7
NT5	762	104.4	97.0 - 111.8	442	105.4	95.6 - 115.2
NT6	467	95.0	86.4 - 103.6	254	88.8	77.9 - 99.7
NT7	464	95.8	87.1 - 104.5	268	95.5	84.1 - 106.9
NT8	1116	99.4	93.6 - 105.2	722	104.4	96.8 - 112.0
NT9	181	131.6	112.4 - 150.8	94	109.9	87.7 - 132.1
NT10	706	102.3	94.7 - 109.8	406	100.7	90.9 - 110.5
NT11	97	77.8	62.3 - 93.3	64	82.5	62.3 - 102.7
NT12	631	98.7	91.0 - 106.4	374	96.1	86.4 - 105.8
NT13	147	109.6	91.9 - 127.3	62	70.6	53.0 - 88.2
NT14	79	109.7	85.5 - 133.9	40	83.7	57.8 - 109.7
NT15	829	114.1	106.4 - 121.9	486	100.9	91.9 - 109.9
NT16	1904	104.5	99.8 - 109.2	1284	101.6	96.1 - 107.2
NT17	406	89.5	80.8 - 98.3	241	80.0	69.9 - 90.1
NT18	145	123.4	103.3 - 143.5	87	116.5	92.0 - 141.0
NT19	179	123.0	105.0 - 141.1	115	124.9	102.1 - 147.8

ALL CANCERS

Sex-Age specific mortality rate (1/100,000) of all cancers in Hong Kong (1989–1993)

	Male		Female	
Age	No. of deaths	Mortality rate	No. of deaths	Mortality rate
0–4	35	3.67	29	3.28
5–9	31	2.93	38	3.89
10–14	46	4.21	36	3.57
15–19	68	6.23	47	4.69
20–24	81	7.09	68	6.00
25–29	169	11.72	132	8.92
30–34	382	24.50	267	17.57
35–39	606	45.26	414	32.90
40–44	985	89.44	606	62.34
45–49	1177	161.10	542	90.77
50–54	1897	273.42	834	146.47
55–59	3122	446.77	1372	225.25
60–64	4217	683.14	1825	315.80
65+	14653	1322.83	10659	758.70
TOTAL	27469	187.82	16869	120.56

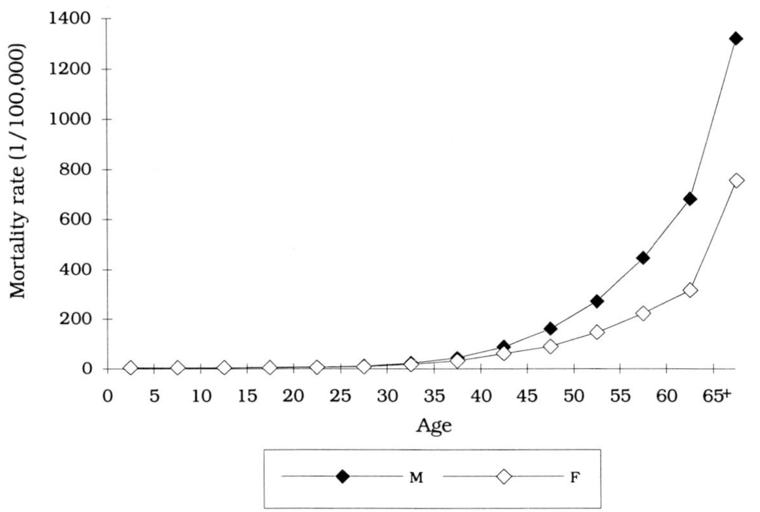

Number of communities on map by category based on standardized mortality ratio (SMR) during 1989–1993

	Number of communities	
Category	Male	Female
SMR significantly high, in top 20%	10	6
SMR significantly high , not in top 20%	3	1
SMR not significantly high, in top 20%	3	7
SMR not significantly low, in bottom 20%	3	3
SMR significantly low, not in bottom 20%	5	3
SMR significantly low, in bottom 20%	10	10
other communities	31	35

Values of the standardized mortality ratio (SMR) which divide the 65 communities into quintile

Percentile	Male	Female
20th	80.91	84.42
40th	93.05	95.50
60th	98.73	100.74
80th	109.04	111.99
Lowest SMR	49.20	58.36
Highest SMR	165.33	162.13
No. of communities with zero cases	0	0

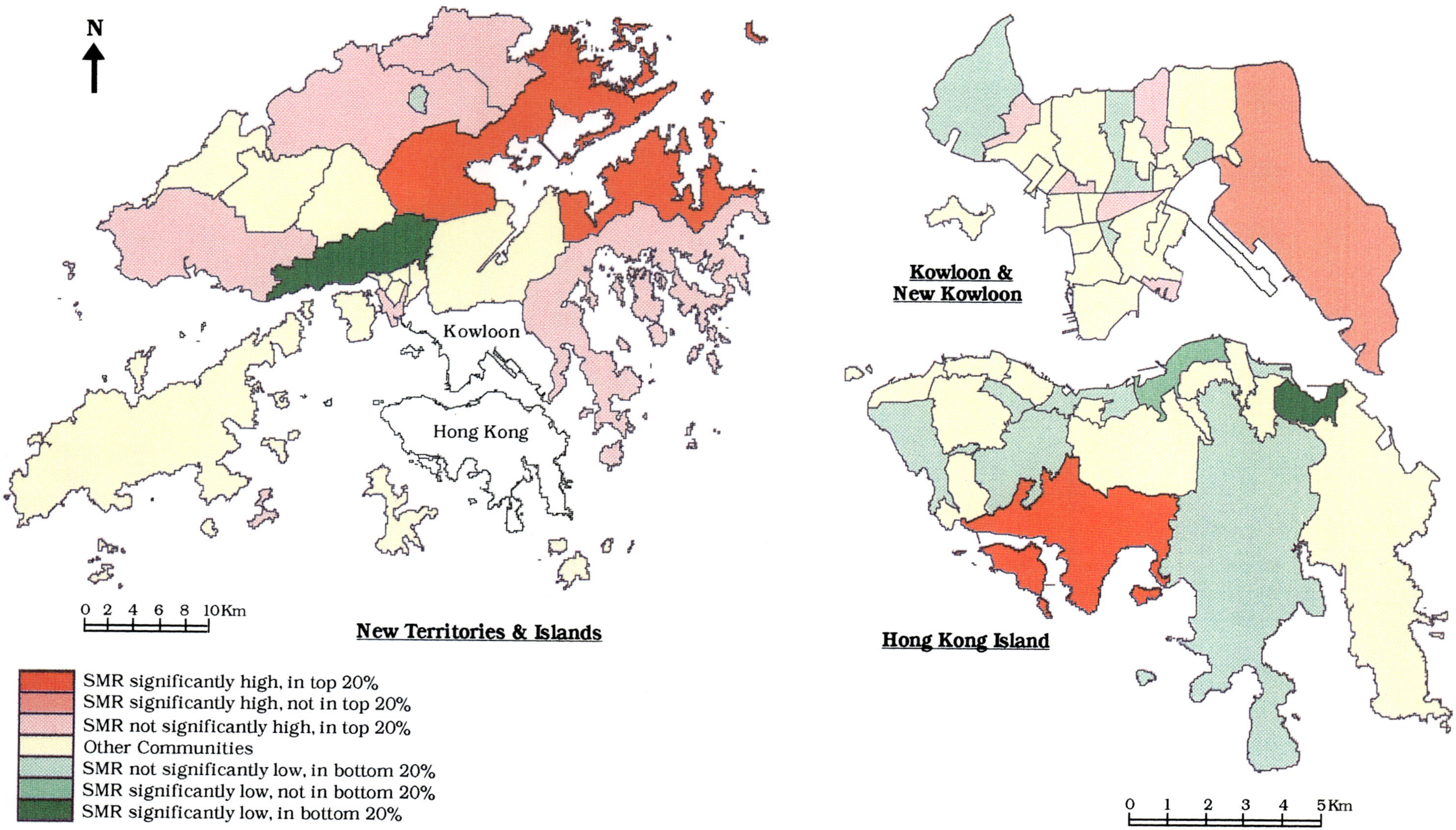

NPC (Male, 1979 - 1983)

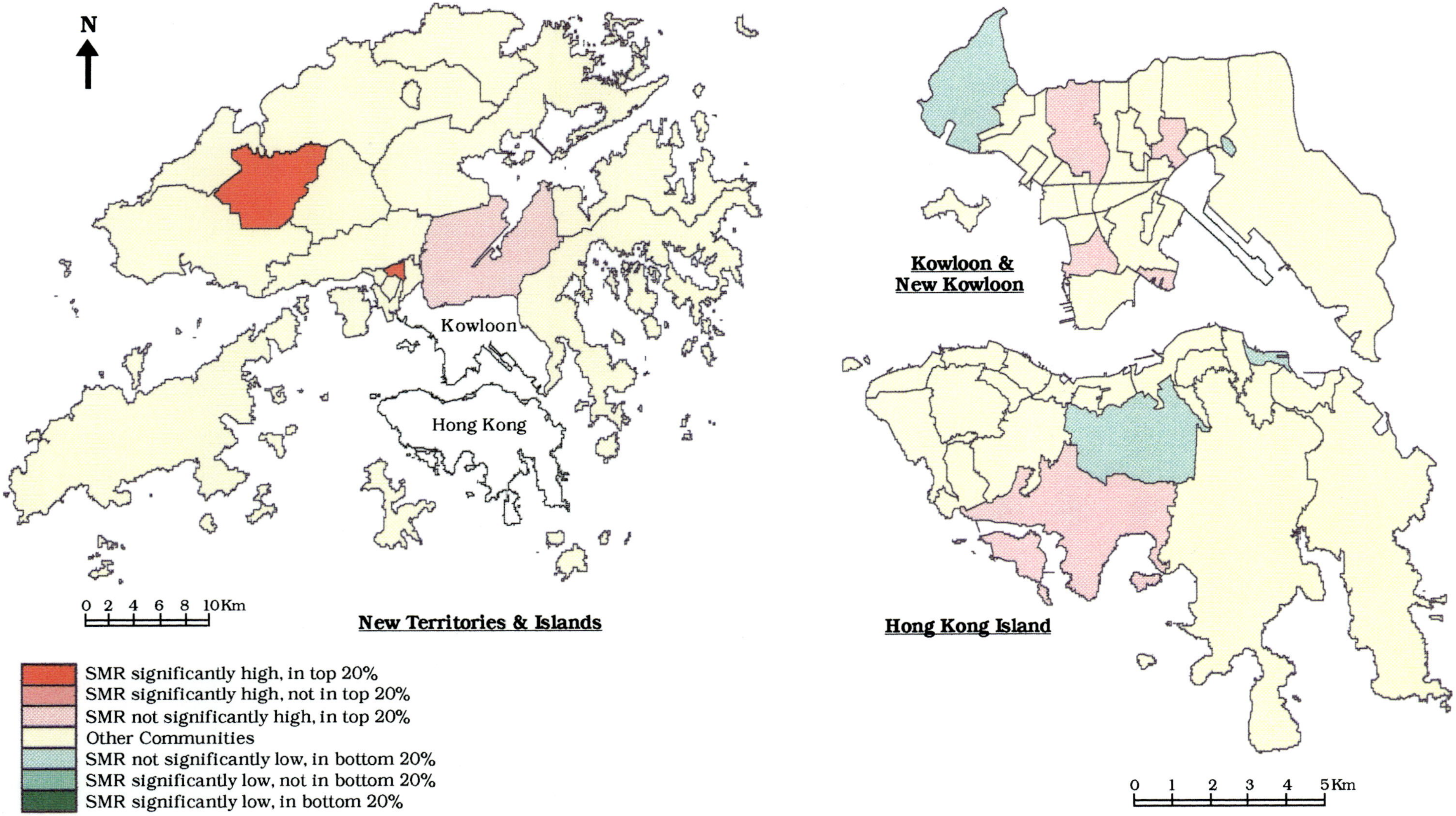

NPC (Female, 1979 – 1983)

Number of Deaths, Standardised Mortality Ratio (SMR) and 95% Confidence Interval of NPC by 65 Communities in 1979–1983

Community	Male			Female		
	Number of deaths	SMR	95% C.I.	Number of deaths	SMR	95% C.I.
HK1	32	107.9	70.5 - 145.3	12	121.2	62.5 - 211.5
HK2	43	98.8	69.3 - 128.3	7	53.9	21.6 - 111.2
HK3	15	88.8	49.6 - 146.5	4	89.7	24.4 - 229.4
HK4	19	64.6	38.9 - 101.0	6	68.6	25.1 - 149.5
HK5	23	86.0	54.5 - 129.2	10	129.9	62.4 - 238.8
HK6	18	78.2	42.1 - 114.3	3	30.6	6.3 - 89.4
HK7	4	83.8	22.8 - 214.2	1	47.0	1.2 - 261.3
HK8	4	44.6	12.1 - 114.0	1	25.3	0.6 - 140.4
HK9	2	42.6	5.2 - 153.9	0	0.0	...
HK10	46	71.0	50.5 - 91.5	20	82.0	50.0 - 126.7
HK11	5	80.7	26.1 - 188.5	2	93.6	11.3 - 337.9
HK12	5	87.9	28.4 - 205.3	0	0.0	...
HK13	9	110.8	50.8 - 210.2	2	67.7	8.2 - 244.5
HK14	11	56.9	28.4 - 101.7	3	42.9	8.8 - 125.5
HK15	7	79.7	32.0 - 164.4	0	0.0	...
HK16	21	61.2	37.3 - 94.5	11	99.6	49.8 - 178.1
HK17	41	119.9	83.2 - 156.6	10	87.3	42.0 - 160.5
HK18	0	0.0	...	1	47.5	1.2 - 263.9
HK19	21	105.0	64.0 - 162.2	4	55.8	15.2 - 142.8
HK20	63	166.3	125.2 - 207.3	20	156.3	95.3 - 241.6
HK21	4	62.6	17.0 - 160.0	2	101.1	12.2 - 364.9
KL1	22	85.6	53.5 - 129.7	10	126.0	60.6 - 231.7
KL2	54	97.9	71.8 - 124.1	16	107.5	61.4 - 174.6
KL3	17	111.2	64.6 - 177.9	6	124.6	45.6 - 271.5
KL4	45	102.9	72.9 - 133.0	14	119.8	65.5 - 201.0
KL5	41	118.0	81.9 - 154.2	14	148.6	81.2 - 249.3
KL6	10	128.2	61.6 - 235.6	3	84.2	17.4 - 246.1
KL7	2	30.6	3.7 - 110.4	4	149.7	40.8 - 382.8
KL8	24	95.9	61.5 - 142.7	10	126.5	60.8 - 232.6
KL9	84	92.4	72.6 - 112.1	29	94.8	60.3 - 129.3
KL10	13	137.8	73.3 - 235.6	5	151.3	49.0 - 353.5
KL11	14	60.3	32.9 - 101.2	4	48.0	13.1 - 122.7
KL12	10	144.8	69.6 - 266.2	0	0.0	...

Community	Male			Female		
	Number of deaths	SMR	95% C.I.	Number of deaths	SMR	95% C.I.
KL13	84	97.7	76.8 - 118.6	27	106.6	66.4 - 146.8
KL14	42	100.6	70.2 - 131.0	19	137.7	82.9 - 215.1
KL15	3	66.7	13.7 - 194.9	3	253.0	52.2 - 739.6
KL16	30	144.8	93.0 - 196.6	5	84.4	27.3 - 197.3
KL17	3	49.3	10.2 - 144.2	2	72.5	8.8 - 261.8
KL18	4	85.2	23.2 - 217.9	1	62.6	1.6 - 347.8
KL19	77	102.8	79.9 - 125.8	26	101.5	62.5 - 140.6
KL20	29	124.1	78.9 - 169.3	10	123.4	59.3 - 226.9
KL21	35	96.5	64.5 - 128.4	18	141.9	83.9 - 224.1
KL22	4	52.9	14.4 - 135.2	0	0.0	...
KL23	23	101.6	64.3 - 152.6	7	103.3	41.5 - 213.0
KL24	16	108.6	62.1 - 176.3	2	37.4	4.5 - 135.2
KL25	255	114.9	100.8 - 129.0	63	88.3	66.5 - 110.1
NT1	4	34.1	9.3 - 87.2	2	56.9	6.9 - 205.4
NT2	24	136.4	87.5 - 203.0	5	92.6	30.0 - 216.2
NT3	29	83.0	52.8 - 113.2	9	93.5	42.9 - 177.4
NT4	15	70.6	39.4 - 116.5	16	239.1	136.7 - 388.2
NT5	73	114.8	88.5 - 141.1	24	118.3	75.8 - 176.0
NT6	23	69.0	43.7 - 103.6	8	74.8	32.2 - 147.2
NT7	9	76.1	34.9 - 144.4	3	82.4	17.0 - 240.9
NT8	42	121.0	84.4 - 157.6	9	90.8	41.7 - 172.3
NT9	9	99.7	45.7 - 189.1	4	145.7	39.7 - 372.6
NT10	29	76.4	48.6 - 104.2	20	170.9	104.2 - 264.1
NT11	7	89.2	35.8 - 184.0	3	130.1	26.8 - 380.4
NT12	47	135.2	96.5 - 173.8	9	84.3	38.7 - 159.9
NT13	3	45.3	9.3 - 132.3	4	190.8	52.0 - 488.0
NT14	10	174.7	84.0 - 321.1	1	49.9	1.3 - 277.0
NT15	36	149.3	100.5 - 198.1	6	74.4	27.2 - 162.0
NT16	33	94.6	62.3 - 126.8	18	155.6	92.0 - 245.7
NT17	20	144.8	88.3 - 223.8	6	129.5	47.4 - 282.2
NT18	11	180.6	90.3 - 323.1	2	87.6	10.6 - 316.2
NT19	12	104.9	54.1 - 183.0	3	88.1	18.2 - 257.6

NPC

Sex-Age specific mortality rate (1/100,000) of NPC in Hong Kong (1979–1983)

	Male		Female	
Age	No. of deaths	Mortality rate	No. of deaths	Mortality rate
0–4	0	0.00	0	0.00
5–9	0	0.00	0	0.00
10–14	2	0.17	1	0.09
15–19	11	0.77	1	0.08
20–24	18	1.18	4	0.29
25–29	38	2.88	20	1.72
30–34	94	8.52	24	2.62
35–39	123	17.04	33	5.94
40–44	189	26.86	54	9.76
45–49	285	39.51	89	14.71
50–54	285	41.48	91	14.92
55–59	276	48.52	75	14.02
60–64	213	46.61	61	13.37
65+	236	34.62	118	11.69
TOTAL	1770	13.42	571	4.69

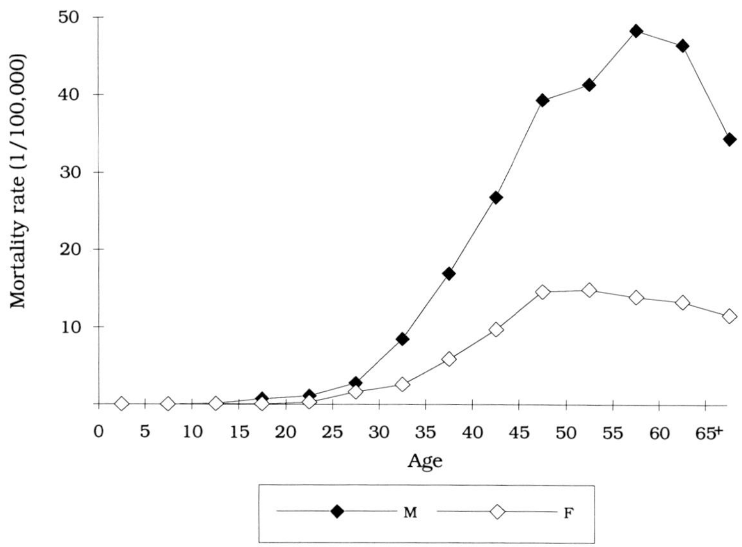

Number of communities on map by category based on standardized mortality ratio (SMR) during 1979–1983

Category	Number of communities Male	Female
SMR significantly high, in top 20%	2	2
SMR significantly high , not in top 20%	1	0
SMR not significantly high, in top 20%	11	6
SMR not significantly low, in bottom 20%	11	4
SMR significantly low, not in bottom 20%	1	0
SMR significantly low, in bottom 20%	2	0
other communities	37	53

Values of the standardized mortality ratio (SMR) which divide the 65 communities into quintile

Percentile	Male	Female
20th	64.62	49.87
40th	85.57	84.28
60th	100.61	101.09
80th	119.92	129.89
Lowest SMR	0.00	0.00
Highest SMR	180.64	252.95
No. of communities with zero death	1	5

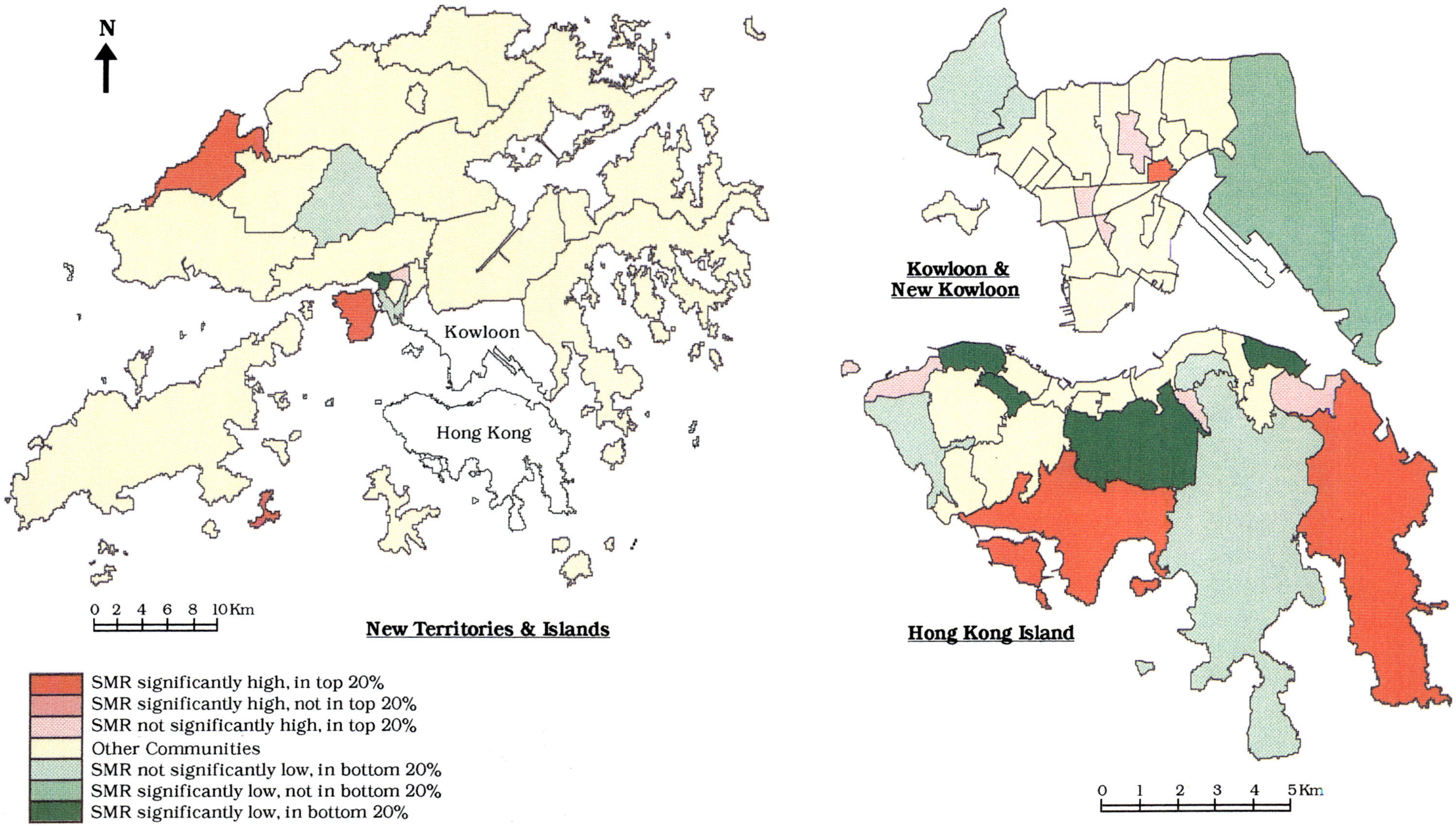

NPC (Male, 1984 – 1988)

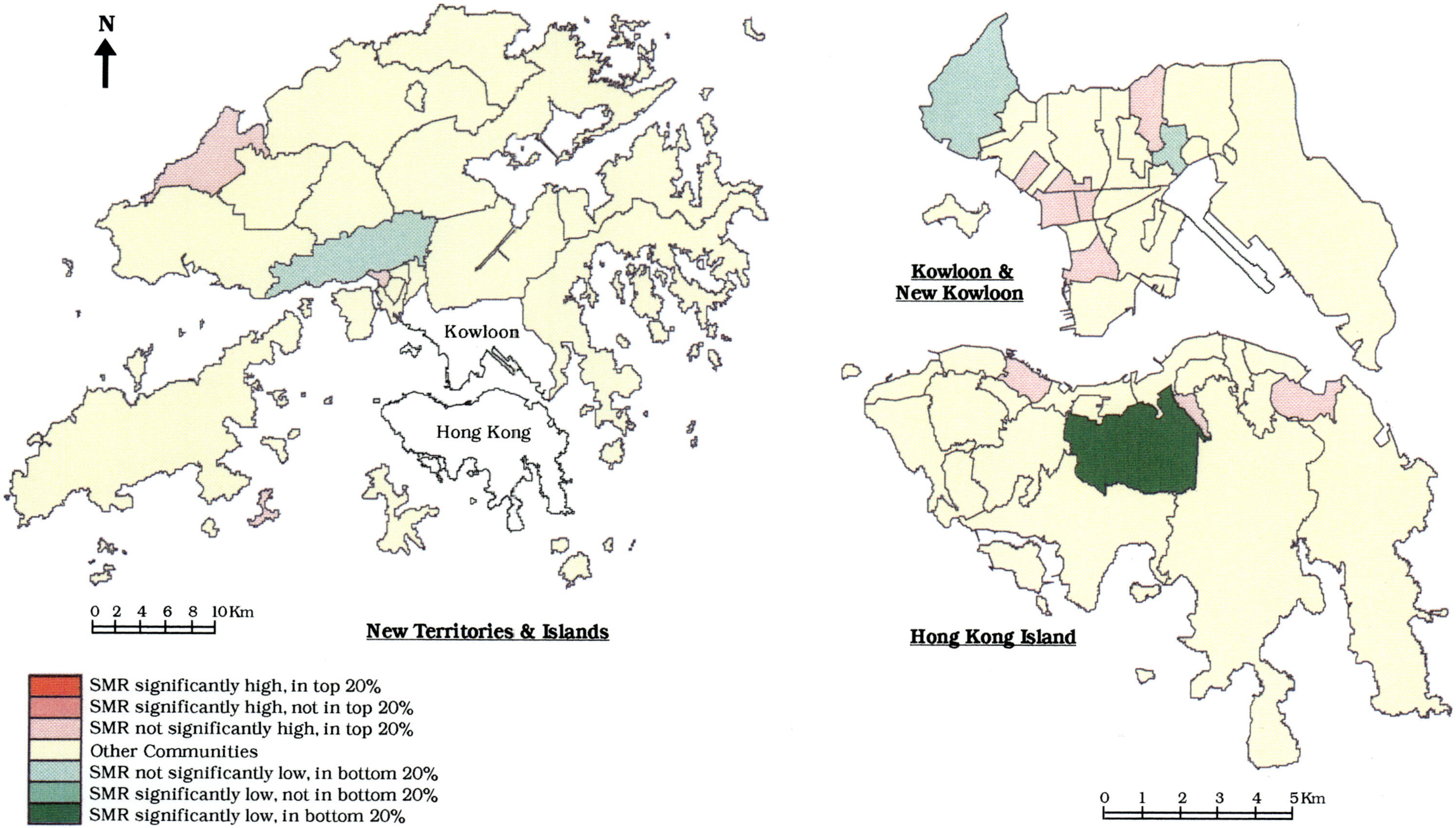

NPC (Female, 1984 – 1988)

Number of Deaths, Standardised Mortality Ratio (SMR) and 95% Confidence Interval of NPC by 65 Communities in 1984–1988

	Male			Female				Male			Female		
Community	Number of deaths	SMR	95% C.I.	Number of deaths	SMR	95% C.I.	Community	Number of deaths	SMR	95% C.I.	Number of deaths	SMR	95% C.I.
HK1	30	119.4	76.7 - 162.1	8	100.3	43.2 - 197.4	KL13	76	117.9	91.4 - 144.4	23	126.6	80.1 - 190.1
HK2	24	68.3	40.9 - 95.6	9	85.7	39.3 - 162.6	KL14	39	107.7	73.9 - 141.5	11	93.7	46.9 - 167.7
HK3	9	70.2	32.2 - 133.2	6	175.9	64.4 - 383.1	KL15	7	89.5	35.9 - 184.6	4	155.3	42.3 - 397.2
HK4	15	69.9	39.0 - 115.3	7	109.5	44.0 - 225.8	KL16	13	78.1	41.5 - 133.5	6	133.8	49.0 - 291.6
HK5	19	99.1	59.7 - 154.9	5	86.7	28.0 - 202.5	KL17	4	70.3	19.2 - 179.9	2	68.4	8.3 - 246.9
HK6	11	55.5	27.8 - 99.3	2	25.4	3.1 - 91.6	KL18	5	140.6	45.5 - 328.6	0	0.0	...
HK7	3	75.9	15.7 - 222.0	0	0.0	...	KL19	60	97.5	72.8 - 122.2	18	89.9	53.2 - 142.0
HK8	0	0.0	...	0	0.0	...	KL20	11	75.7	37.8 - 135.4	7	142.5	57.2 - 293.8
HK9	1	25.9	0.7 - 143.7	1	54.6	1.4 - 303.1	KL21	24	105.9	67.9 - 157.6	4	54.0	14.7 - 138.1
HK10	57	98.8	73.2 - 124.5	18	85.6	50.7 - 135.3	KL22	6	96.6	35.4 - 210.5	0	0.0	...
HK11	7	143.3	57.6 - 295.5	4	235.1	64.1 - 601.2	KL23	24	159.4	102.2 - 237.2	5	114.0	36.9 - 266.4
HK12	1	19.5	0.5 - 108.6	2	100.5	12.2 - 362.9	KL24	12	99.6	51.3 - 173.7	5	125.5	40.6 - 293.3
HK13	5	78.4	25.4 - 183.1	0	0.0	...	KL25	190	85.8	73.6 - 98.0	76	108.5	84.1 - 132.9
HK14	12	56.2	29.0 - 98.1	7	87.6	35.2 - 180.7	NT1	10	72.0	34.6 - 132.3	2	45.7	5.5 - 165.0
HK15	8	106.0	45.7 - 208.7	2	71.4	8.6 - 257.8	NT2	10	62.2	29.9 - 114.4	5	100.1	32.4 - 233.8
HK16	38	134.6	91.8 - 177.4	12	136.6	70.4 - 238.4	NT3	20	67.3	37.8 - 96.8	12	140.9	72.7 - 246.0
HK17	50	146.0	105.5 - 186.4	8	71.8	31.0 - 141.4	NT4	36	129.2	87.0 - 171.4	8	90.7	39.1 - 178.6
HK18	2	44.0	5.3 - 158.8	1	58.5	1.5 - 325.1	NT5	51	100.0	72.6 - 127.5	20	127.7	77.8 - 197.3
HK19	17	86.3	50.2 - 138.2	8	116.0	50.0 - 228.3	NT6	33	110.1	72.5 - 147.6	10	107.0	51.4 - 196.7
HK20	56	152.2	112.3 - 192.0	14	114.1	62.3 - 191.4	NT7	31	177.1	120.3 - 251.6	5	96.3	31.2 - 225.0
HK21	2	33.8	4.1 - 122.2	0	0.0	...	NT8	67	110.2	83.8 - 136.6	20	109.2	66.6 - 168.9
KL1	23	114.2	72.3 - 171.4	5	82.5	26.7 - 192.8	NT9	19	220.0	132.6 - 343.8	4	153.9	41.9 - 393.6
KL2	41	101.3	70.3 - 132.3	15	136.1	76.0 - 224.6	NT10	41	108.4	75.2 - 141.5	8	70.1	30.2 - 137.9
KL3	14	125.3	68.5 - 210.2	5	137.6	44.5 - 321.6	NT11	4	57.9	15.8 - 148.1	1	43.9	1.1 - 244.2
KL4	27	76.5	47.6 - 105.3	11	122.1	61.0 - 218.4	NT12	36	106.0	71.4 - 140.6	7	66.3	26.6 - 136.7
KL5	24	94.7	56.8 - 132.6	10	142.1	68.3 - 261.2	NT13	8	91.4	39.4 - 179.9	1	39.2	1.0 - 217.5
KL6	7	107.0	43.0 - 220.6	3	108.7	22.4 - 317.7	NT14	6	113.5	41.6 - 247.2	1	61.3	1.6 - 340.5
KL7	7	127.8	51.3 - 263.6	2	95.4	11.6 - 344.6	NT15	40	118.4	81.7 - 155.1	7	62.3	25.0 - 128.4
KL8	20	102.3	62.4 - 158.1	7	117.3	47.1 - 241.9	NT16	94	108.8	86.8 - 130.8	39	131.7	90.4 - 173.1
KL9	77	103.6	80.5 - 126.8	21	86.3	53.3 - 132.0	NT17	10	78.7	37.8 - 144.6	4	95.8	26.1 - 245.1
KL10	7	85.4	34.3 - 176.1	0	0.0	...	NT18	12	209.9	108.2 - 366.4	4	202.9	55.3 - 518.9
KL11	13	59.7	31.8 - 102.0	4	52.6	14.3 - 134.4	NT19	9	98.2	45.0 - 186.4	3	110.5	22.8 - 323.0
KL12	4	69.6	19.0 - 177.9	3	220.3	45.4 - 644.2							

NPC

Sex-Age specific mortality rate (1/100,000) of NPC in Hong Kong (1984–1988)

	Male		Female	
	No. of	Mortality	No. of	Mortality
Age	deaths	rate	deaths	rate
0–4	0	0.00	0	0.00
5–9	0	0.00	0	0.00
10–14	0	0.00	1	0.10
15–19	6	0.50	1	0.09
20–24	9	0.62	4	0.29
25–29	29	1.85	7	0.47
30–34	71	5.25	27	2.18
35–39	135	12.17	41	4.23
40–44	148	20.19	52	8.67
45–49	198	28.13	67	11.48
50–54	286	39.02	54	8.55
55–59	267	40.20	72	11.85
60–64	191	35.36	54	10.09
65+	315	34.89	145	11.75
TOTAL	1655	11.61	525	3.91

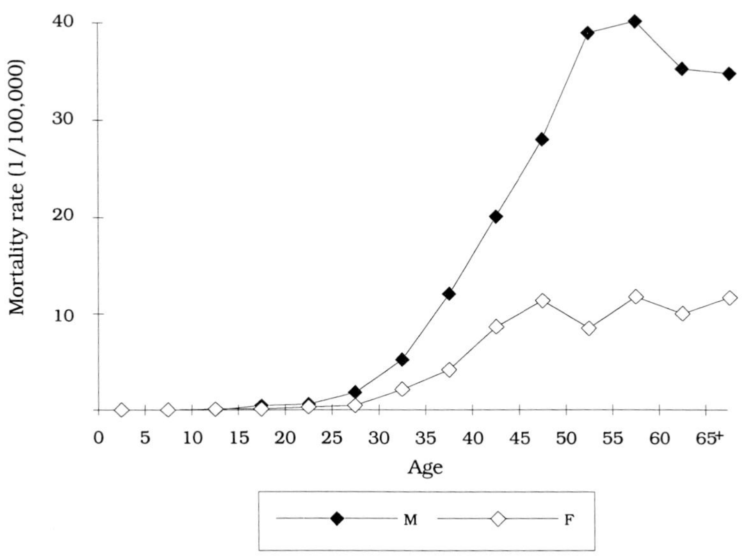

Number of communities on map by category based on standardized mortality ratio (SMR) during 1984–1988

	Number of communities	
Category	Male	Female
SMR significantly high, in top 20%	6	0
SMR significantly high , not in top 20%	0	0
SMR not significantly high, in top 20%	7	12
SMR not significantly low, in bottom 20%	7	3
SMR significantly low, not in bottom 20%	1	0
SMR significantly low, in bottom 20%	5	1
other communities	39	49

Values of the standardized mortality ratio (SMR) which divide the 65 communities into quintile

Percentile	Male	Female
20th	69.55	54.01
40th	86.35	86.32
60th	103.62	108.53
80th	118.43	131.72
Lowest SMR	0.00	0.00
Highest SMR	220.04	235.07
No. of communities with zero death	1	7

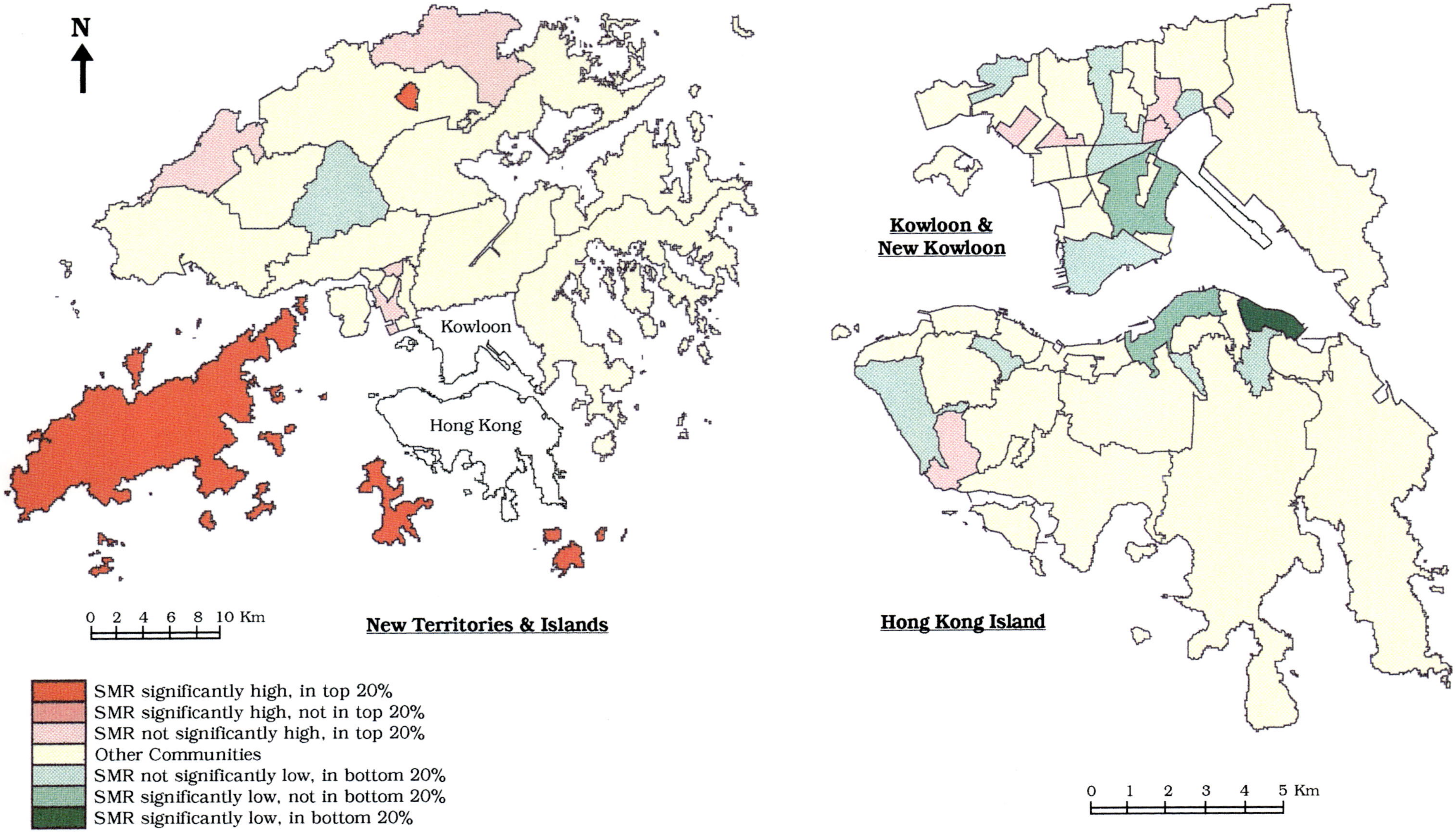

NPC (Male, 1989 -1993)

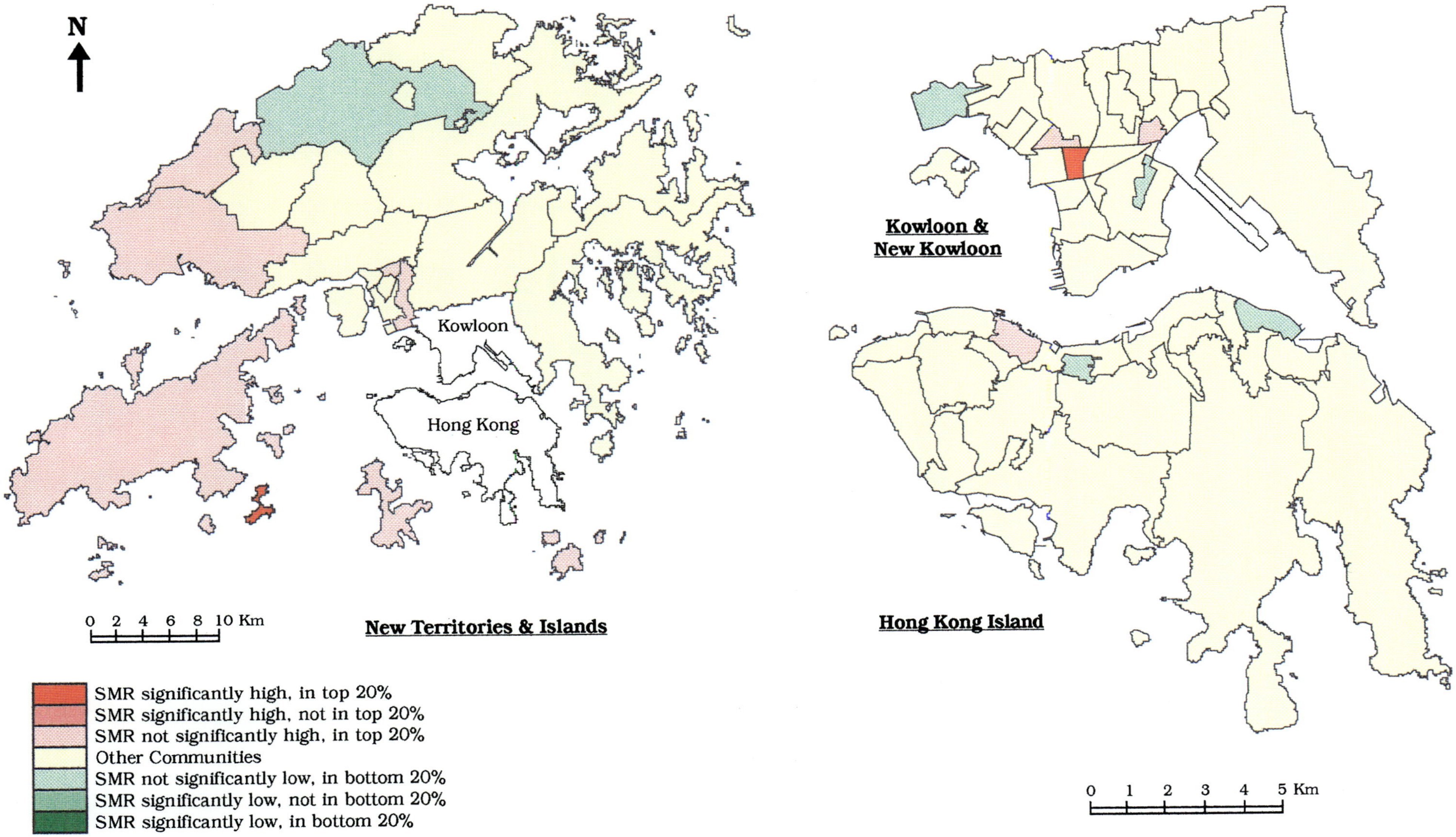

NPC (Female, 1989 -1993)

Number of Deaths, Standardised Mortality Ratio (SMR) and 95% Confidence Interval of NPC by 65 Communities in 1989–1993

Community	Male			Female		
	Number of deaths	SMR	95% C.I.	Number of deaths	SMR	95% C.I.
HK1	16	68.4	39.1 - 110.9	8	104.0	44.8 - 204.9
HK2	25	78.7	50.9 - 116.5	6	64.6	23.7 - 140.8
HK3	9	85.7	39.3 - 162.9	5	178.3	57.8 - 415.5
HK4	15	84.2	47.2 - 139.0	5	99.1	32.1 - 230.9
HK5	14	83.8	45.7 - 140.7	2	42.8	5.2 - 154.5
HK6	10	78.2	37.5 - 143.9	5	65.7	21.3 - 153.2
HK7	3	66.0	13.6 - 192.7	1	53.2	1.3 - 296.6
HK8	4	57.5	15.6 - 147.2	0	0.0	...
HK9	2	51.8	6.3 - 186.9	1	59.7	1.5 - 332.5
HK10	44	76.7	54.0 - 80.3	25	121.5	78.6 - 179.8
HK11	1	20.2	0.5 - 112.4	0	0.0	...
HK12	4	78.2	21.3 - 200.2	2	104.3	12.6 - 376.4
HK13	7	130.0	52.1 - 267.8	2	110.7	13.4 - 399.5
HK14	14	58.3	31.8 - 98.0	3	35.3	7.3 - 103.2
HK15	8	52.6	22.7 - 103.5	3	54.3	11.2 - 158.6
HK16	20	89.8	54.9 - 138.3	7	98.5	39.5 - 202.9
HK17	47	101.8	72.7 - 130.9	14	92.1	50.3 - 154.7
HK18	1	19.8	0.5 - 110.3	1	53.8	1.4 - 512.7
HK19	26	132.6	81.6 - 183.6	4	60.1	16.3 - 153.8
HK20	49	118.6	85.4 - 151.8	16	120.3	68.8 - 194.9
HK21	6	106.0	38.9 - 231.0	0	0.0	...
KL1	8	54.7	23.6 - 107.8	3	67.2	13.8 - 196.2
KL2	35	97.4	65.2 - 129.7	5	54.2	17.6 - 126.2
KL3	12	126.0	65.1 - 220.5	8	270.5	116.6 - 532.9
KL4	28	100.2	63.1 - 137.3	5	69.9	22.6 - 162.9
KL5	25	126.0	81.6 - 186.5	4	75.9	20.7 - 194.4
KL6	4	64.2	17.5 - 164.3	2	78.1	9.5 - 282.0
KL7	5	93.0	30.1 - 216.6	1	48.3	1.2 - 269.1
KL8	17	94.8	55.3 - 151.7	2	37.6	4.6 - 135.9
KL9	54	78.5	57.6 - 99.5	25	114.2	73.9 - 169.1
KL10	10	70.5	33.9 - 129.8	4	79.4	21.6 - 203.4
KL11	12	74.9	38.7 - 131.1	2	35.8	4.3 - 129.4
KL12	3	59.1	12.2 - 172.6	0	0.0	...

Community	Male			Female		
	Number of deaths	SMR	95% C.I.	Number of deaths	SMR	95% C.I.
KL13	61	101.6	76.1 - 127.1	17 #	102.7	59.9 - 164.3
KL14	29	92.7	59.0 - 126.5	7 #	65.5	26.3 - 134.9
KL15	10	132.1	63.4 - 243.1	2 #	86.8	10.5 - 313.2
KL16	21	145.3	90.0 - 222.4	7 #	182.4	73.1 - 375.8
KL17	2	39.4	4.8 - 142.3	3 #	134.4	27.7 - 392.3
KL18	2	65.4	7.9 - 236.0	2 #	184.5	22.3 - 666.1
KL19	53	93.7	68.5 - 118.9	14 #	73.6	40.2 - 123.7
KL20	13	95.4	50.8 - 163.1	4 #	84.9	23.1 - 217.3
KL21	26	136.6	84.1 - 189.2	5 #	74.9	24.3 - 174.6
KL22	1	20.3	0.5 - 112.8	0 0	0.0	...
KL23	16	168.0	96.1 - 272.1	5 #	181.9	58.9 - 423.9
KL24	15	139.2	78.0 - 229.7	2 #	53.3	6.4 - 192.4
KL25	200	100.5	86.6 - 114.5	62 #	98.1	73.7 - 122.5
NT1	23	114.0	72.3 - 171.1	7	109.1	43.8 - 224.8
NT2	24	141.8	90.9 - 211.3	6	113.8	41.8 - 248.2
NT3	31	91.9	59.6 - 124.3	8	83.2	35.8 - 163.8
NT4	32	137.3	89.7 - 184.9	13	178.6	95.0 - 305.3
NT5	44	101.7	71.7 - 131.8	17	127.7	74.5 - 204.4
NT6	37	119.3	80.9 - 157.8	13	139.8	74.4 - 239.0
NT7	44	119.7	84.3 - 155.0	11	103.8	51.8 - 185.8
NT8	81	97.0	75.9 - 118.1	36	147.1	99.1 - 151.1
NT9	11	154.5	77.1 - 276.6	5	237.1	76.8 - 552.4
NT10	47	116.9	83.5 - 150.3	16	133.8	76.5 - 216.7
NT11	3	47.0	9.7 - 137.1	3	153.9	31.7 - 449.4
NT12	47	123.9	88.5 - 159.3	6	52.6	19.3 - 114.6
NT13	16	192.8	110.3 - 293.1	2	76.5	9.3 - 276.2
NT14	5	138.4	44.8 - 322.5	2	168.4	20.4 - 607.8
NT15	57	121.5	90.0 - 153.1	11	73.6	36.7 - 131.8
NT16	128	102.7	84.9 - 120.5	46	111.4	79.2 - 143.6
NT17	26	86.4	53.2 - 119.6	11	112.0	55.9 - 200.4
NT18	13	222.4	118.3 - 380.4	9	454.4	208.1 - 863.4
NT19	15	186.6	104.5 - 308.0	5	211.7	68.6 - 493.3

NPC

Sex-Age specific mortality rate (1/100,000) of NPC in Hong Kong (1989–1993)

Age	Male: No. of deaths	Male: Mortality rate	Female: No. of deaths	Female: Mortality rate
0–4	0	0.00	0	0.00
5–9	0	0.00	0	0.00
10–14	2	0.18	0	0.00
15–19	3	0.27	0	0.00
20–24	3	0.26	5	0.44
25–29	26	1.80	7	0.47
30–34	53	3.40	22	1.45
35–39	127	9.49	39	3.10
40–44	188	17.07	56	5.76
45–49	183	25.05	41	6.87
50–54	222	32.00	64	11.24
55–59	262	37.49	70	11.49
60–64	259	41.96	63	10.90
65+	343	30.97	161	11.46
TOTAL	1671	11.43	528	3.77

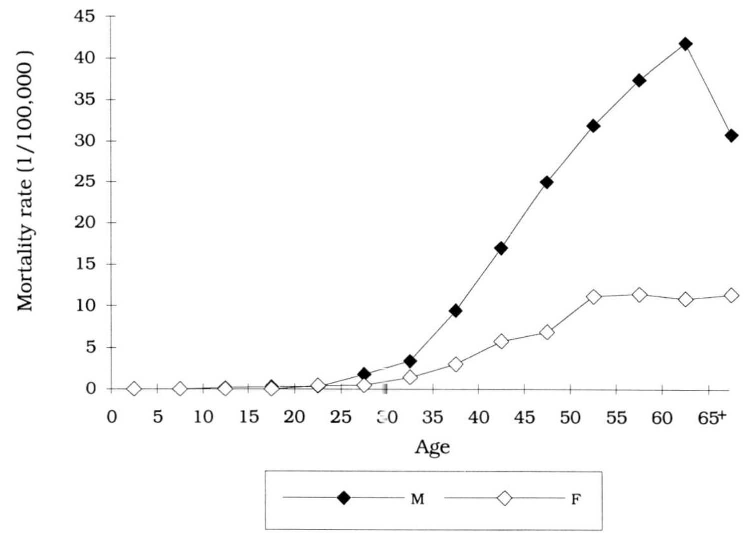

Number of communities on map by category based on standardized mortality ratio (SMR) during 1989–1993

Category	Number of communities: Male	Number of communities: Female
SMR significantly high, in top 20%	3	2
SMR significantly high , not in top 20%	0	0
SMR not significantly high, in top 20%	10	8
SMR not significantly low, in bottom 20%	10	5
SMR significantly low, not in bottom 20%	2	0
SMR significantly low, in bottom 20%	1	0
other communities	39	50

Values of the standardized mortality ratio (SMR) which divide the 65 communities into quintile

Percentile	Male	Female
20th	65.37	53.30
40th	86.38	74.94
60th	101.72	103.79
80th	129.99	134.35
Lowest SMR	[illegible]9.81	0.00
Highest SMR	222.44	454.40
No. of communities with zero cases	0	1

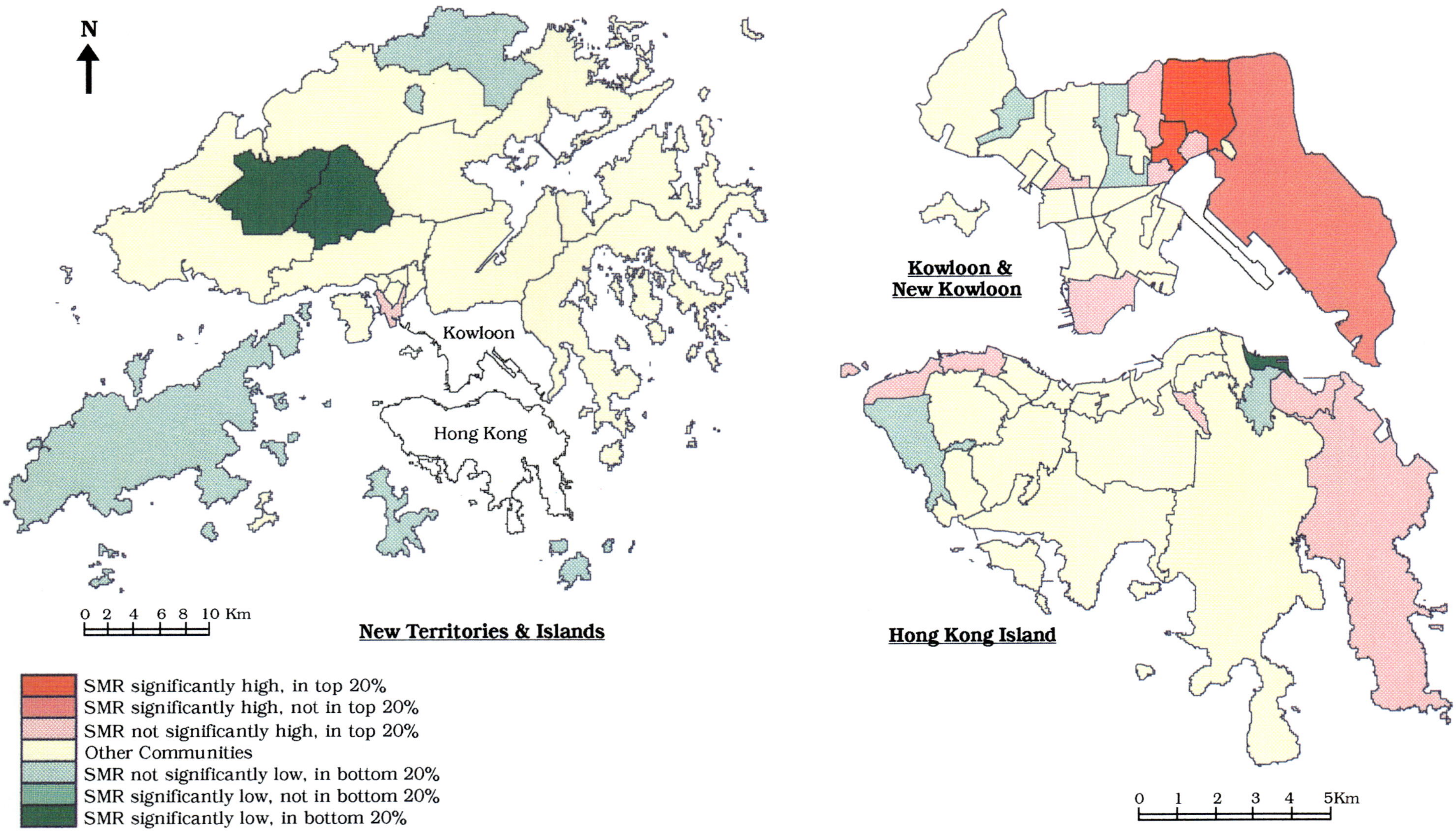

Oesophageal Cancer (Male, 1979 –1983)

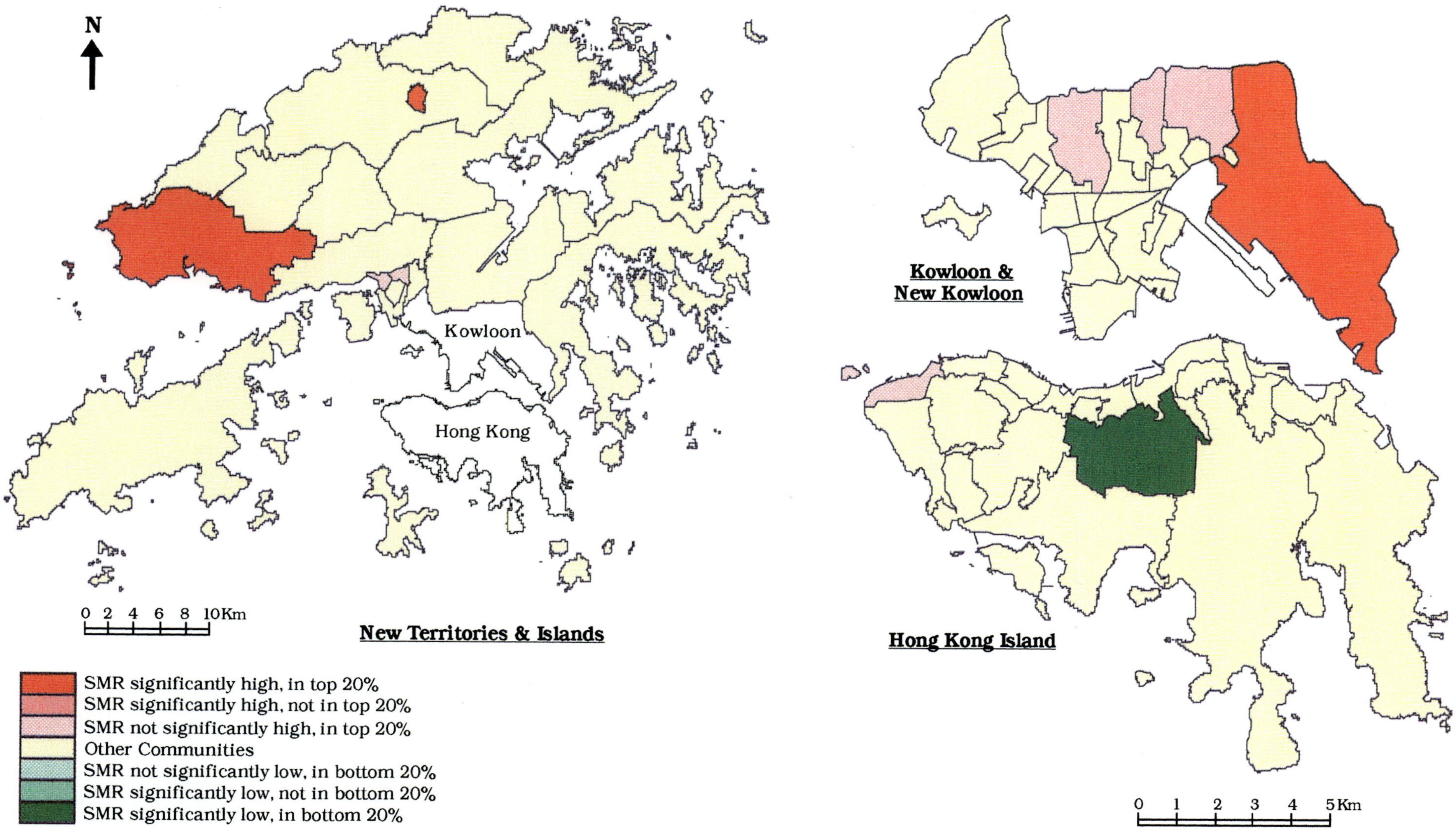

Oesophageal Cancer (Female, 1979 - 1983)

Number of Deaths, Standardised Mortality Ratio (SMR) and 95% Confidence Interval of Oesophageal Cancer by 65 Communities in 1979–1983

Community	Male			Female		
	Number of deaths	SMR	95% C.I.	Number of deaths	SMR	95% C.I.
HK1	30	129.7	83.3 - 176.1	7	127.8	51.3 - 263.6
HK2	49	134.1	96.6 - 171.7	9	113.0	51.8 - 214.4
HK3	11	76.5	38.2 - 136.8	0	0.0	...
HK4	16	71.3	40.8 - 115.8	3	58.7	12.1 - 171.6
HK5	24	110.9	71.1 - 165.0	5	103.5	33.5 - 241.8
HK6	13	72.6	38.6 - 124.2	1	17.6	0.4 - 97.7
HK7	4	114.4	31.2 - 292.5	0	0.0	...
HK8	8	115.3	49.7 - 227.0	0	0.0	...
HK9	0	0.0	...	0	0.0	...
HK10	42	86.0	60.0 - 112.0	13	92.9	49.4 - 158.7
HK11	9	191.1	87.7 - 362.7	1	103.0	2.6 - 572.0
HK12	2	54.1	6.5 - 195.2	1	76.9	1.9 - 427.4
HK13	0	0.0	...	1	66.4	1.7 - 369.0
HK14	6	43.4	15.9 - 94.6	1	27.0	0.7 - 149.9
HK15	2	35.5	4.3 - 128.1	1	63.3	1.6 - 351.7
HK16	35	130.6	87.4 - 173.9	6	99.9	36.6 - 217.7
HK17	40	138.6	95.7 - 181.6	3	44.5	9.2 - 130.2
HK18	2	50.4	6.1 - 182.0	0	0.0	...
HK19	8	57.9	25.0 - 114.0	1	29.4	0.7 - 163.1
HK20	27	88.9	55.4 - 122.4	4	57.3	15.6 - 146.7
HK21	4	101.6	27.7 - 259.9	2	245.9	29.8 - 887.7
KL1	25	128.6	78.2 - 179.0	5	114.4	37.0 - 267.3
KL2	35	87.0	58.2 - 115.8	6	65.9	24.1 - 143.6
KL3	8	69.3	29.9 - 136.3	1	33.7	0.9 - 187.2
KL4	25	76.3	46.4 - 106.3	3	41.9	8.6 - 122.5
KL5	18	66.1	39.1 - 104.5	3	51.0	10.5 - 149.0
KL6	5	74.6	24.1 - 174.2	1	43.2	1.1 - 240.1
KL7	4	81.7	22.3 - 208.9	1	63.9	1.6 - 354.9
KL8	11	62.1	31.0 - 111.0	4	93.4	25.5 - 238.9
KL9	61	94.1	70.5 - 117.7	18	111.7	66.1 - 176.4
KL10	4	64.6	17.6 - 165.2	1	57.4	1.5 - 319.1
KL11	13	77.2	41.1 - 132.0	3	63.9	13.2 - 186.9
KL12	0	0.0	...	0	0.0	...
KL13	55	82.0	60.4 - 103.7	14	94.7	51.7 - 158.9
KL14	45	116.6	82.5 - 150.6	11	129.9	65.0 - 232.5
KL15	3	95.2	19.6 - 278.5	2	279.7	33.9 - 1009.8
KL16	20	129.9	79.2 - 200.7	3	81.3	16.8 - 237.6
KL17	2	44.9	5.4 - 162.1	0	0.0	...
KL18	1	35.0	0.9 - 194.4	0	0.0	...
KL19	77	131.6	102.2 - 161.1	21	147.2	90.9 - 225.1
KL20	29	142.0	90.3 - 193.7	9	185.3	85.0 - 351.6
KL21	57	174.1	128.9 - 219.3	9	113.8	52.2 - 215.9
KL22	8	144.8	62.4 - 284.9	2	174.2	21.1 - 628.8
KL23	22	129.0	80.7 - 195.5	3	77.1	15.9 - 225.6
KL24	11	93.6	46.8 - 167.4	3	126.1	26.0 - 368.6
KL25	201	124.9	107.6 - 142.1	56	152.6	112.6 - 192.5
NT1	6	77.1	28.3 - 168.0	3	152.9	31.7 - 446.9
NT2	15	129.4	72.3 - 213.5	1	38.9	1.0 - 216.1
NT3	25	104.7	63.7 - 145.8	6	132.2	48.4 - 288.0
NT4	16	124.4	71.1 - 201.9	5	167.1	54.1 - 390.5
NT5	53	116.4	85.1 - 147.8	11	108.0	54.0 - 193.2
NT6	19	84.3	50.8 - 131.7	5	96.4	31.2 - 225.1
NT7	6	81.5	29.8 - 177.5	1	60.6	1.5 - 336.4
NT8	22	93.0	58.1 - 141.0	13	246.0	130.9 - 420.5
NT9	5	66.0	21.4 - 154.2	1	60.8	1.5 - 337.7
NT10	13	41.7	22.2 - 71.3	7	103.7	41.6 - 213.8
NT11	1	15.5	0.4 - 86.2	0	0.0	...
NT12	25	83.9	51.0 - 116.8	8	121.1	52.2 - 238.4
NT13	1	18.0	0.5 - 100.1	5	379.6	122.8 - 886.8
NT14	2	39.0	4.7 - 140.7	0	0.0	...
NT15	17	84.1	48.9 - 134.6	6	117.8	43.1 - 256.6
NT16	28	112.1	70.6 - 153.6	7	111.3	44.7 - 229.5
NT17	10	85.0	40.9 - 156.2	1	34.1	0.9 - 189.3
NT18	5	86.9	28.1 - 203.1	0	0.0	...
NT19	5	49.8	16.1 - 116.3	1	38.9	1.0 - 215.9

OESOPHAGEAL CANCER

Sex-Age specific mortality rate (1/100,000) of oesophageal cancer in Hong Kong (1979–1983)

	Male		Female	
Age	No. of deaths	Mortality rate	No. of deaths	Mortality rate
0–4	0	0.00	0	0.00
5–9	0	0.00	0	0.00
10–14	0	0.00	0	0.00
15–19	0	0.00	0	0.00
20–24	1	0.07	0	0.00
25–29	0	0.00	1	0.09
30–34	4	0.36	4	0.44
35–39	8	1.11	0	0.00
40–44	25	3.55	0	0.00
45–49	98	13.59	7	1.16
50–54	175	25.47	19	3.12
55–59	264	46.41	40	7.48
60–64	274	59.96	49	10.74
65+	497	72.90	199	19.71
TOTAL	1346	10.21	319	2.62

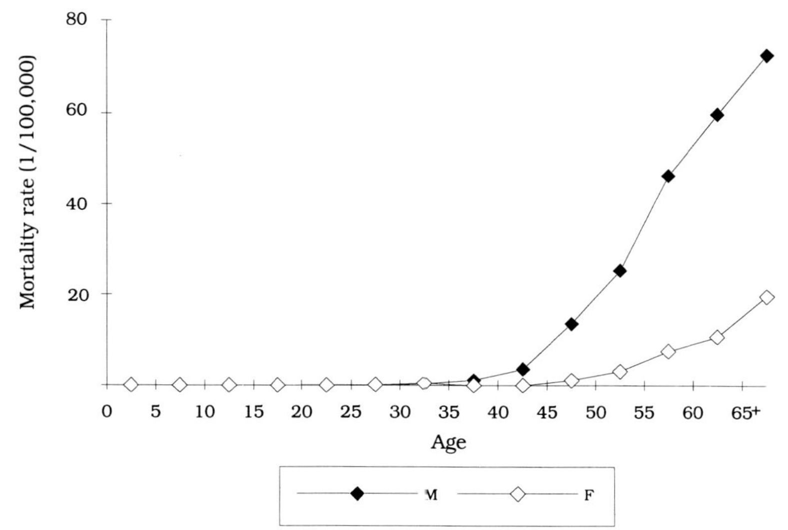

Number of communities on map by category based on standardized mortality ratio (SMR) during 1979–1983

Category	Number of communities Male	Female
SMR significantly high, in top 20%	2	3
SMR significantly high , not in top 20%	1	0
SMR not significantly high, in top 20%	11	6
SMR not significantly low, in bottom 20%	7	0
SMR significantly low, not in bottom 20%	0	0
SMR significantly low, in bottom 20%	3	1
other communities	41	55

Values of the standardized mortality ratio (SMR) which divide the 65 communities into quintile

Percentile	Male	Female
20th	50.40	26.99
40th	77.13	60.55
60th	93.03	96.36
80th	124.88	126.07
Lowest SMR	0.00	0.00
Highest SMR	191.14	379.57
No. of communities with zero death	3	11

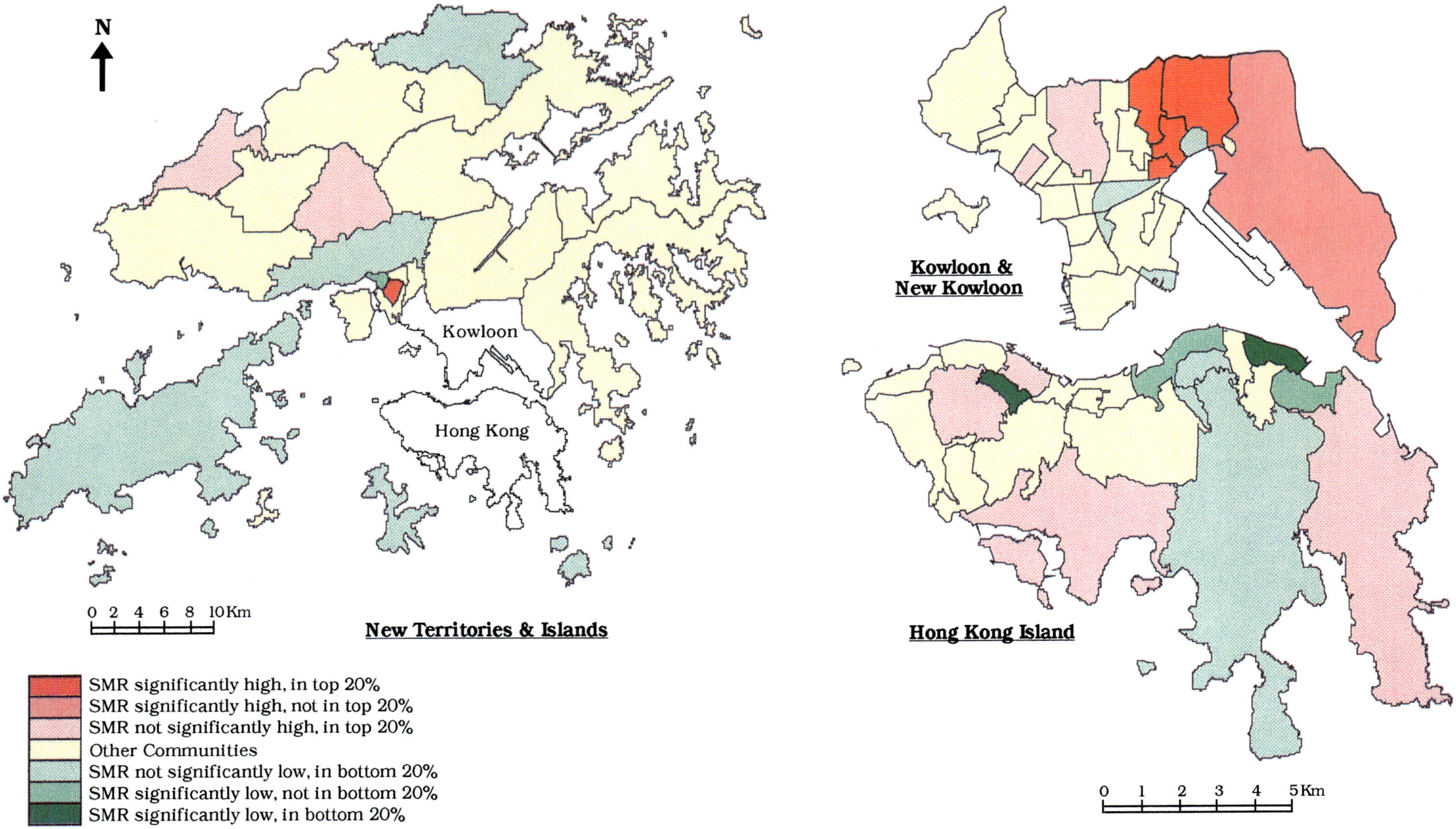

Oesophageal Cancer (Male, 1984 – 1988)

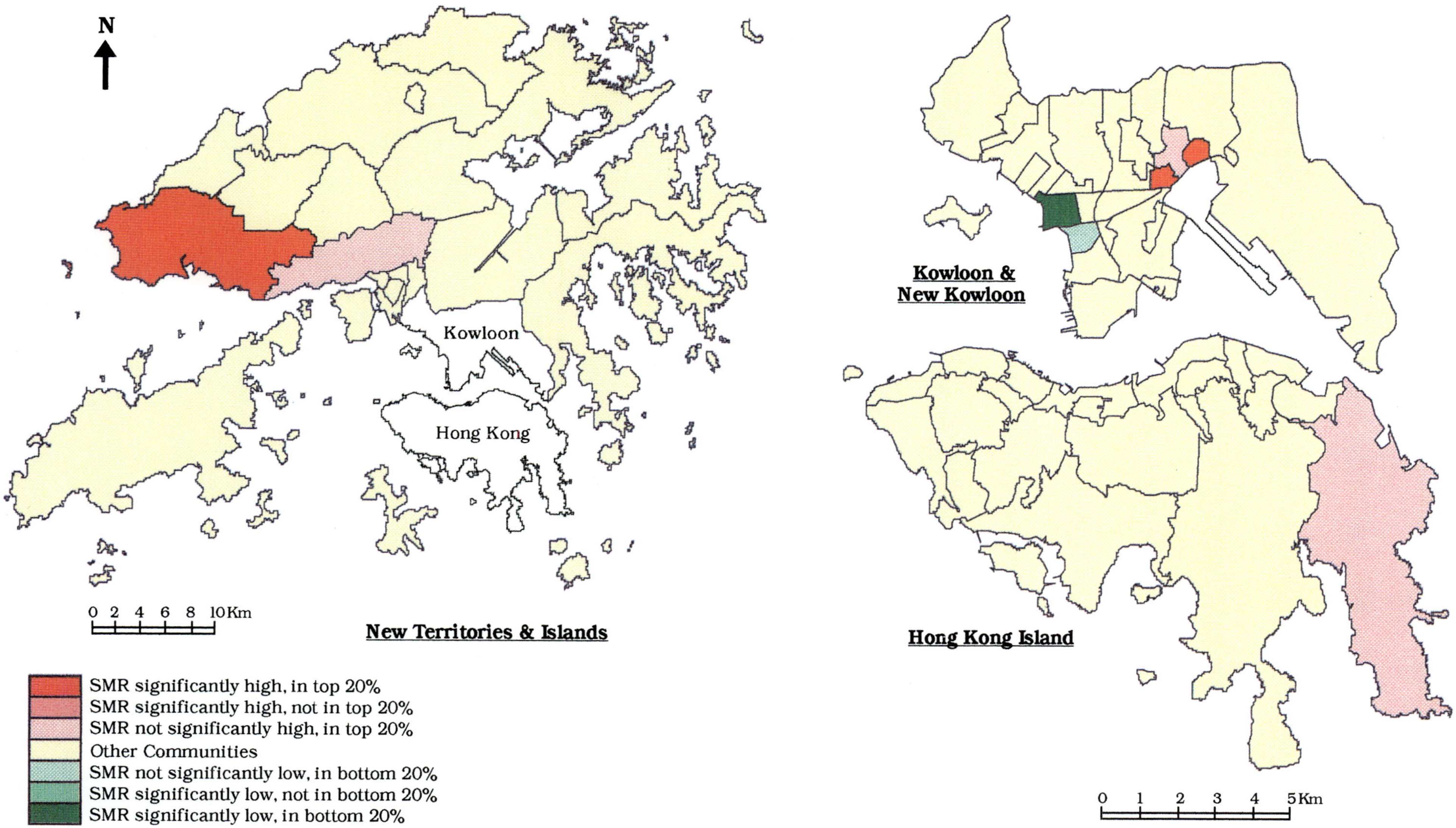

Oesophageal Cancer (Female, 1984 - 1988)

Number of Deaths, Standardised Mortality Ratio (SMR) and 95% Confidence Interval of Oesophageal Cancer by 65 Communities in 1984–1988

Community	Male			Female		
	Number of deaths	SMR	95% C.I.	Number of deaths	SMR	95% C.I.
HK1	23	93.5	59.2 - 140.3	3	62.5	12.9 - 182.6
HK2	31	89.5	58.0 - 121.0	7	103.4	41.5 - 213.2
HK3	17	128.6	74.8 - 205.7	0	0.0	...
HK4	16	77.0	44.0 - 125.0	2	49.1	5.9 - 177.3
HK5	11	57.2	28.6 - 102.4	1	26.1	0.7 - 145.1
HK6	16	86.3	49.3 - 140.0	2	42.7	5.2 - 154.0
HK7	5	136.8	44.3 - 319.6	1	107.1	2.7 - 595.1
HK8	1	14.3	0.4 - 79.4	1	58.5	1.5 - 325.2
HK9	1	31.9	0.8 - 177.3	0	0.0	...
HK10	38	73.5	50.1 - 96.8	12	97.0	50.0 - 169.3
HK11	1	20.5	0.5 - 113.8	2	242.3	29.3 - 874.9
HK12	1	23.4	0.6 - 130.2	0	0.0	...
HK13	4	62.8	17.1 - 160.6	2	168.8	20.4 - 609.2
HK14	9	48.1	22.1 - 91.3	6	136.6	50.0 - 297.5
HK15	3	49.1	10.1 - 143.5	3	206.2	42.5 - 602.8
HK16	18	67.1	36.1 - 98.1	8	151.4	65.3 - 298.0
HK17	46	132.1	93.9 - 170.3	13	183.0	97.3 - 312.8
HK18	2	53.2	6.4 - 192.2	0	0.0	...
HK19	15	87.3	48.8 - 144.1	3	85.7	17.7 - 250.7
HK20	50	138.0	99.7 - 176.2	7	96.1	38.6 - 198.1
HK21	1	22.3	0.6 - 124.0	0	0.0	...
KL1	16	85.0	48.6 - 138.0	2	56.6	6.9 - 204.3
KL2	41	110.8	76.9 - 144.7	1	14.3	0.4 - 79.4
KL3	8	74.0	31.9 - 145.7	2	83.0	10.0 - 299.5
KL4	29	84.4	53.7 - 115.1	2	33.9	4.1 - 122.2
KL5	21	83.5	47.8 - 119.2	4	86.9	23.7 - 222.4
KL6	3	43.2	8.9 - 126.4	2	112.0	13.6 - 404.3
KL7	2	40.8	4.9 - 147.3	0	0.0	...
KL8	16	89.3	51.0 - 145.0	1	29.4	0.7 - 163.4
KL9	57	82.8	61.3 - 104.3	10	72.1	34.7 - 132.6
KL10	3	45.1	9.3 - 132.0	0	0.0	...
KL11	14	71.7	39.2 - 120.4	2	48.8	5.9 - 176.1
KL12	4	71.3	19.4 - 182.3	2	202.5	24.5 - 731.0
KL13	67	107.2	81.5 - 132.9	10	85.1	40.9 - 156.4
KL14	56	132.9	98.1 - 167.7	8	95.3	41.1 - 187.7
KL15	12	156.6	80.7 - 273.2	2	122.6	14.8 - 442.8
KL16	10	65.2	31.4 - 119.9	1	35.5	0.9 - 197.4
KL17	4	64.4	17.6 - 164.8	1	43.7	1.1 - 242.5
KL18	3	102.8	21.2 - 300.7	1	175.0	4.4 - 972.5
KL19	81	127.9	100.1 - 155.8	19	149.8	90.3 - 234.1
KL20	29	186.2	125.0 - 267.5	5	151.2	48.9 - 353.2
KL21	41	156.3	108.5 - 204.2	8	160.0	69.0 - 315.0
KL22	2	34.9	4.2 - 126.1	4	392.7	107.0 - 1004.4
KL23	25	182.8	118.0 - 269.7	9	352.1	161.5 - 668.0
KL24	17	124.8	72.5– - 199.6	1	44.1	1.1 - 245.1
KL25	235	115.5	100.8 - 130.3	49	127.2	91.6 - 162.9
NT1	5	46.2	15.0 - 108.0	4	179.2	48.8 - 458.4
NT2	14	101.3	55.3 - 169.9	1	38.8	1.0 - 215.4
NT3	17	67.1	35.2 - 99.0	3	74.2	15.3 - 216.8
NT4	25	110.8	71.5 - 163.4	3	72.8	15.0 - 212.8
NT5	63	135.3	101.9 - 168.7	7	85.3	34.2 - 175.8
NT6	22	80.9	47.1 - 114.7	3	62.6	12.9 - 182.9
NT7	15	113.6	63.5 - 187.5	1	45.9	1.2 - 255.0
NT8	38	87.7	59.8 - 115.5	16	175.8	100.5 - 285.4
NT9	12	142.9	73.6 - 249.4	0	0.0	...
NT10	34	89.5	59.4 - 119.6	6	83.4	30.5 - 181.6
NT11	9	129.9	59.6 - 246.5	1	68.0	1.7 - 377.8
NT12	36	108.3	72.9 - 143.7	5	71.6	23.2 - 167.3
NT13	6	70.8	25.9 - 154.2	2	132.9	16.1 - 479.7
NT14	2	35.7	4.3 - 128.9	3	261.4	53.9 - 764.2
NT15	27	89.4	55.7 - 123.1	5	72.6	23.5 - 169.6
NT16	77	113.9	88.4 - 139.3	18	115.1	68.1 - 181.8
NT17	8	62.9	27.1 - 123.9	2	75.9	9.2 - 273.9
NT18	6	94.8	34.7 - 206.5	3	208.6	43.0 - 609.9
NT19	4	41.4	11.3 - 105.8	3	144.3	29.7 - 421.9

OESOPHAGEAL CANCER

Sex-Age specific mortality rate (1/100,000) of oesophageal cancer in Hong Kong (1984–1988)

	Male		Female	
Age	No. of deaths	Mortality rate	No. of deaths	Mortality rate
0–4	0	0.00	0	0.00
5–9	0	0.00	0	0.00
10–14	0	0.00	0	0.00
15–19	0	0.00	0	0.00
20–24	0	0.00	0	0.00
25–29	0	0.00	0	0.00
30–34	1	0.07	0	0.00
35–39	7	0.63	2	0.21
40–44	25	3.41	1	0.17
45–49	84	11.93	6	1.03
50–54	170	23.20	13	2.06
55–59	277	41.70	33	5.43
60–64	312	57.77	26	4.86
65+	662	73.32	225	18.23
TOTAL	1538	10.79	306	2.28

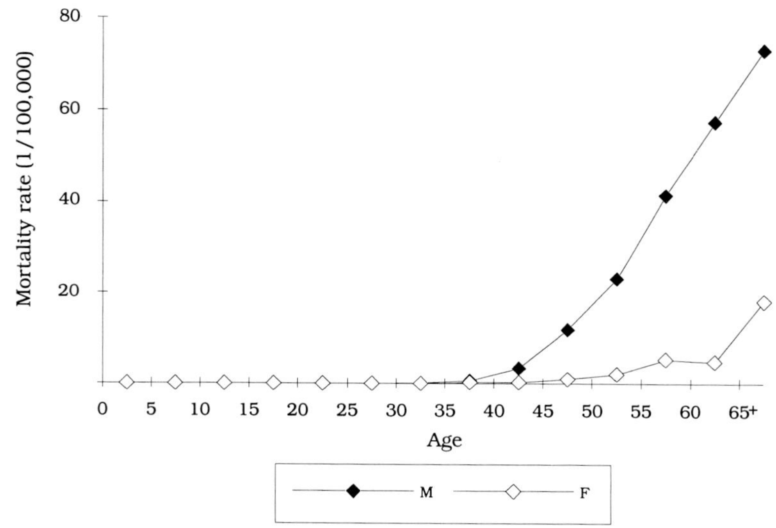

Number of communities on map by category based on standardized mortality ratio (SMR) during 1984–1988

Category	Number of communities Male	Female
SMR significantly high, in top 20%	5	3
SMR significantly high , not in top 20%	1	0
SMR not significantly high, in top 20%	8	3
SMR not significantly low, in bottom 20%	10	1
SMR significantly low, not in bottom 20%	3	0
SMR significantly low, in bottom 20%	2	1
other communities	36	57

Values of the standardized mortality ratio (SMR) which divide the 65 communities into quintile

Percentile	Male	Female
20th	48.11	35.53
40th	73.45	71.62
60th	89.46	96.06
80th	124.76	151.40
Lowest SMR	14.30	0.00
Highest SMR	186.21	392.71
No. of communities with zero death	0	8

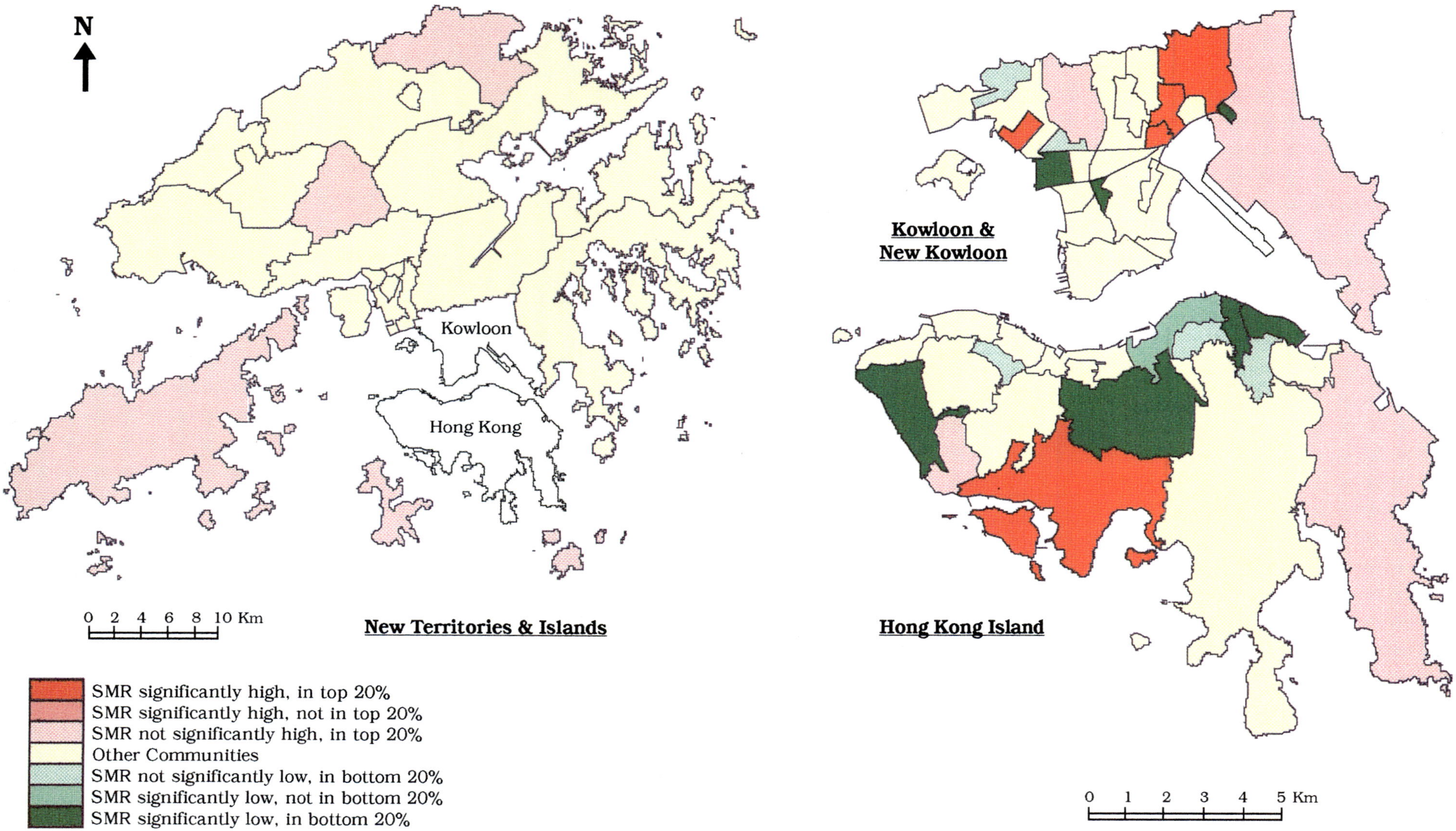

Oesophageal Cancer (Male, 1989 -1993)

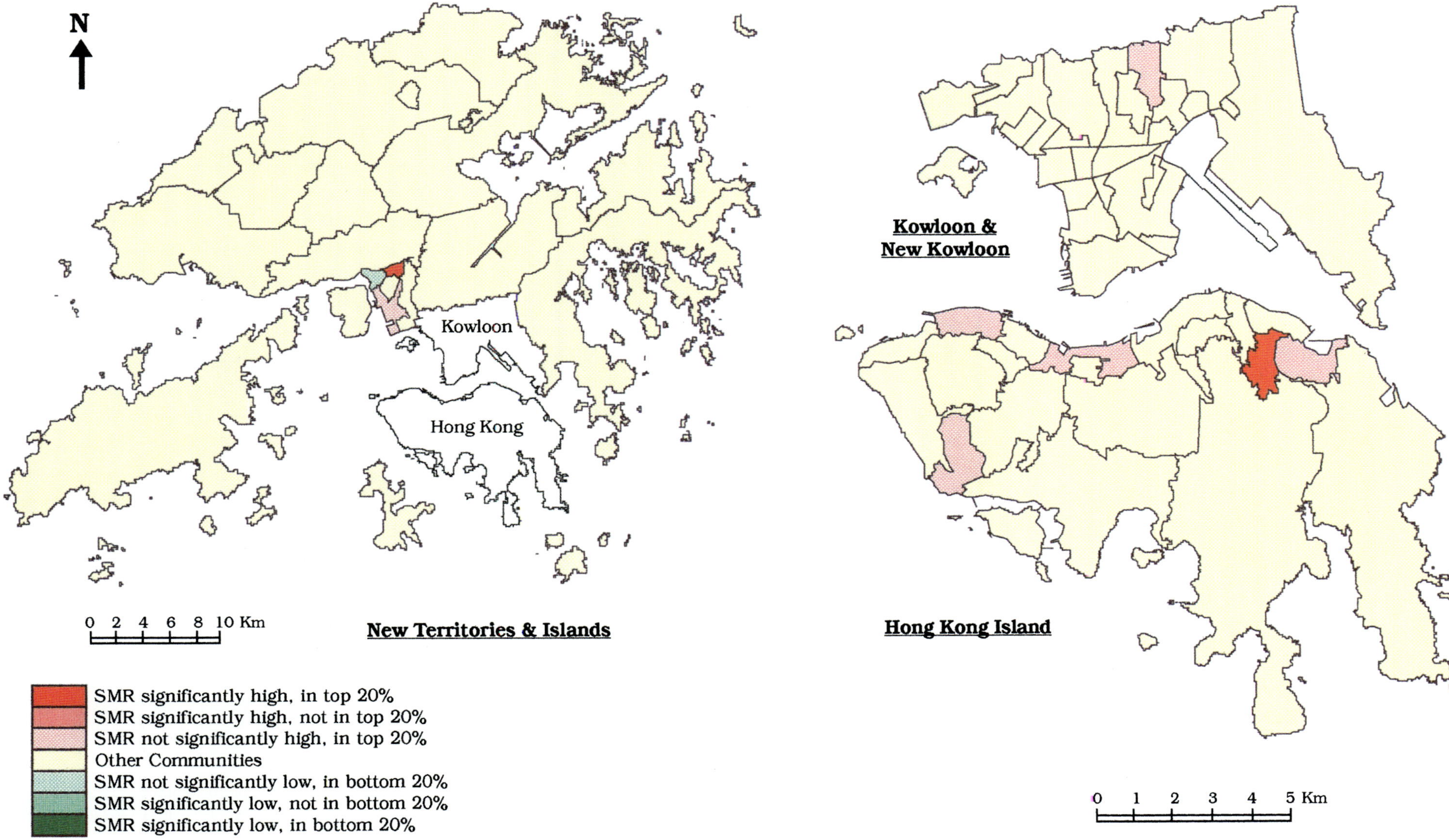

Oesophageal Cancer (Female, 1989 -1993)

Number of Deaths, Standardised Mortality Ratio (SMR) and 95% Confidence Interval
of Oesophageal Cancer by 65 Communities in 1989–1993

Community	Male			Female		
	Number of deaths	SMR	95% C.I.	Number of deaths	SMR	95% C.I.
HK1	25	109.0	70.5 - 161.3	5	111.2	36.0 - 259.9
HK2	31	99.7	64.6 - 134.8	10	183.3	88.1 - 337.0
HK3	8	74.3	32.0 - 146.3	0	0.0	...
HK4	12	67.5	34.9 - 118.2	6	190.4	69.7 - 414.8
HK5	19	112.3	67.6 - 175.1	3	100.5	20.7 - 293.9
HK6	6	33.2	12.2 - 72.4	2	46.2	5.6 - 166.7
HK7	1	25.3	0.6 - 141.0	3	294.1	60.6 - 859.9
HK8	2	31.3	3.8 - 113.1	0	0.0	...
HK9	2	66.6	8.1 - 240.4	2	292.8	35.4 - 1057.1
HK10	34	64.7	43.0 - 86.5	11	91.3	45.6 - 163.3
HK11	4	77.3	21.0 - 197.8	0	0.0	...
HK12	2	47.2	5.7 - 170.2	1	105.8	2.7 - 587.6
HK13	1	17.5	0.4 - 97.4	1	92.2	2.3 - 512.3
HK14	10	48.8	23.4 - 89.8	1	23.4	0.6 - 129.8
HK15	6	49.1	18.0 - 107.0	11	421.5	210.7 - 754.0
HK16	25	113.8	73.7 - 168.5	7	169.4	68.0 - 349.2
HK17	57	128.5	95.1 - 161.8	10	112.1	53.9 - 206.0
HK18	0	0.0	...	1	86.8	2.2 - 482.4
HK19	27	142.6	88.8 - 196.3	7	201.3	80.9 - 415.1
HK20	55	137.2	100.9 - 173.4	5	62.9	20.4 - 147.0
HK21	4	104.2	28.4 - 266.8	0	0.0	...
KL1	9	64.4	29.5 - 122.4	2	78.1	9.4 - 281.8
KL2	21	62.1	38.4 - 95.0	3	52.4	10.8 - 152.9
KL3	6	63.1	23.2 - 137.5	0	0.0	...
KL4	31	112.4	72.8 - 151.9	4	90.3	24.5 - 231.1
KL5	14	69.8	38.1 - 117.3	3	87.1	17.9 - 254.4
KL6	7	101.4	40.7 - 208.9	1	53.1	1.3 - 295.6
KL7	0	0.0	...	0	0.0	...
KL8	18	104.8	62.2 - 165.6	2	66.1	8.0 - 238.5
KL9	59	88.2	65.7 - 110.8	12	96.5	49.9 - 168.9
KL10	8	73.1	31.5 - 143.9	4	162.5	44.2 - 416.1
KL11	10	68.7	33.0 - 126.5	2	64.4	7.8 - 232.3
KL12	1	20.6	0.5 - 115.0	0	0.0	...
KL13	49	79.8	57.5 - 102.2	11	104.1	51.9 - 186.3
KL14	44	120.6	85.0 - 156.2	3	38.9	8.0 - 113.6
KL15	17	228.3	133.1 - 365.3	0	0.0	...
KL16	8	58.9	25.4 - 115.9	2	84.8	10.3 - 306.3
KL17	6	114.0	41.8 - 248.5	0	0.0	...
KL18	2	74.2	9.0 - 267.7	0	0.0	...
KL19	95	153.5	122.6 - 184.3	15	115.1	64.5 - 189.9
KL20	15	105.4	59.0 - 173.9	5	182.0	59.0 - 424.0
KL21	42	188.7	131.6 - 245.8	7	151.7	60.8 - 312.5
KL22	3	64.1	13.2 - 187.3	1	117.1	3.0 - 652.4
KL23	24	257.0	164.8 - 383.0	3	170.6	35.1 - 498.0
KL24	6	44.8	16.4 - 97.6	1	45.3	1.1 - 252.5
KL25	222	114.8	99.7 - 129.9	41	110.9	77.0 - 144.9
NT1	11	74.2	37.0 - 132.9	1	33.0	0.8 - 183.7
NT2	16	101.6	58.1 - 164.6	5	164.1	53.2 - 382.2
NT3	25	85.3	55.2 - 126.3	1	21.3	0.5 - 118.6
NT4	19	90.4	54.4 - 141.0	10	262.7	126.1 - 483.4
NT5	46	108.0	65.0 - 168.5	8	104.8	45.2 - 143.6
NT6	22	76.3	47.8 - 115.2	2	38.7	4.7 - 139.7
NT7	21	79.5	49.2 - 121.6	6	129.2	47.4 - 281.6
NT8	58	98.0	72.8 - 123.2	12	103.8	53.7 - 181.7
NT9	7	89.6	35.9 - 184.6	0	0.0	...
NT10	43	111.9	78.5 - 145.4	3	41.0	8.4 - 119.7
NT11	9	129.0	59.1 - 245.1	1	67.8	1.7 - 377.6
NT12	35	98.9	66.1 - 131.6	8	112.9	48.7 - 222.4
NT13	7	93.7	37.6 - 193.0	2	125.8	15.2 - 454.3
NT14	6	145.1	53.3 - 316.4	0	0.0	...
NT15	37	94.4	64.0 - 124.9	10	116.6	56.0 - 214.6
NT16	103	102.8	83.0 - 122.7	17	76.4	44.5 - 122.2
NT17	23	93.4	59.2 - 140.1	6	113.0	41.5 - 246.4
NT18	10	152.1	73.0 - 279.9	3	212.7	43.8 - 621.0
NT19	13	162.8	86.6 - 278.4	3	170.9	35.2 - 499.1

OESOPHAGEAL CANCER

Sex-Age specific mortality rate (1/100,000) of oesophageal cancer in Hong Kong (1989–1993)

	Male		Female	
Age	No. of deaths	Mortality rate	No. of deaths	Mortality rate
0–4	0	0.00	0	0.00
5–9	0	0.00	0	0.00
10–14	0	0.00	0	0.00
15–19	0	0.00	0	0.00
20–24	0	0.00	0	0.00
25–29	0	0.00	0	0.00
30–34	5	0.32	1	0.07
35–39	7	0.52	0	0.00
40–44	24	2.18	3	0.31
45–49	62	8.49	5	0.84
50–54	121	17.44	16	2.81
55–59	227	32.48	19	3.12
60–64	318	51.51	29	5.02
65+	795	71.77	233	16.58
TOTAL	1559	10.66	306	2.19

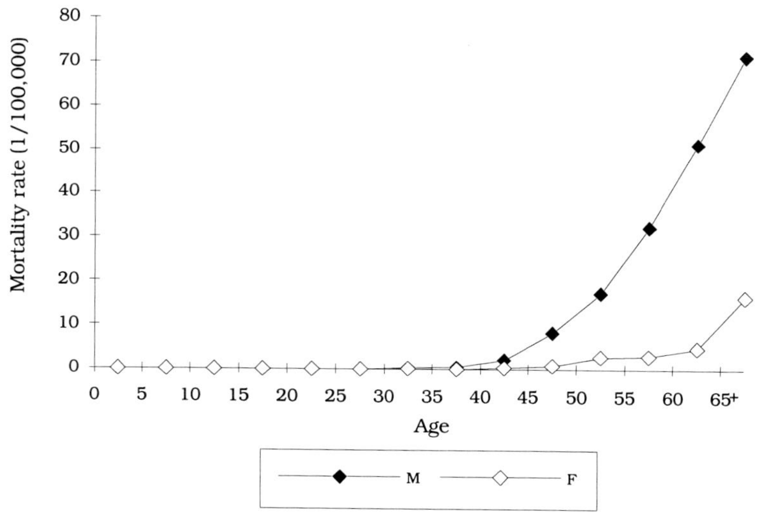

Number of communities on map by category based on standardized Mortality ratio (SMR) during 1989–1993

Category	Number of communities Male	Female
SMR significantly high, in top 20%	5	2
SMR significantly high , not in top 20%	0	0
SMR not significantly high, in top 20%	8	6
SMR not significantly low, in bottom 20%	5	1
SMR significantly low, not in bottom 20%	1	0
SMR significantly low, in bottom 20%	7	0
other communities	39	56

Values of the standardized mortality ratio (SMR) which divide the 65 communities into quintile

Percentile	Male	Female
20th	62.07	21.29
40th	76.27	67.79
60th	99.71	104.83
80th	113.97	162.55
Lowest SMR	0.00	0.00
Highest SMR	257.03	421.49
No. of communities with zero cases	2	12

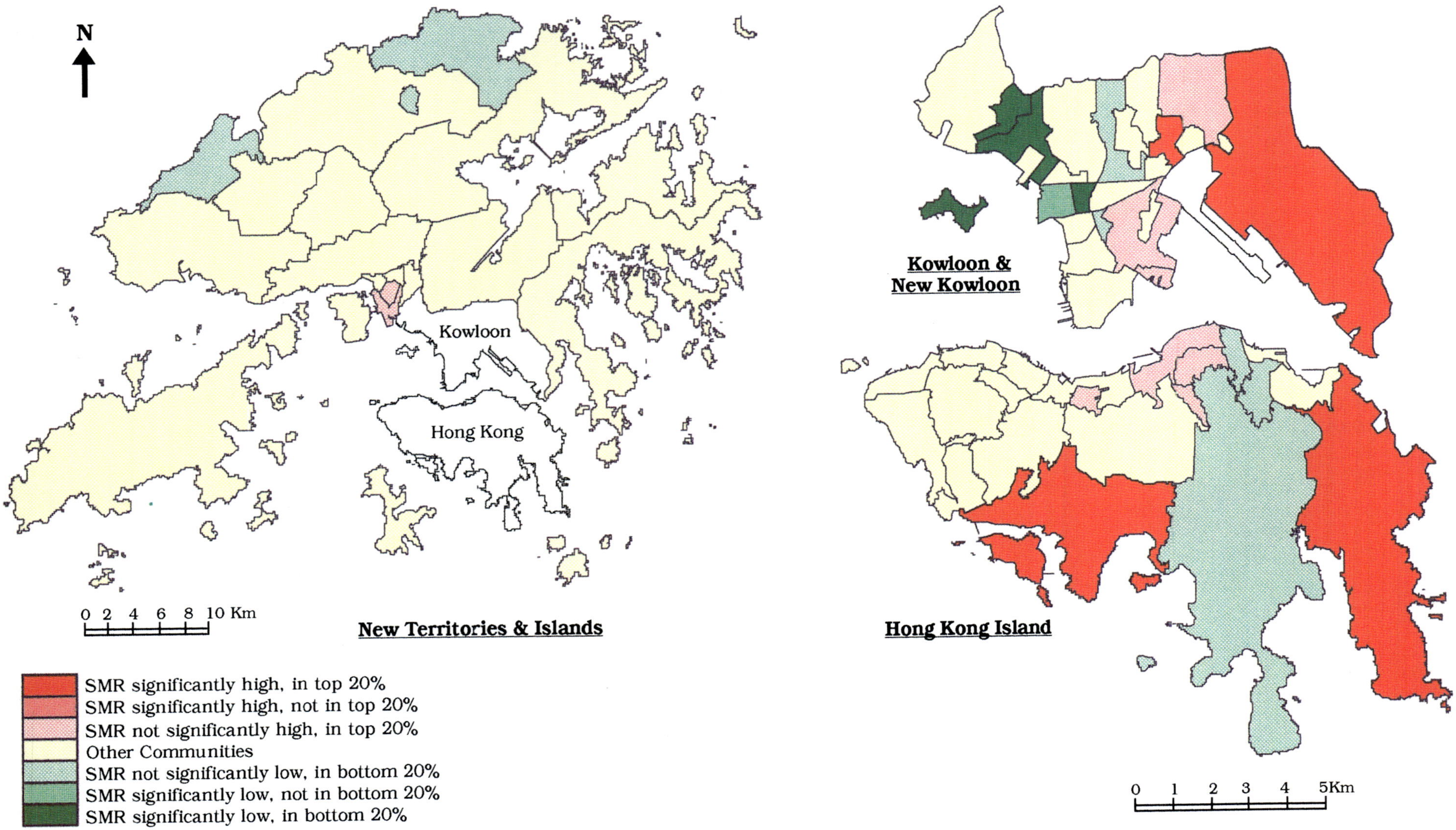

Gastric Cancer (Male, 1979 -1983)

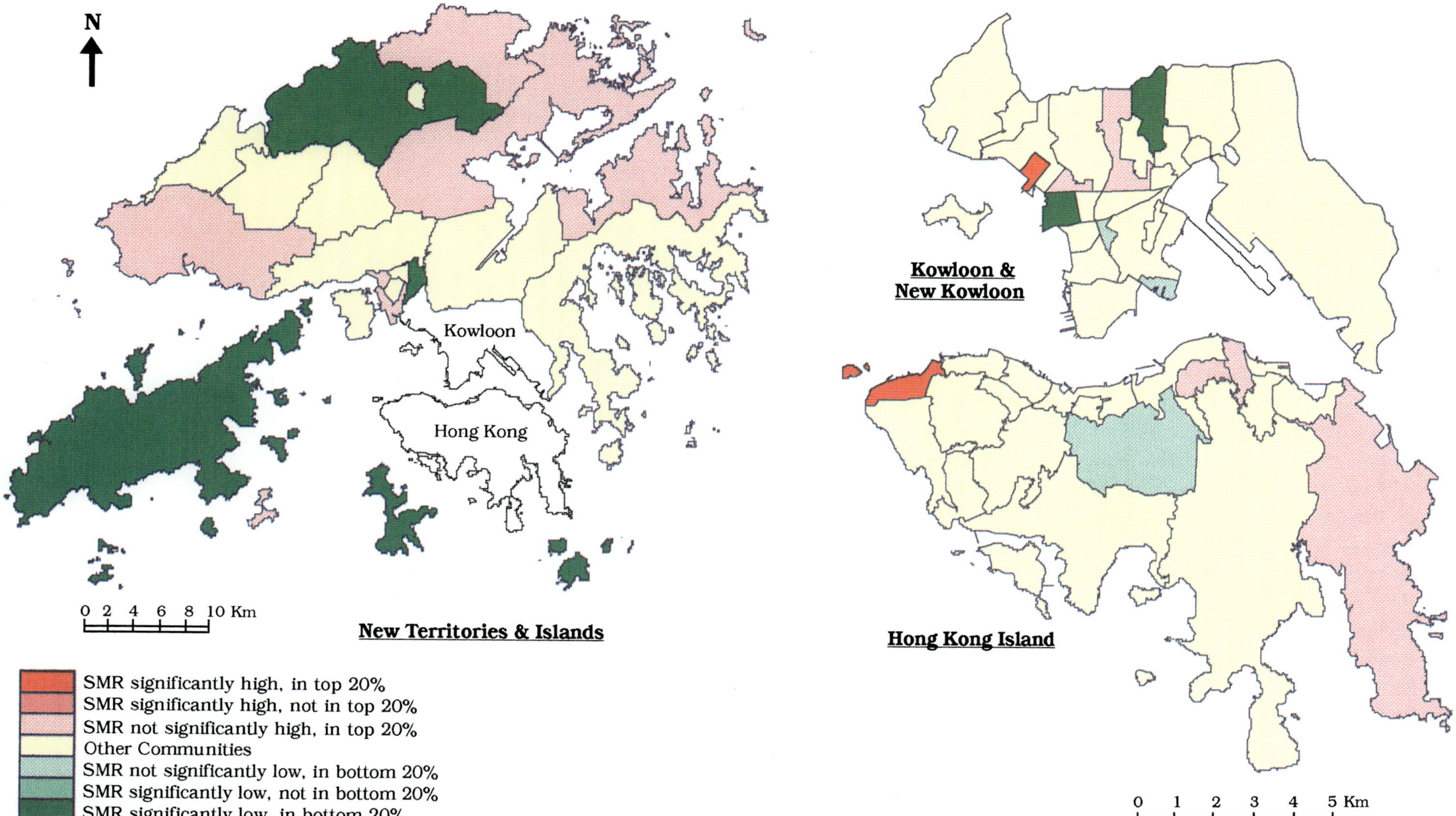

Gastric Cancer (Female, 1979 -1983)

Number of Deaths, Standardised Mortality Ratio (SMR) and 95% Confidence Interval of Gastric Cancer by 65 Communities in 1979–1983

Community	Male			Female		
	Number of deaths	SMR	95% C.I.	Number of deaths	SMR	95% C.I.
HK1	25	100.5	61.1 - 139.9	30	195.8	125.7 - 265.9
HK2	43	107.7	75.5 - 139.9	27	123.7	77.1 - 170.4
HK3	16	101.6	58.1 - 165.0	10	126.2	60.7 - 232.0
HK4	23	94.6	59.9 - 142.1	11	77.7	38.8 - 138.9
HK5	35	148.6	99.4 - 197.8	13	98.6	52.5 - 168.6
HK6	15	77.2	43.2 - 127.5	9	57.0	26.2 - 108.2
HK7	0	0.0	...	2	60.8	7.4 - 219.6
HK8	6	78.2	28.6 - 170.4	4	61.7	16.8 - 157.8
HK9	0	0.0	...	1	33.0	0.8 - 183.3
HK10	66	123.4	93.6 - 153.2	41	105.8	73.4 - 138.2
HK11	7	147.2	59.1 - 303.5	1	35.2	0.9 - 195.4
HK12	5	126.5	41.0 - 295.7	8	214.3	92.4 - 421.8
HK13	3	48.0	9.9 - 140.4	6	138.3	50.7 - 301.3
HK14	10	65.6	31.5 - 120.5	9	85.6	39.3 - 162.4
HK15	2	32.4	3.9 - 117.1	3	65.5	13.5 - 191.5
HK16	29	101.6	64.6 - 138.6	20	118.8	72.4 - 183.6
HK17	45	144.9	102.5 - 187.2	25	136.4	82.9 - 189.9
HK18	3	67.9	14.0 - 198.6	1	30.5	0.8 - 169.7
HK19	15	102.2	57.1 - 168.6	9	88.9	40.8 - 168.7
HK20	47	143.9	102.7 - 185.0	23	117.3	74.2 - 176.1
HK21	1	24.2	0.6 - 134.7	2	78.7	9.5 - 284.3
KL1	15	71.6	40.0 - 118.2	15	121.9	68.1 - 201.2
KL2	30	69.8	44.8 - 94.7	13	51.7	27.5 - 88.3
KL3	5	39.9	12.9 - 93.1	6	73.0	26.8 - 159.1
KL4	26	74.4	45.8 - 103.0	18	91.3	54.0 - 144.2
KL5	22	74.9	46.8 - 113.5	13	80.7	42.9 - 137.9
KL6	5	68.0	22.0 - 158.8	4	63.8	17.4 - 163.1
KL7	3	55.6	11.5 - 162.5	1	22.8	0.6 - 126.8
KL8	19	102.6	61.8 - 160.3	9	73.7	33.8 - 139.9
KL9	81	118.3	92.6 - 144.1	49	106.8	76.9 - 136.7
KL10	9	132.1	60.6 - 250.7	2	40.5	4.9 - 146.2
KL11	17	90.9	52.9 - 145.5	11	82.8	41.4 - 148.1
KL12	1	17.2	0.4 - 95.8	4	130.1	35.4 - 332.6

Community	Male			Female		
	Number of deaths	SMR	95% C.I.	Number of deaths	SMR	95% C.I.
KL13	44	62.5	44.1 - 81.0	35	85.6	57.2 - 113.9
KL14	47	112.0	80.0 - 144.1	29	128.4	81.7 - 175.2
KL15	3	90.5	18.7 - 264.5	6	299.4	109.7 - 652.4
KL16	14	84.2	46.0 - 141.2	15	147.6	82.5 - 243.5
KL17	1	20.9	0.5 - 116.3	6	134.0	49.1 - 291.9
KL18	2	64.7	7.8 - 233.4	2	85.8	10.4 - 309.9
KL19	73	119.8	92.4 - 147.3	36	90.5	61.0 - 120.1
KL20	23	107.4	68.0 - 161.2	6	45.8	16.8 - 99.7
KL21	52	149.6	108.9 - 190.2	19	89.9	54.1 - 140.4
KL22	6	100.8	36.9 - 219.6	4	124.0	33.8 - 317.2
KL23	16	87.0	49.7 - 141.2	10	92.9	44.7 - 170.7
KL24	12	107.2	55.3 - 187.1	7	101.7	40.9 - 209.7
KL25	201	119.2	102.8 - 135.7	117	111.1	90.9 - 131.2
NT1	9	104.1	47.7 - 197.5	5	88.3	28.6 - 206.3
NT2	16	128.8	73.6 - 209.1	12	157.8	81.4 - 275.4
NT3	27	107.4	66.9 - 147.9	18	134.5	79.6 - 212.5
NT4	12	90.1	46.4 - 157.2	8	86.0	13.1 - 169.3
NT5	55	115.4	84.9 - 145.9	37	124.9	84.7 - 165.1
NT6	20	86.1	52.5 - 133.0	7	45.6	18.4 - 94.0
NT7	6	75.2	27.5 - 163.8	3	59.7	12.3 - 174.7
NT8	23	88.0	55.7 - 132.1	20	131.4	80.1 - 203.1
NT9	3	36.7	7.6 - 107.3	4	88.7	24.2 - 226.9
NT10	39	115.2	79.0 - 151.4	19	101.1	60.9 - 158.0
NT11	7	99.3	39.9 - 204.7	1	26.9	0.7 - 149.5
NT12	27	83.8	52.2 - 115.4	9	49.7	22.8 - 94.4
NT13	3	49.8	10.3 - 145.5	1	27.8	0.7 - 154.5
NT14	3	53.6	11.1 - 156.8	5	136.4	44.1 - 318.7
NT15	16	71.9	41.1 - 116.7	20	143.9	87.8 - 222.4
NT16	27	99.7	62.1 - 137.3	17	94.8	55.1 - 151.7
NT17	9	68.3	31.3 - 129.5	10	124.6	59.9 - 229.1
NT18	5	77.2	25.0 - 180.3	6	146.0	53.5 - 318.1
NT19	9	80.9	37.1 - 153.5	1	14.7	0.4 - 81.7

GASTRIC CANCER

Sex-Age specific mortality rate (1/100,000) of gastric cancer in Hong Kong (1979–1983)

	Male		Female	
Age	No. of deaths	Mortality rate	No. of deaths	Mortality rate
0–4	0	0.00	0	0.00
5–9	0	0.00	0	0.00
10–14	0	0.00	0	0.00
15–19	0	0.00	1	0.08
20–24	7	0.46	5	0.36
25–29	8	0.61	8	0.69
30–34	18	1.63	22	2.40
35–39	24	3.32	29	5.22
40–44	47	6.68	39	7.05
45–49	63	8.73	31	5.12
50–54	131	19.07	71	11.64
55–59	185	32.52	82	15.33
60–64	218	47.71	100	21.92
65+	738	108.25	507	50.23
TOTAL	1439	10.91	895	7.35

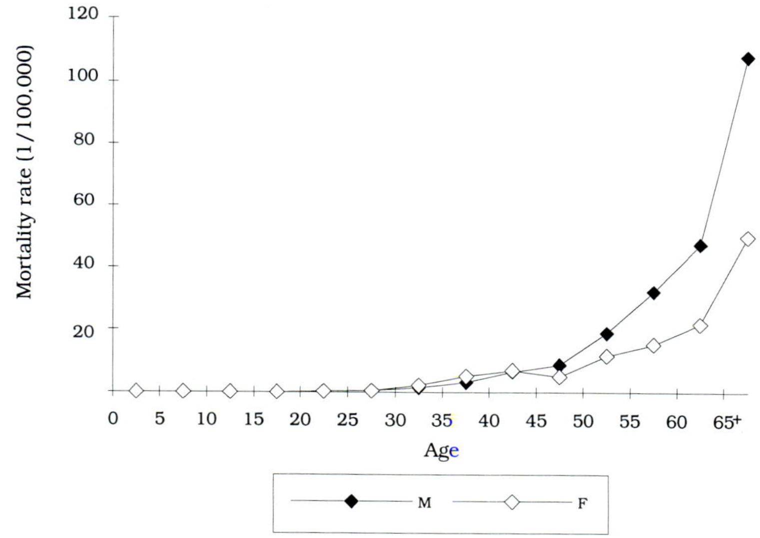

Number of communities on map by category based on standardized mortality ratio (SMR) during 1979–1983

Category	Number of communities Male	Number of communities Female
SMR significantly high, in top 20%	4	2
SMR significantly high , not in top 20%	0	0
SMR not significantly high, in top 20%	9	11
SMR not significantly low, in bottom 20%	8	3
SMR significantly low, not in bottom 20%	1	0
SMR significantly low, in bottom 20%	3	5
other communities	40	44

Values of the standardized mortality ratio (SMR) which divide the 65 communities into quintile

Percentile	Male	Female
20th	62.54	57.04
40th	77.24	85.59
60th	99.73	101.73
80th	115.20	130.05
Lowest SMR	0.00	14.71
Highest SMR	149.55	299.43
No. of communities with zero death	2	0

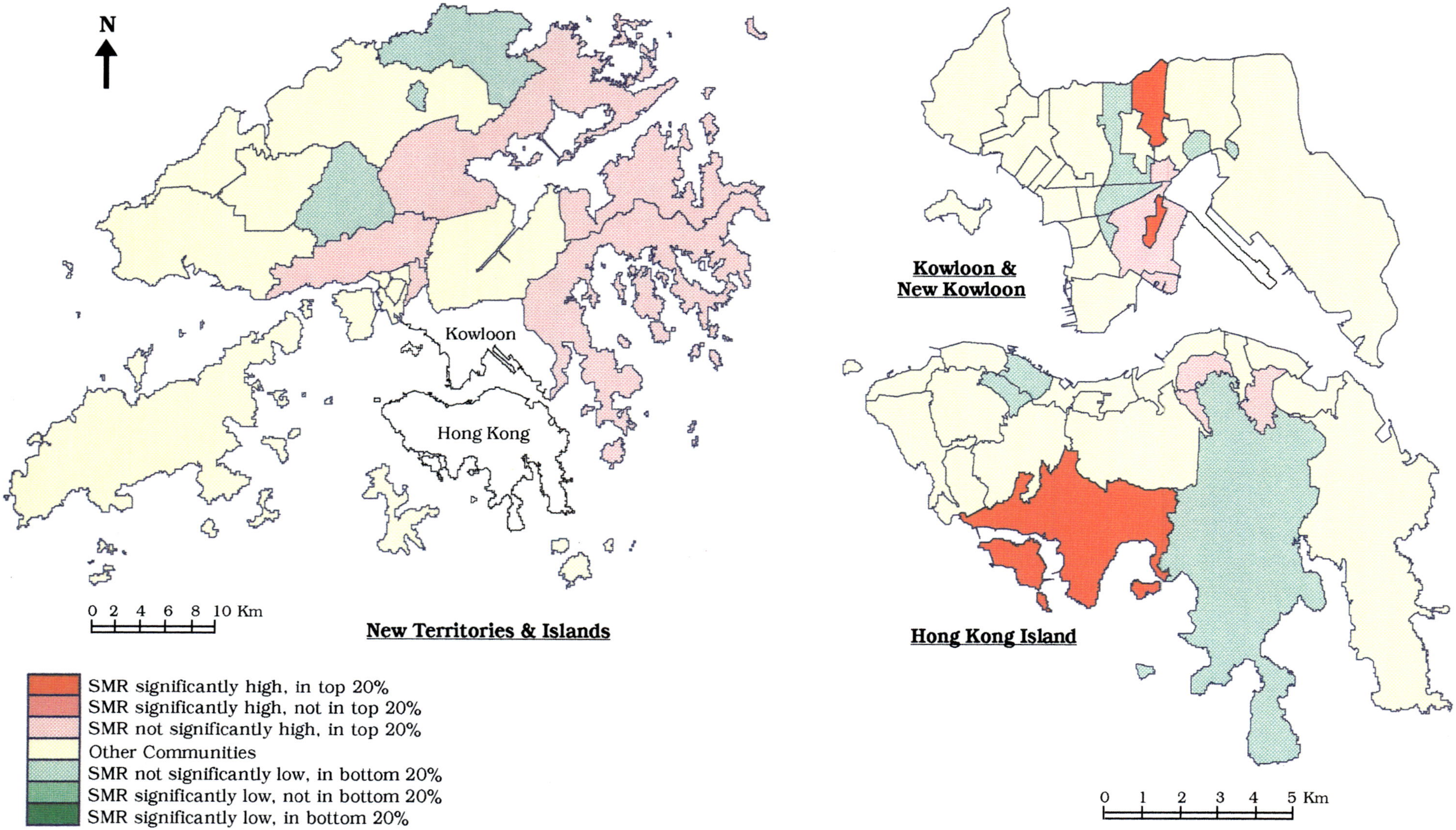

Gastric Cancer (Male, 1984 –1988)

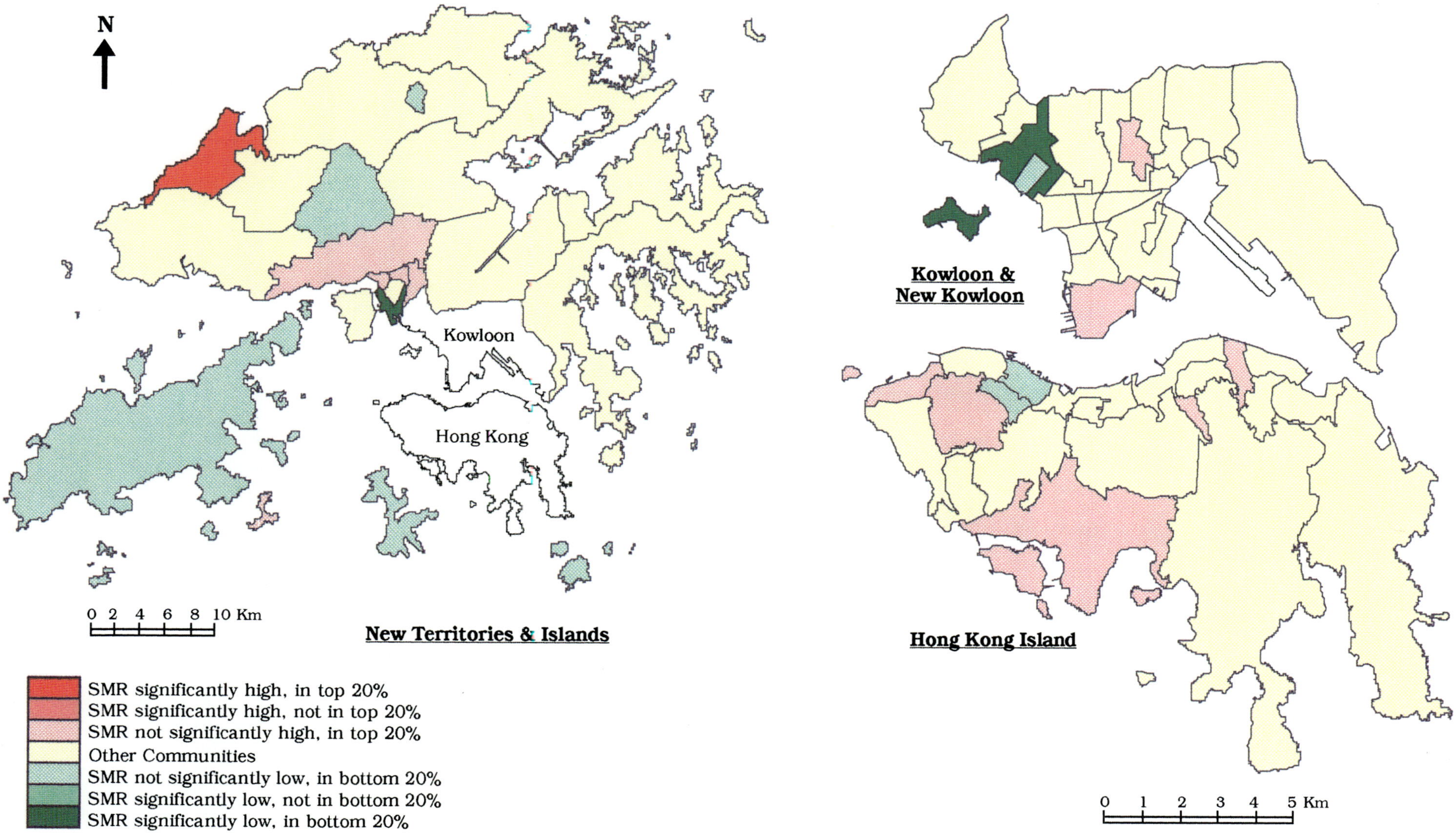

Gastric Cancer (Female, 1984 -1988)

Number of Deaths, Standardised Mortality Ratio (SMR) and 95% Confidence Interval of Gastric Cancer by 65 Communities in 1984–1988

	Male			Female				Male			Female		
Community	Number of deaths	SMR	95% C.I.	Number of deaths	SMR	95% C.I.	Community	Number of deaths	SMR	95% C.I.	Number of deaths	SMR	95% C.I.
HK1	22	91.1	56.9 - 138.0	22	143.0	89.4 - 216.7	KL13	47	78.5	56.1 - 100.9	25	68.2	41.5 - 94.9
HK2	31	90.9	58.9 - 122.8	26	121.9	79.7 - 178.8	KL14	47	108.2	77.3 - 139.2	30	116.6	74.9 - 158.4
HK3	6	46.8	17.1 - 101.9	4	57.1	15.5 - 145.9	KL15	5	68.3	22.1 - 159.6	3	59.4	12.2 - 173.5
HK4	15	73.6	41.1 - 121.4	13	101.4	53.9 - 173.3	KL16	17	113.5	66.0 - 181.5	7	78.6	31.6 - 162.1
HK5	18	97.9	57.9 - 154.6	10	83.9	40.3 - 154.3	KL17	4	60.2	16.4 - 153.9	7	102.1	41.0 - 210.5
HK6	15	80.9	45.2 - 133.5	12	79.5	41.0 - 138.7	KL18	3	107.6	22.2 - 314.5	4	198.9	54.2 - 508.6
HK7	0	0.0	...	4	129.4	35.3 - 330.9	KL19	65	105.8	80.0 - 131.5	47	118.4	84.5 - 152.2
HK8	4	57.9	15.8 - 148.2	2	36.1	4.4 - 130.5	KL20	26	171.9	112.4 - 252.1	8	78.8	34.0 - 155.1
HK9	3	98.8	20.4 - 288.8	2	69.5	8.4 - 250.9	KL21	19	73.1	40.2 - 105.9	12	78.1	40.3 - 136.3
HK10	44	85.9	60.5 - 111.2	47	118.2	84.4 - 152.0	KL22	2	37.3	4.5 - 134.8	2	61.7	7.5 - 222.9
HK11	7	150.4	60.4 - 310.1	5	180.8	58.5 - 422.3	KL23	21	157.5	97.2 - 240.8	9	109.0	50.0 - 206.8
HK12	6	141.4	51.8 - 308.0	3	87.6	18.1 - 256.0	KL24	7	55.0	22.1 - 113.4	5	69.6	22.5 - 162.7
HK13	4	64.6	17.6 - 165.1	6	156.7	57.4 - 341.5	KL25	203	104.2	89.9 - 118.5	119	94.3	77.4 - 111.3
HK14	18	95.3	56.4 - 150.5	12	82.0	42.3 - 143.1	NT1	18	166.9	98.8 - 263.7	11	142.2	71.1 - 254.4
HK15	10	165.5	79.6 - 304.2	6	122.5	44.9 - 266.8	NT2	13	96.2	51.2 - 164.5	2	23.1	2.8 - 83.6
HK16	29	110.6	70.4 - 150.9	17	100.5	58.4 - 160.8	NT3	25	102.7	66.3 - 151.5	20	143.7	87.6 - 222.1
HK17	33	94.7	62.4 - 127.0	22	98.3	61.4 - 148.9	NT4	21	101.7	62.7 - 155.4	18	127.3	75.3 - 201.2
HK18	2	53.0	6.4 - 191.2	1	32.1	0.8 - 178.2	NT5	45	102.5	72.6 - 132.5	24	88.5	53.1 - 124.0
HK19	17	103.1	60.0 - 165.0	12	102.5	52.9 - 179.0	NT6	31	120.1	77.8 - 162.4	21	131.8	81.3 - 201.5
HK20	50	139.3	100.7 - 177.9	30	128.1	86.6 - 183.0	NT7	9	70.3	32.3 - 133.4	8	99.4	42.8 - 195.6
HK21	2	45.3	5.5 - 163.4	3	92.0	19.0 - 269.1	NT8	46	104.1	74.0 - 134.2	27	83.3	51.9 - 114.7
KL1	21	113.7	70.2 - 173.9	15	131.8	73.6 - 217.5	NT9	9	111.9	51.3 - 212.3	12	227.6	117.3 - 397.2
KL2	27	76.3	47.5 - 105.0	18	81.9	48.5 - 129.4	NT10	36	95.3	64.1 - 126.4	21	92.2	56.9 - 140.9
KL3	8	74.8	32.2 - 147.1	8	106.8	46.0 - 210.3	NT11	4	59.6	16.2 - 152.4	2	43.2	5.2 - 156.0
KL4	28	84.5	53.2 - 115.9	20	108.5	66.1 - 167.6	NT12	28	84.5	53.2 - 115.7	17	77.7	45.2 - 124.3
KL5	21	85.8	53.0 - 131.3	12	83.7	43.2 - 146.1	NT13	4	46.6	12.7 - 119.2	3	61.1	12.6 - 178.5
KL6	3	43.6	9.0 - 127.4	4	71.9	19.6 - 183.9	NT14	2	36.1	4.4 - 130.4	1	28.5	0.7 - 158.3
KL7	1	20.3	0.5 - 112.6	1	27.6	0.7 - 153.5	NT15	42	137.9	96.2 - 179.6	23	102.9	65.1 - 154.4
KL8	26	153.1	100.0 - 224.4	9	82.2	37.7 - 156.0	NT16	80	120.1	93.8 - 146.4	62	116.6	87.6 - 145.6
KL9	80	120.4	94.0 - 146.8	49	109.5	78.8 - 140.2	NT17	18	137.3	81.3 - 216.9	10	118.6	57.0 - 218.0
KL10	9	138.3	63.4 - 262.4	4	82.1	22.4 - 210.1	NT18	5	76.8	24.8 - 179.4	6	136.7	50.1 - 297.9
KL11	14	72.1	39.4 - 121.0	15	109.8	61.4 - 181.2	NT19	9	90.6	41.6 - 171.9	3	48.2	9.9 - 140.8
KL12	5	92.5	29.9 - 216.1	3	98.9	20.4 - 289.3							

GASTRIC CANCER

Sex-Age specific mortality rate (1/100,000) of gastric cancer in Hong Kong (1984–1988)

	Male		Female	
Age	No. of deaths	Mortality rate	No. of deaths	Mortality rate
0–4	0	0.00	0	0.00
5–9	0	0.00	0	0.00
10–14	0	0.00	0	0.00
15–19	0	0.00	1	0.09
20–24	3	0.21	6	0.43
25–29	4	0.25	17	1.15
30–34	14	1.03	31	2.51
35–39	20	1.80	33	3.40
40–44	40	5.46	30	5.00
45–49	60	8.52	36	6.17
50–54	105	14.33	56	8.87
55–59	176	26.50	87	14.32
60–64	263	48.69	103	19.24
65+	820	90.82	589	47.72
TOTAL	1505	10.55	989	7.37

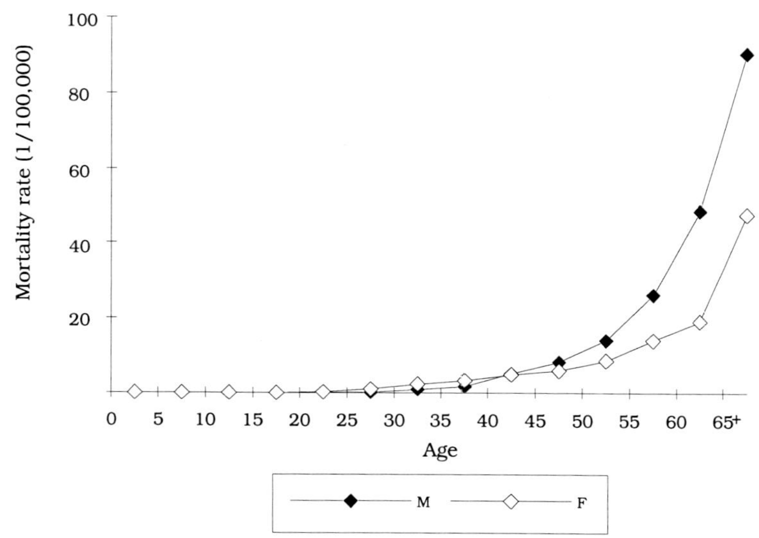

Number of communities on map by category based on standardized mortality ratio (SMR) during 1984–1988

Category	Number of communities Male	Female
SMR significantly high, in top 20%	3	1
SMR significantly high , not in top 20%	0	0
SMR not significantly high, in top 20%	10	12
SMR not significantly low, in bottom 20%	11	6
SMR significantly low, not in bottom 20%	0	0
SMR significantly low, in bottom 20%	0	2
other communities	41	44

Values of the standardized mortality ratio (SMR) which divide the 65 communities into quintile

Percentile	Male	Female
20th	60.19	69.50
40th	84.54	83.74
60th	101.65	102.54
80th	120.12	122.48
Lowest SMR	0.00	23.15
Highest SMR	171.92	227.61
No. of communities with zero death	1	0

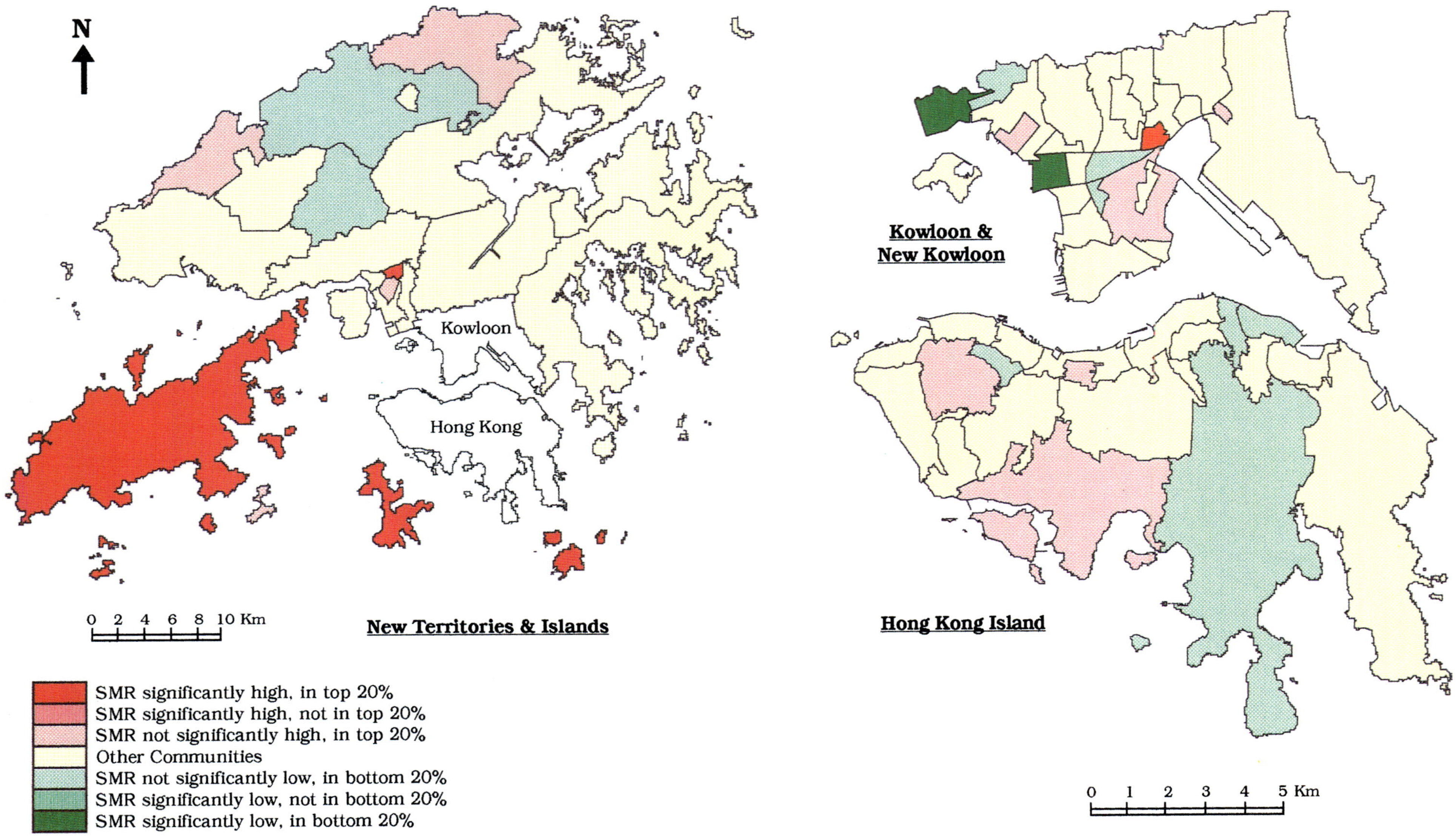

Gastric Cancer (Male, 1989 -1993)

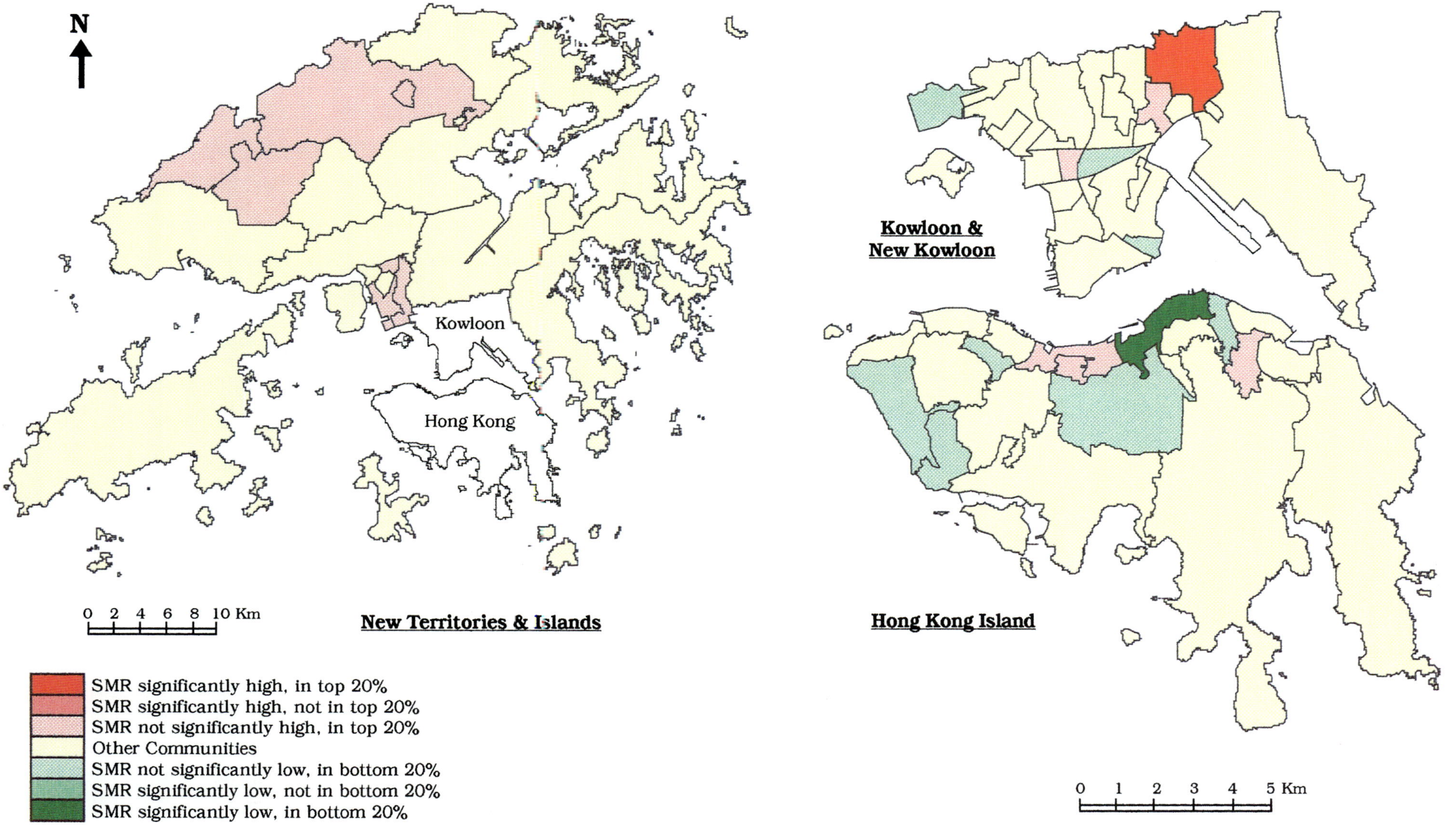

Gastric Cancer (Female, 1989 -1993)

Number of Deaths, Standardised Mortality Ratio (SMR) and 95% Confidence Interval of Gastric Cancer by 65 Communities in 1989–1993

Community	Male			Female		
	Number of deaths	SMR	95% C.I.	Number of deaths	SMR	95% C.I.
HK1	28	105.9	66.7 - 145.1	15	100.8	56.5 - 166.4
HK2	33	92.2	60.8 - 123.7	19	105.3	63.4 - 164.3
HK3	9	73.0	33.4 - 138.7	4	70.2	19.1 - 179.7
HK4	15	74.4	41.7 - 122.7	13	125.2	66.6 - 214.0
HK5	24	124.7	79.9 - 185.8	12	124.0	64.1 - 217.1
HK6	20	81.2	49.6 - 125.1	8	53.7	23.1 - 105.8
HK7	6	127.1	46.6 - 277.0	4	111.6	30.4 - 285.8
HK8	4	52.3	14.2 - 134.0	2	40.8	4.9 - 147.2
HK9	1	29.0	0.7 - 161.4	2	80.8	9.8 - 291.8
HK10	51	83.6	60.7 - 106.6	21	52.9	32.8 - 81.0
HK11	5	87.8	28.5 - 204.6	3	105.0	21.6 - 306.7
HK12	4	81.2	22.1 - 208.0	4	120.0	32.6 - 307.2
HK13	3	45.5	9.4 - 132.8	2	56.8	6.9 - 204.9
HK14	17	70.8	41.3 - 113.3	17	115.7	67.5 - 185.1
HK15	17	120.0	70.0 - 192.0	14	154.3	84.2 - 259.2
HK16	26	104.9	64.6 - 145.2	14	102.6	56.0 - 172.3
HK17	53	102.5	74.9 - 130.1	31	106.5	69.0 - 144.0
HK18	4	72.0	19.6 - 184.4	1	24.6	0.6 - 137.3
HK19	24	113.6	72.8 - 169.3	8	69.3	29.9 - 136.5
HK20	57	122.6	90.8 - 154.5	22	82.4	51.7 - 124.4
HK21	2	43.8	5.3 - 158.3	3	101.8	21.0 - 297.3
KL1	18	112.8	66.9 - 178.2	8	93.9	40.5 - 185.0
KL2	25	67.2	43.5 - 99.5	15	79.9	44.7 - 131.8
KL3	11	101.4	50.6 - 181.5	8	128.4	55.4 - 253.0
KL4	26	83.8	51.6 - 116.0	17	117.8	68.7 - 188.5
KL5	27	119.2	74.3 - 164.2	11	98.7	49.3 - 176.7
KL6	3	35.6	7.3 - 104.0	2	32.2	3.9 - 116.4
KL7	3	50.9	10.5 - 148.6	5	119.3	38.7 - 277.9
KL8	16	85.1	48.7 - 137.8	7	70.5	28.3 - 145.2
KL9	90	120.5	95.6 - 145.4	39	95.6	65.6 - 125.6
KL10	11	87.7	43.8 - 157.0	3	34.8	7.2 - 101.8
KL11	8	47.2	20.3 - 92.9	6	57.6	21.1 - 125.5
KL12	3	54.8	11.3 - 160.1	1	35.4	0.9 - 197.0

Community	Male			Female		
	Number of deaths	SMR	95% C.I.	Number of deaths	SMR	95% C.I.
KL13	56	81.6	60.2 - 102.9	34	99.6	66.1 - 133.1
KL14	48	108.7	78.0 - 139.5	18	74.0	43.9 - 116.9
KL15	12	142.5	73.7 - 249.3	5	104.9	38.5 - 244.4
KL16	13	84.6	45.0 - 144.7	8	103.2	44.5 - 203.2
KL17	7	105.1	42.1 - 216.4	6	108.8	39.9 - 237.1
KL18	1	31.9	0.8 - 177.7	0	0.0	...
KL19	82	115.5	90.5 - 140.5	59	141.6	105.4 - 177.7
KL20	17	105.1	61.3 - 168.2	11	122.8	61.3 - 219.9
KL21	30	116.8	75.0 - 158.6	22	151.4	94.9 - 228.6
KL22	5	94.3	34.6 - 205.7	2	71.5	8.6 - 258.0
KL23	20	185.4	113.3 - 285.5	7	121.4	48.7 - 250.0
KL24	18	123.7	73.3 - 195.4	8	116.6	50.3 - 229.8
KL25	203	93.8	80.9 - 106.7	114	93.8	76.6 - 111.0
NT1	19	110.9	66.8 - 173.0	10	90.9	43.6 - 167.2
NT2	14	78.4	42.8 - 131.7	14	136.5	74.5 - 229.3
NT3	30	91.8	59.0 - 124.7	15	93.0	52.1 - 153.4
NT4	35	155.3	103.8 - 206.7	18	140.0	83.0 - 221.2
NT5	61	128.8	96.5 - 161.1	25	100.0	60.8 - 139.2
NT6	33	104.8	69.0 - 140.5	23	134.3	85.1 - 201.4
NT7	27	90.0	56.0 - 123.9	17	99.7	58.1 - 159.6
NT8	72	102.2	78.6 - 125.8	43	100.1	70.2 - 130.0
NT9	12	130.0	67.2 - 227.5	8	149.8	64.6 - 295.0
NT10	44	97.2	68.5 - 125.9	35	141.4	94.5 - 188.2
NT11	6	71.4	26.2 - 155.8	6	123.7	45.4 - 269.6
NT12	30	71.8	46.1 - 107.0	32	133.1	87.0 - 179.2
NT13	9	104.0	47.6 - 197.6	8	147.7	63.6 - 290.9
NT14	6	124.0	45.5 - 270.3	2	68.1	8.2 - 245.8
NT15	54	115.0	84.4 - 145.7	29	96.9	61.6 - 132.1
NT16	127	109.5	90.4 - 128.5	82	105.3	82.5 - 128.1
NT17	23	79.2	50.2 - 118.8	14	75.3	41.1 - 126.6
NT18	10	125.9	60.5 - 231.7	3	65.5	13.5 - 191.1
NT19	18	185.0	109.7 - 292.2	6	104.1	38.2 - 226.8

GASTRIC CANCER

Sex-Age specific mortality rate (1/100,000) of gastric cancer in Hong Kong (1989–1993)

	Male		Female	
Age	No. of deaths	Mortality rate	No. of deaths	Mortality rate
0–4	0	0.00	0	0.00
5–9	0	0.00	0	0.00
10–14	0	0.00	0	0.00
15–19	0	0.00	1	0.10
20–24	5	0.44	4	0.35
25–29	7	0.49	8	0.54
30–34	17	1.09	34	2.24
35–39	20	1.49	33	2.62
40–44	57	5.18	43	4.42
45–49	60	8.21	27	4.52
50–54	102	14.70	42	7.38
55–59	200	28.62	55	9.03
60–64	218	35.32	100	17.30
65+	1100	99.30	678	48.26
TOTAL	1786	12.21	1025	7.33

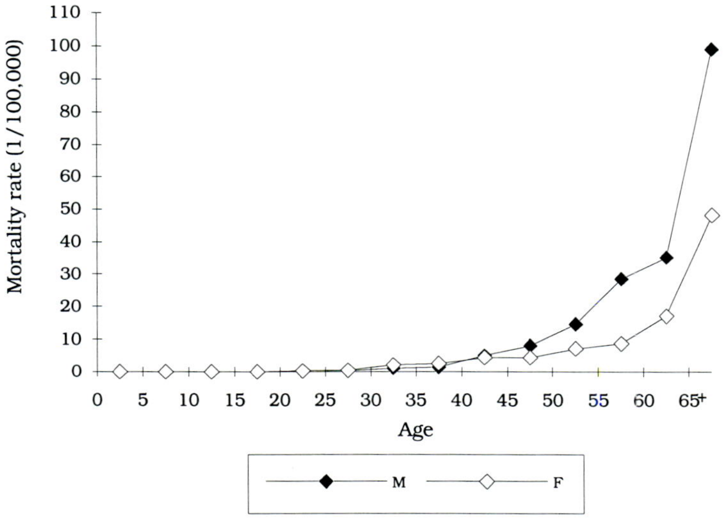

Number of communities on map by category based on standardized mortality ratio (SMR) during 1989–1993

Category	Number of communities Male	Female
SMR significantly high, in top 20%	3	1
SMR significantly high , not in top 20%	0	0
SMR not significantly high, in top 20%	10	12
SMR not significantly low, in bottom 20%	9	8
SMR significantly low, not in bottom 20%	0	0
SMR significantly low, in bottom 20%	2	1
other communities	41	43

Values of the standardized mortality ratio (SMR) which divide the 65 communities into quintile

Percentile	Male	Female
20th	71.84	69.28
40th	87.69	95.61
60th	104.90	105.04
80th	120.02	123.68
Lowest SMR	28.98	0.00
Highest SMR	185.37	154.27
No. of communities with zero cases	0	1

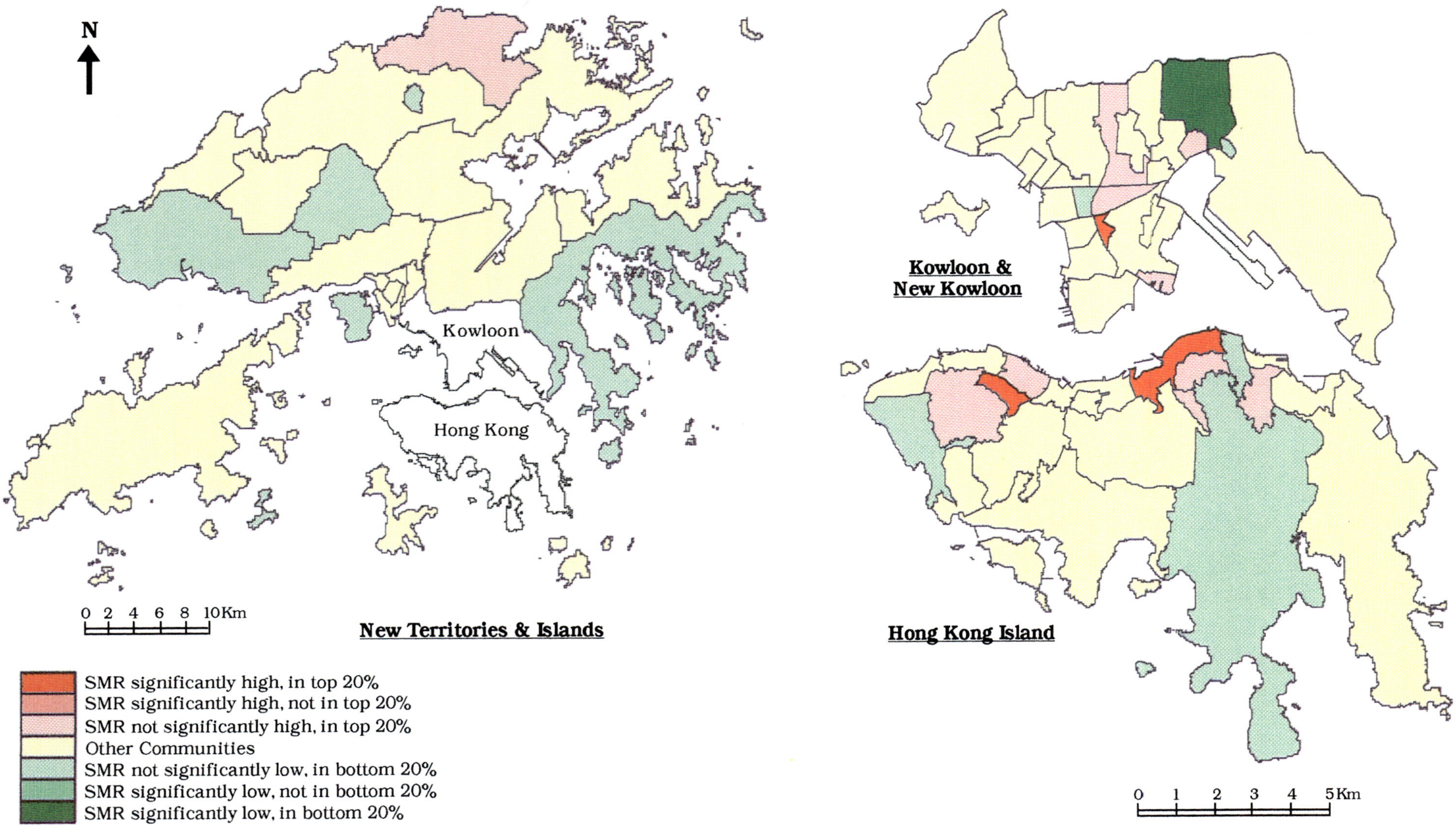

Colorectal Cancer (Male, 1979 - 1983)

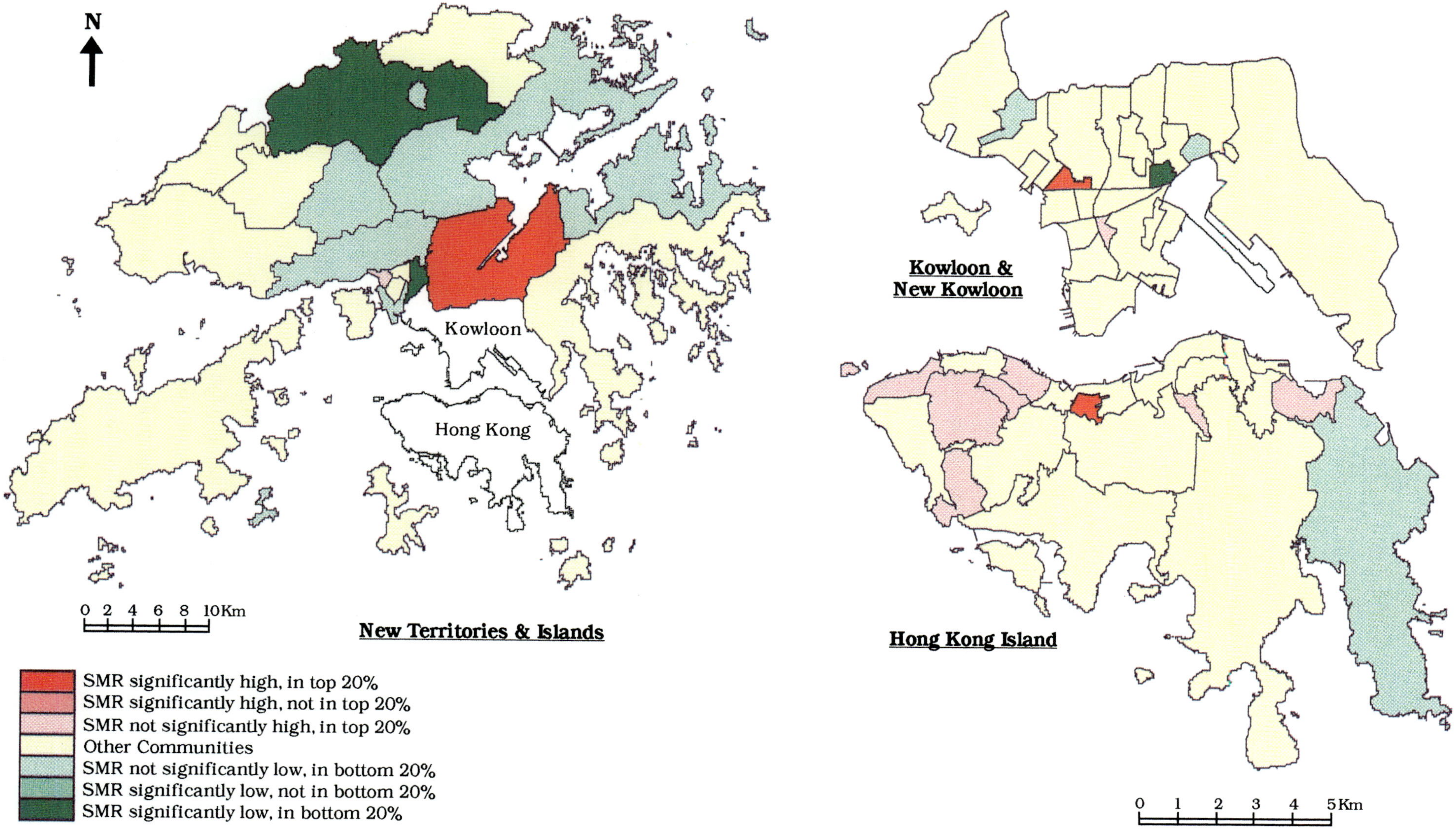

Colorectal Cancer (Female, 1979 - 1983)

Number of Deaths, Standardised Mortality Ratio (SMR) and 95% Confidence Interval of Colorectal Cancer by 65 Communities in 1979–1983

Community	Male			Female		
	Number of deaths	SMR	95% C.I.	Number of deaths	SMR	95% C.I.
HK1	28	112.6	70.9 - 154.3	31	135.8	88.0 - 183.7
HK2	40	101.1	69.8 - 132.4	30	91.7	58.9 - 124.5
HK3	21	135.3	83.5 - 206.9	16	134.1	76.7 - 217.8
HK4	25	103.0	62.7 - 143.4	23	109.0	69.0 - 163.7
HK5	25	107.0	65.1 - 149.0	31	156.5	101.4 - 211.6
HK6	19	98.5	59.3 - 153.9	22	94.0	58.7 - 142.4
HK7	7	179.7	72.2 - 370.6	7	145.6	58.5 - 300.3
HK8	17	223.3	129.8 - 357.3	13	135.4	72.0 - 231.5
HK9	3	86.5	17.8 - 252.8	4	91.5	24.9 - 234.1
HK10	70	130.9	100.2 - 161.6	59	102.3	76.2 - 128.4
HK11	6	126.5	46.3 - 275.5	6	143.4	52.5 - 312.4
HK12	8	200.2	86.3 - 394.1	6	110.5	40.5 - 240.7
HK13	4	64.0	17.4 - 163.7	8	124.9	53.8 - 245.8
HK14	17	110.3	64.1 - 176.5	16	103.5	59.1 - 168.0
HK15	12	189.9	97.9 - 331.3	8	119.9	51.7 - 236.1
HK16	34	119.5	79.3 - 159.6	37	147.0	99.6 - 194.4
HK17	27	87.6	54.5 - 120.6	19	68.5	41.3 - 107.1
HK18	2	45.1	5.5 - 163.0	4	84.1	22.9 - 215.0
HK19	18	121.4	71.8 - 191.8	22	149.9	93.7 - 227.1
HK20	26	79.8	49.1 - 110.4	31	105.9	68.6 - 143.2
HK21	1	23.7	0.6 - 131.6	2	55.8	6.8 - 201.3
KL1	26	124.4	76.6 - 172.3	19	104.4	62.9 - 163.1
KL2	40	92.7	64.0 - 121.5	36	95.7	64.4 - 126.9
KL3	6	47.9	17.5 - 104.3	13	106.1	56.4 - 181.4
KL4	36	102.9	69.3 - 136.6	26	88.1	54.2 - 121.9
KL5	36	123.2	82.9 - 163.4	26	107.7	66.3 - 149.1
KL6	12	166.1	85.6 - 289.9	8	85.2	36.7 - 167.6
KL7	11	204.2	102.1 - 365.2	12	185.3	95.5 - 323.4
KL8	19	102.1	61.5 - 159.6	23	127.3	80.5 - 191.1
KL9	78	113.3	88.2 - 138.4	84	123.6	97.2 - 150.0
KL10	9	129.3	59.3 - 245.3	9	123.5	56.7 - 234.4
KL11	23	122.4	77.5 - 183.8	24	123.0	78.8 - 183.0
KL12	4	69.4	18.9 - 177.5	1	21.5	0.5 - 119.6
KL13	63	90.0	67.7 - 112.2	53	86.1	62.9 - 109.3
KL14	38	92.0	62.7 - 121.2	33	95.9	63.2 - 128.6
KL15	3	89.5	18.5 - 261.8	4	134.2	36.6 - 343.3
KL16	21	126.0	77.8 - 192.6	26	170.7	105.1 - 236.4
KL17	9	189.0	86.7 - 358.7	6	90.5	33.1 - 197.1
KL18	2	63.3	7.7 - 228.6	3	89.5	18.5 - 261.7
KL19	36	59.2	39.9 - 78.6	62	103.7	77.9 - 129.6
KL20	24	113.5	72.8 - 168.9	19	95.2	57.3 - 148.7
KL21	27	78.9	49.1 - 108.7	27	83.7	52.1 - 115.2
KL22	8	134.1	57.8 - 264.0	3	62.6	12.9 - 183.1
KL23	22	119.3	74.6 - 180.8	6	37.2	13.6 - 81.1
KL24	5	45.1	14.6 - 105.4	10	96.0	46.2 - 176.5
KL25	182	107.6	91.9 - 123.2	142	91.0	76.0 - 105.9
NT1	6	67.9	24.9 - 147.9	6	72.0	26.4 - 156.8
NT2	12	95.3	49.1 - 166.3	5	45.2	14.6 - 105.6
NT3	26	102.3	63.0 - 141.6	28	142.5	89.7 - 195.3
NT4	11	80.9	40.5 - 144.8	12	90.5	46.6 - 157.9
NT5	56	117.1	86.5 - 147.8	35	80.4	53.7 - 107.0
NT6	18	76.7	45.4 - 121.2	12	53.5	27.6 - 93.4
NT7	4	49.1	13.4 - 125.6	6	83.1	30.4 - 181.1
NT8	18	67.8	40.1 - 107.2	18	80.5	47.6 - 127.2
NT9	8	99.0	42.7 - 194.8	9	132.3	60.7 - 251.0
NT10	27	80.3	50.0 - 110.6	26	92.3	56.8 - 127.8
NT11	2	28.6	3.5 - 103.1	4	71.9	19.6 - 184.0
NT12	23	72.3	45.8 - 108.6	14	51.3	28.0 - 86.1
NT13	4	67.0	18.3 - 171.4	3	55.3	11.4 - 161.7
NT14	7	127.5	51.2 - 262.9	5	90.0	29.1 - 210.2
NT15	17	77.1	44.8 - 123.3	14	66.8	36.5 - 112.1
NT16	29	106.1	67.5 - 144.8	39	147.0	100.9 - 193.1
NT17	8	61.2	26.4 - 120.5	11	91.3	45.7 - 163.3
NT18	4	62.9	17.1 - 160.9	3	48.1	9.9 - 140.6
NT19	8	72.8	31.4 - 143.3	13	125.7	66.8 - 214.8

COLORECTAL CANCER

Sex-Age specific mortality rate (1/100,000) of colorectal cancer in Hong Kong (1979–1983)

Age	Male No. of deaths	Male Mortality rate	Female No. of deaths	Female Mortality rate
0–4	0	0.00	0	0.00
5–9	0	0.00	0	0.00
10–14	0	0.00	0	0.00
15–19	8	0.56	3	0.23
20–24	9	0.59	11	0.79
25–29	22	1.67	15	1.29
30–34	35	3.17	17	1.85
35–39	28	3.88	20	3.60
40–44	54	7.67	27	4.88
45–49	79	10.95	65	10.74
50–54	112	16.30	95	15.58
55–59	180	31.64	136	25.43
60–64	212	46.40	166	36.39
65+	699	102.53	778	77.07
TOTAL	1438	10.91	1333	10.95

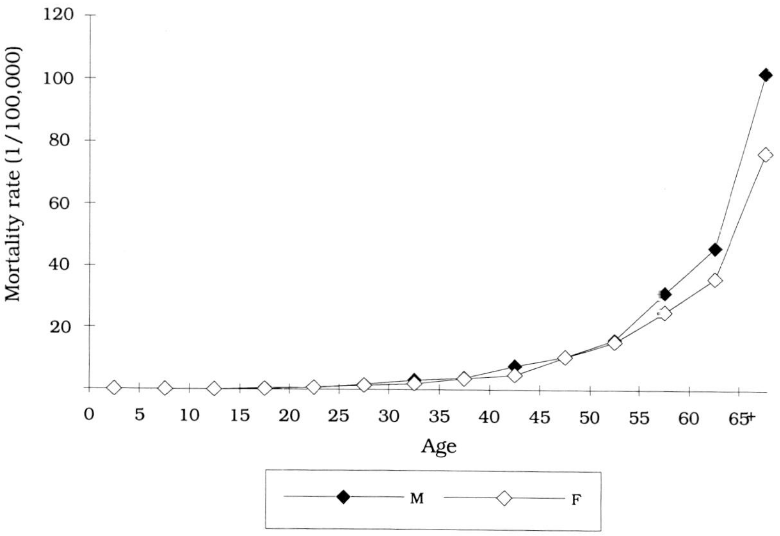

Number of communities on map by category based on standardized mortality ratio (SMR) during 1979–1983

Category	Number of communities Male	Number of communities Female
SMR significantly high, in top 20%	3	3
SMR significantly high , not in top 20%	0	0
SMR not significantly high, in top 20%	10	9
SMR not significantly low, in bottom 20%	11	9
SMR significantly low, not in bottom 20%	0	0
SMR significantly low, in bottom 20%	1	3
other communities	40	41

Values of the standardized mortality ratio (SMR) which divide the 65 communities into quintile

Percentile	Male	Female
20th	67.84	71.97
40th	89.52	90.96
60th	107.05	104.36
80th	125.97	132.30
Lowest SMR	23.69	21.53
Highest SMR	223.29	185.33
No. of communities with zero death	0	0

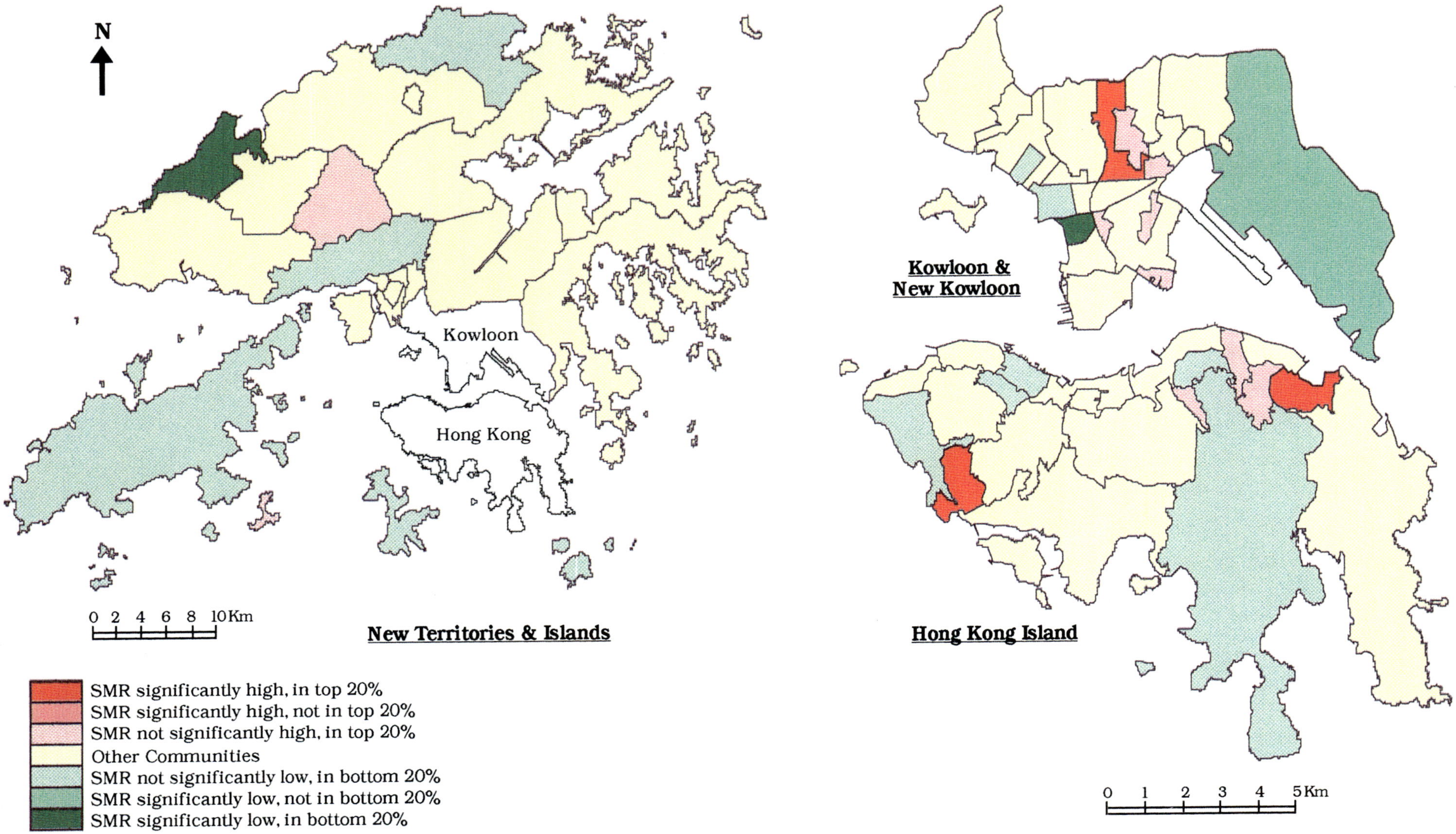

Colorectal Cancer (Male, 1984 - 1988)

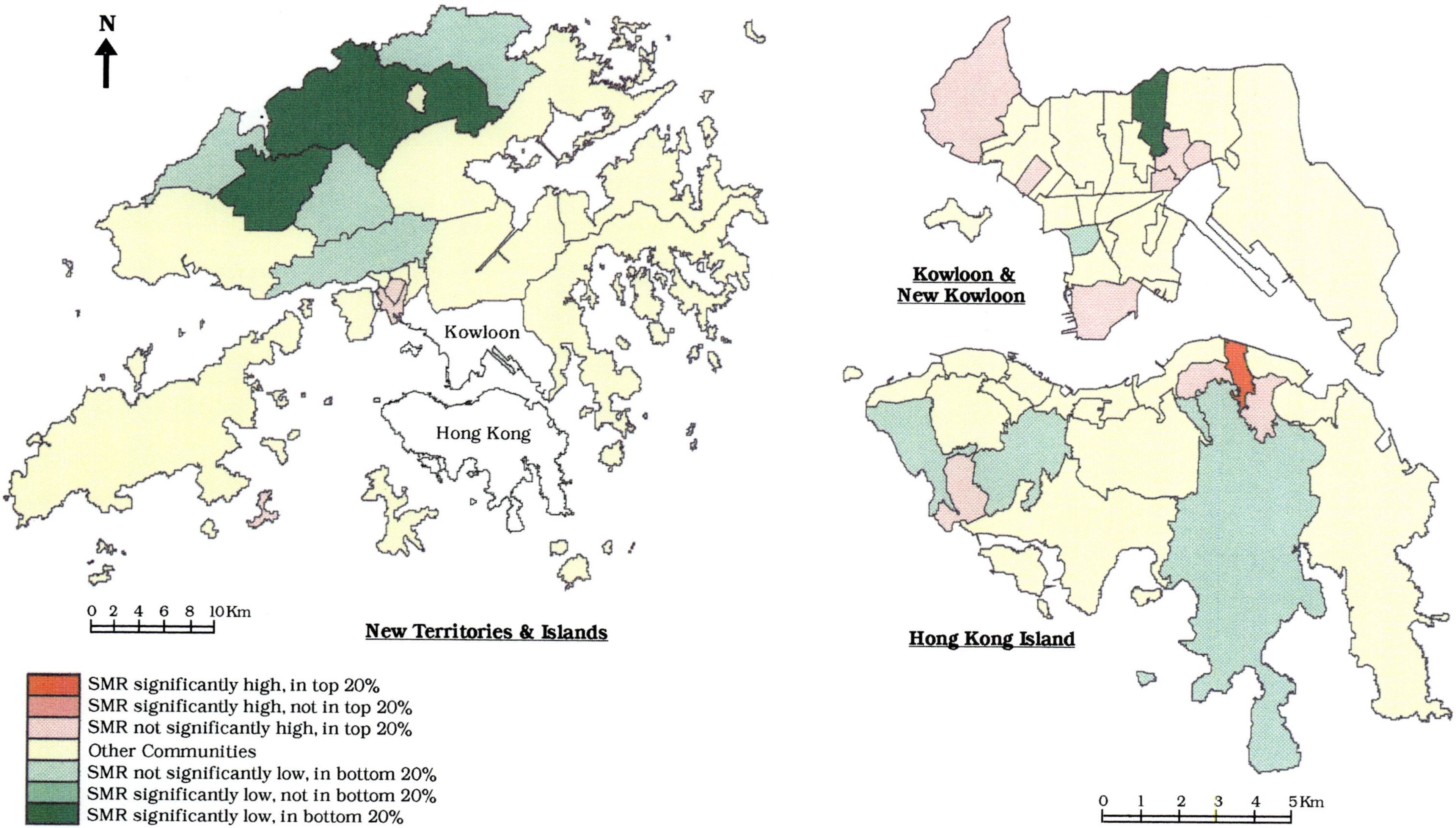

Colorectal Cancer (Female, 1984 – 1988)

Number of Deaths, Standardised Mortality Ratio (SMR) and 95% Confidence Interval of Colorectal Cancer by 65 Communities in 1984–1988

	Male			Female		
Community	Number of deaths	SMR	95% C.I.	Number of deaths	SMR	95% C.I.
HK1	34	108.0	71.7 - 144.3	22	80.6	46.9 - 114.2
HK2	40	89.8	62.0 - 117.7	36	95.1	64.0 - 126.1
HK3	11	66.1	33.0 - 118.2	13	103.5	55.0 - 176.9
HK4	26	97.7	60.1 - 135.2	27	118.5	77.9 - 172.5
HK5	26	109.3	71.4 - 160.2	18	84.4	50.0 - 133.4
HK6	25	103.9	67.0 - 153.2	26	97.9	60.3 - 135.5
HK7	4	82.2	22.4 - 210.1	5	92.6	30.0 - 216.4
HK8	7	77.9	31.3 - 160.7	10	102.4	49.2 - 188.2
HK9	1	25.4	0.6 - 141.2	1	20.2	0.5 - 112.3
HK10	78	116.3	90.5 - 142.2	72	102.4	78.7 - 126.0
HK11	11	182.4	91.2 - 326.3	3	60.7	12.5 - 177.3
HK12	4	72.4	19.7 - 185.2	10	169.2	81.4 - 311.0
HK13	12	148.7	76.6 - 259.5	13	191.4	101.8 - 327.1
HK14	28	113.5	75.7 - 164.0	27	105.7	65.8 - 145.5
HK15	13	165.3	87.9 - 282.5	15	176.3	98.5 - 291.0
HK16	56	163.6	120.7 - 206.4	30	100.0	64.2 - 135.8
HK17	40	88.4	61.0 - 115.8	43	107.4	75.3 - 139.6
HK18	3	59.9	12.4 - 175.2	3	55.9	11.5 - 163.5
HK19	34	157.0	108.4 - 219.5	27	132.3	87.0 - 192.6
HK20	45	96.0	67.9 - 124.0	42	101.5	70.8 - 132.1
HK21	3	51.9	10.7 - 151.7	3	53.8	11.1 - 157.3
KL1	22	91.6	57.3 - 138.8	27	134.0	88.2 - 195.1
KL2	35	75.7	50.6 - 100.7	39	99.6	68.3 - 130.8
KL3	17	120.9	70.3 - 193.5	15	112.7	63.0 - 185.9
KL4	32	74.3	48.5 - 100.0	26	79.1	48.7 - 109.5
KL5	38	119.6	81.6 - 157.6	26	101.4	62.4 - 140.4
KL6	10	112.1	53.9 - 206.1	9	90.8	41.6 - 172.2
KL7	12	187.1	96.4 - 326.5	6	95.7	35.0 - 208.4
KL8	31	139.7	94.9 - 198.4	25	129.1	83.3 - 190.4
KL9	93	107.2	85.4 - 129.0	84	105.8	83.2 - 128.5
KL10	12	139.5	71.9 - 243.4	10	117.8	56.6 - 216.5
KL11	27	106.8	66.5 - 147.1	31	130.4	88.6 - 185.3
KL12	6	85.4	31.3 - 186.1	5	92.3	29.9 - 215.6

	Male			Female		
Community	Number of deaths	SMR	95% C.I.	Number of deaths	SMR	95% C.I.
KL13	70	89.7	68.7 - 110.7	66	100.5	76.3 - 124.7
KL14	50	89.3	64.5 - 114.0	40	86.0	59.3 - 112.6
KL15	7	73.8	29.7 - 152.3	12	132.3	68.2 - 231.0
KL16	20	102.2	62.3 - 157.9	15	94.7	52.9 - 156.2
KL17	16	185.2	105.8 - 300.6	12	98.0	50.5 - 171.0
KL18	7	190.6	76.5 - 392.9	0	0.0	...
KL19	71	89.0	68.3 - 109.7	70	98.0	75.0 - 120.9
KL20	24	123.0	78.8 - 183.0	10	54.3	26.1 - 99.8
KL21	38	113.4	77.3 - 149.5	38	136.1	92.8 - 179.4
KL22	8	113.7	49.0 - 223.8	8	139.5	60.1 - 274.5
KL23	23	131.8	83.4 - 197.8	19	130.0	78.3 - 203.1
KL24	21	129.0	79.6 - 197.3	15	115.1	64.3 - 189.9
KL25	219	86.1	74.7 - 97.5	209	93.8	81.0 - 106.5
NT1	9	62.5	28.7 - 118.5	10	75.3	36.2 - 138.3
NT2	18	101.8	60.2 - 160.8	22	145.7	91.1 - 220.8
NT3	27	84.2	52.5 - 116.0	29	119.6	80.3 - 171.9
NT4	28	103.0	64.9 - 141.2	22	90.1	56.3 - 136.5
NT5	60	104.9	78.4 - 131.4	63	131.7	99.2 - 164.2
NT6	29	86.1	54.8 - 117.4	24	85.6	51.3 - 119.8
NT7	14	82.9	45.3 - 139.2	15	110.2	61.6 - 181.9
NT8	50	85.3	61.6 - 108.9	55	99.9	73.5 - 126.3
NT9	3	28.7	5.9 - 84.1	6	63.7	23.3 - 138.8
NT10	42	85.3	59.5 - 111.1	27	66.5	41.4 - 91.5
NT11	12	136.9	70.6 - 238.9	5	60.5	19.6 - 141.3
NT12	40	92.7	63.9 - 121.4	26	66.7	41.0 - 92.3
NT13	10	89.1	42.8 - 163.8	9	103.5	47.5 - 196.4
NT14	5	70.5	22.8 - 164.7	3	47.6	9.8 - 139.2
NT15	38	95.0	64.8 - 125.3	34	86.5	57.4 - 115.6
NT16	106	120.2	97.3 - 143.1	91	99.1	78.7 - 119.4
NT17	19	111.1	66.9 - 173.5	16	107.5	61.4 - 174.4
NT18	15	178.2	99.6 - 294.1	13	164.9	87.7 - 281.8
NT19	10	77.3	37.1 - 142.0	10	88.9	42.8 - 163.5

COLORECTAL CANCER

Sex-Age specific mortality rate (1/100,000) of colorectal cancer in Hong Kong (1984–1988)

	Male		Female	
Age	No. of deaths	Mortality rate	No. of deaths	Mortality rate
0–4	0	0.00	0	0.00
5–9	0	0.00	0	0.00
10–14	0	0.00	0	0.00
15–19	3	0.25	1	0.09
20–24	12	0.83	8	0.58
25–29	27	1.72	16	1.08
30–34	27	1.99	37	2.99
35–39	42	3.79	34	3.51
40–44	31	4.23	35	5.84
45–49	89	12.64	48	8.23
50–54	169	23.06	105	16.63
55–59	218	32.82	190	31.28
60–64	281	52.03	195	36.43
65+	1060	117.40	1081	87.59
TOTAL	1959	13.74	1750	13.04

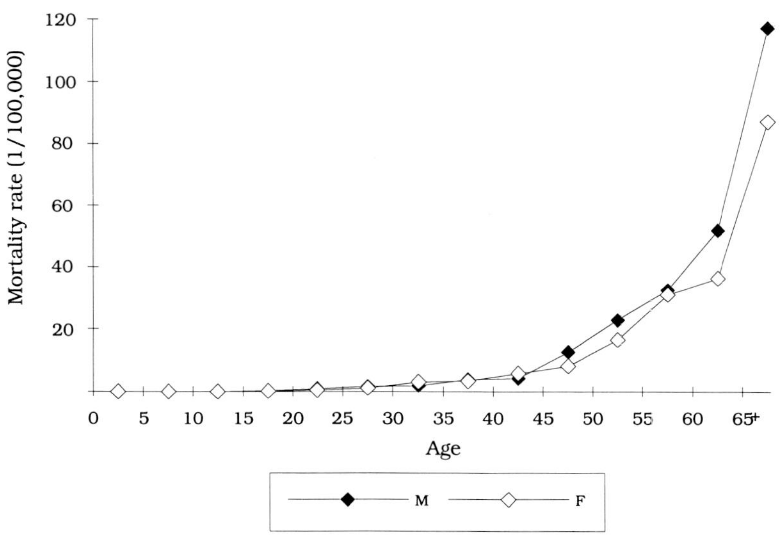

Number of communities on map by category based on standardized mortality ratio (SMR) during 1984–1988

Category	Number of communities Male	Female
SMR significantly high, in top 20%	3	1
SMR significantly high , not in top 20%	0	0
SMR not significantly high, in top 20%	10	12
SMR not significantly low, in bottom 20%	10	9
SMR significantly low, not in bottom 20%	1	0
SMR significantly low, in bottom 20%	2	3
other communities	39	40

Values of the standardized mortality ratio (SMR) which divide the 65 communities into quintile

Percentile	Male	Female
20th	77.94	79.09
40th	89.70	95.07
60th	107.21	102.38
80th	129.01	129.11
Lowest SMR	25.41	0.00
Highest SMR	190.57	191.38
No. of communities with zero death	0	1

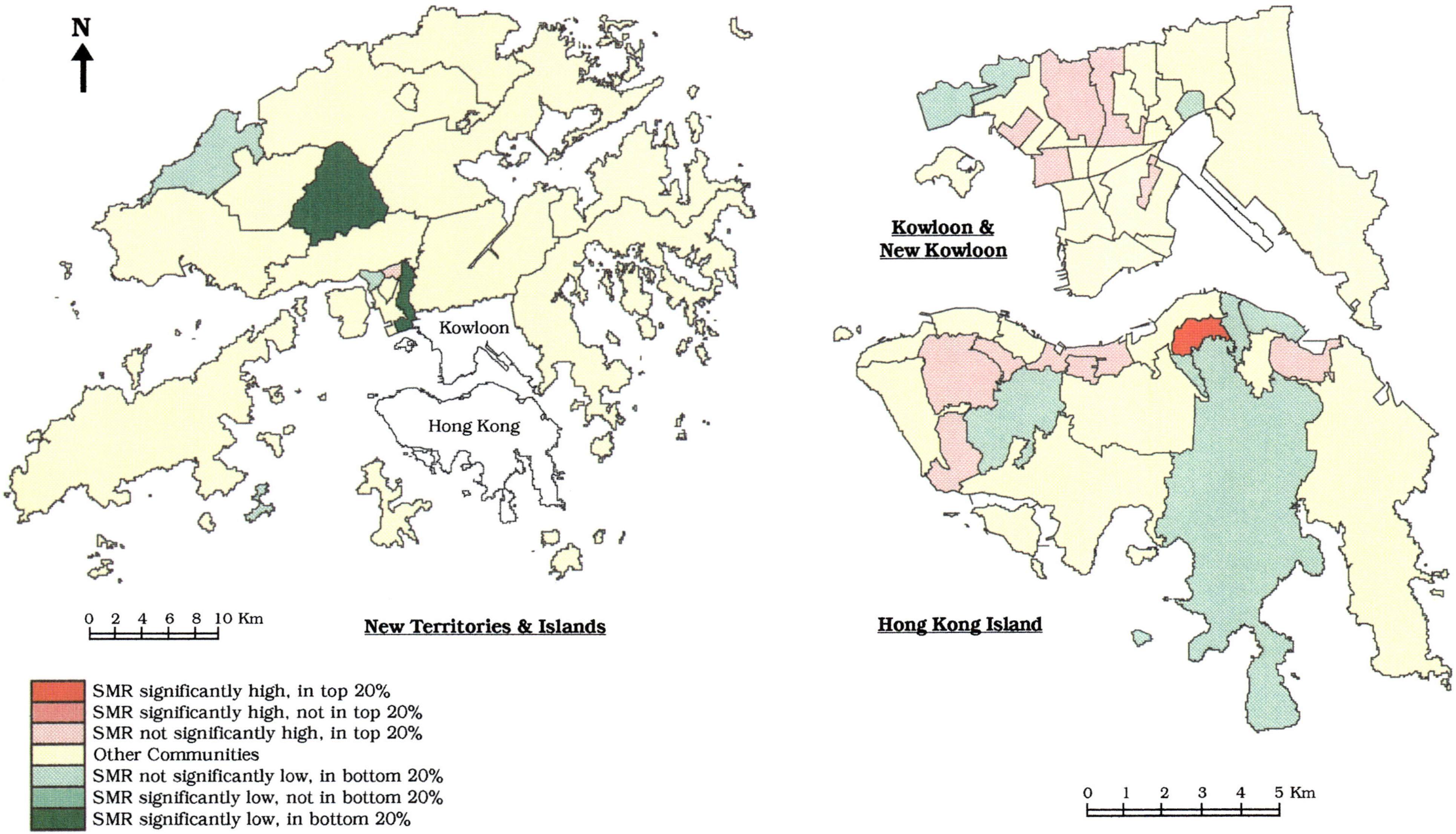

Colorectal Cancer (Male, 1989 -1993)

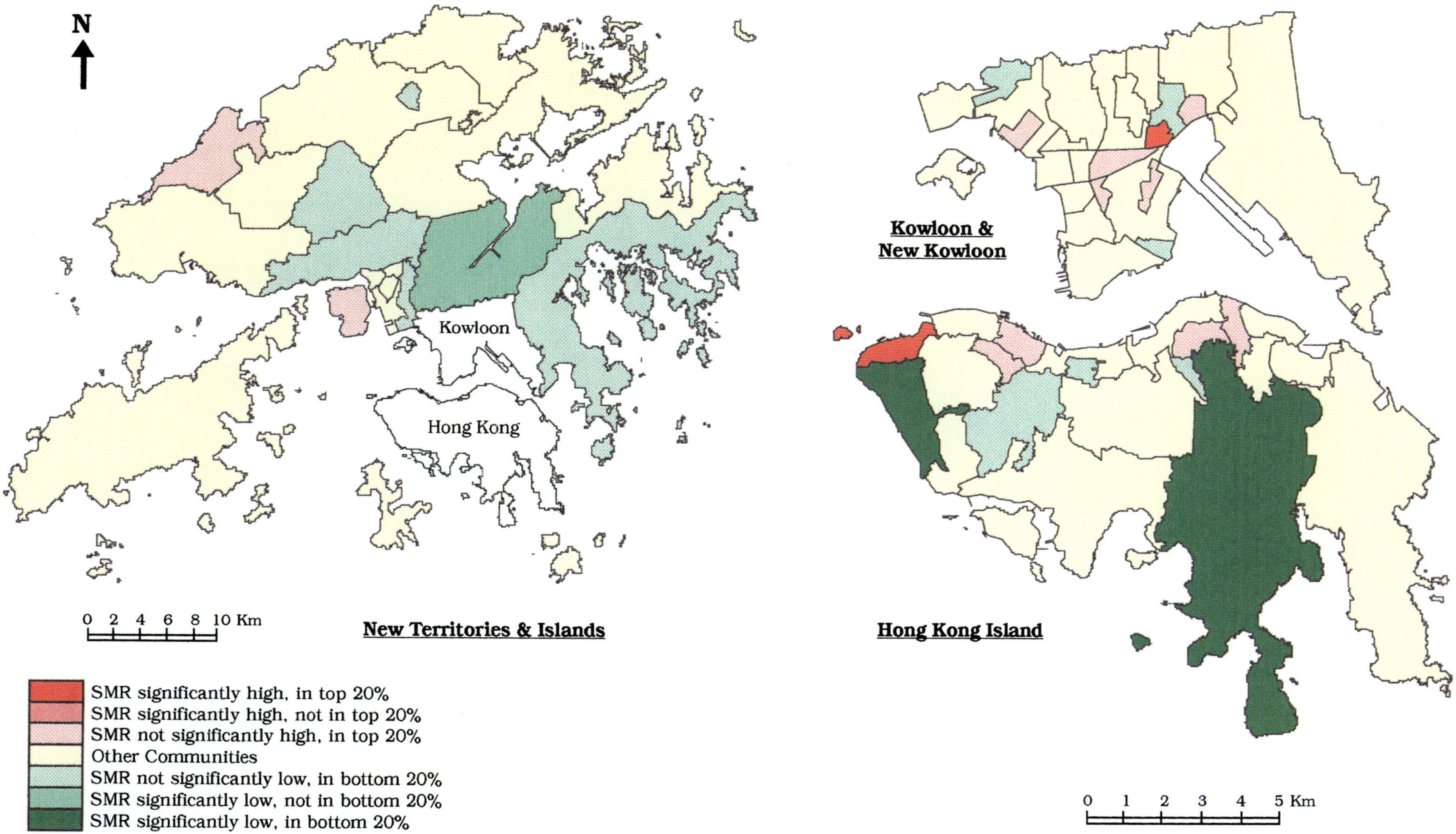

Colorectal Cancer (Female, 1989 -1993)

Number of Deaths, Standardised Mortality Ratio (SMR) and 95% Confidence Interval of Colorectal Cancer by 65 Communities in 1989–1993

Community	Male			Female		
	Number of deaths	SMR	95% C.I.	Number of deaths	SMR	95% C.I.
HK1	43	117.1	82.1 - 152.1	44	145.8	102.7 - 188.9
HK2	43	86.8	60.8 - 112.7	39	106.8	73.3 - 140.4
HK3	17	99.7	58.2 - 159.6	15	127.7	71.5 - 210.8
HK4	33	118.6	78.2 - 159.1	19	90.7	54.6 - 141.5
HK5	37	139.7	94.7 - 184.7	16	81.3	46.5 - 131.6
HK6	26	87.5	53.9 - 121.1	24	81.6	52.3 - 121.6
HK7	12	182.8	94.5 - 319.9	6	85.7	31.4 - 186.8
HK8	13	123.1	65.5 - 210.5	12	122.8	63.5 - 214.9
HK9	4	84.2	22.9 - 215.7	4	81.4	22.1 - 208.4
HK10	90	107.2	85.1 - 129.4	85	105.7	83.2 - 128.1
HK11	5	63.9	20.7 - 148.9	4	67.1	18.3 - 171.8
HK12	13	190.8	101.5 - 326.3	10	152.2	73.0 - 280.0
HK13	6	65.8	24.2 - 143.5	9	124.1	56.9 - 235.9
HK14	26	78.1	48.1 - 108.1	28	95.4	60.0 - 130.7
HK15	22	111.2	69.8 - 168.0	16	88.3	50.5 - 143.0
HK16	42	122.0	85.1 - 158.9	31	111.5	72.2 - 150.7
HK17	64	88.7	66.9 - 110.4	65	108.5	82.1 - 134.9
HK18	8	104.0	44.8 - 204.8	2	25.3	3.1 - 91.5
HK19	41	141.2	98.0 - 184.4	20	84.9	51.9 - 130.7
HK20	70	108.2	82.8 - 133.5	62	115.3	86.6 - 144.0
HK21	4	62.2	16.9 - 159.3	0	0.0	...
KL1	24	109.0	69.9 - 162.4	20	115.9	70.8 - 178.5
KL2	62	120.5	90.5 - 150.5	38	99.6	68.0 - 131.3
KL3	16	107.1	61.3 - 173.5	13	102.7	54.6 - 175.5
KL4	48	112.1	80.4 - 143.8	31	105.4	68.3 - 142.6
KL5	35	112.4	75.1 - 149.6	22	96.9	60.8 - 146.3
KL6	12	103.6	53.5 - 181.3	18	144.7	85.8 - 228.7
KL7	8	98.4	42.4 - 193.8	11	131.0	65.4 - 234.5
KL8	35	135.0	90.3 - 179.8	25	123.0	79.6 - 182.1
KL9	96	93.2	74.6 - 111.8	82	98.1	76.8 - 119.3
KL10	15	85.5	47.9 - 141.0	13	76.2	40.5 - 130.3
KL11	16	68.3	39.1 - 110.7	20	95.5	58.3 - 147.0
KL12	5	66.1	21.4 - 153.9	3	53.3	11.0 - 155.8
KL13	103	108.4	87.5 - 129.4	74	105.7	81.6 - 129.7
KL14	77	125.7	97.6 - 153.8	48	96.0	68.8 - 123.2
KL15	16	137.0	78.4 - 222.0	14	144.1	78.7 - 242.1
KL16	18	84.7	50.2 - 133.9	15	95.4	53.4 - 157.4
KL17	15	163.5	91.6 - 269.8	13	119.2	63.4 - 203.8
KL18	5	116.2	37.7 - 270.8	5	118.6	38.4 - 276.3
KL19	93	94.2	75.1 - 113.4	95	110.9	88.6 - 133.3
KL20	16	107.0	61.2 - 173.4	19	103.1	62.0 - 160.8
KL21	42	118.0	82.3 - 153.6	23	76.3	48.3 - 114.4
KL22	6	82.4	30.3 - 179.7	10	175.6	84.3 - 323.1
KL23	16	107.0	61.2 - 173.4	24	205.6	131.8 - 306.3
KL24	19	94.0	56.6 - 146.7	15	102.4	57.4 - 169.0
KL25	290	96.7	85.5 - 107.8	247	99.5	87.1 - 111.9
NT1	26	107.4	66.1 - 148.7	14	64.9	35.5 - 109.1
NT2	28	113.5	71.5 - 155.6	21	101.5	62.8 - 155.3
NT3	34	75.0	49.8 - 100.2	30	91.9	59.0 - 124.8
NT4	42	135.6	94.6 - 176.7	30	114.6	73.6 - 155.7
NT5	66	100.9	76.6 - 125.3	51	99.3	72.1 - 126.6
NT6	32	73.7	48.2 - 99.3	27	77.1	48.0 - 106.2
NT7	40	94.8	65.4 - 124.2	40	120.1	82.9 - 157.3
NT8	109	109.3	88.8 - 129.9	97	117.3	94.0 - 140.7
NT9	9	70.4	32.2 - 133.8	15	138.9	77.8 - 229.1
NT10	55	86.8	63.9 - 109.8	47	94.7	67.6 - 121.7
NT11	5	42.8	13.9 - 99.8	7	71.6	28.7 - 147.5
NT12	50	85.4	61.8 - 109.1	41	85.4	59.3 - 111.6
NT13	11	90.5	45.1 - 161.9	7	64.8	26.0 - 133.6
NT14	7	104.8	42.0 - 215.9	5	83.3	27.0 - 194.2
NT15	59	89.2	66.5 - 112.0	52	88.2	64.2 - 112.2
NT16	140	86.2	71.9 - 100.4	129	83.9	69.4 - 98.4
NT17	40	97.8	67.5 - 128.1	25	68.2	44.1 - 100.9
NT18	6	54.3	19.9 - 118.5	10	107.5	51.6 - 197.7
NT19	15	110.6	61.9 - 182.4	11	94.8	47.3 - 169.7

COLORECTAL CANCER

Sex-Age specific mortality rate (1/100,000) of colorectal cancer in Hong Kong (1989–1993)

	Male		Female	
Age	No. of deaths	Mortality rate	No. of deaths	Mortality rate
0–4	0	0.00	0	0.00
5–9	0	0.00	0	0.00
10–14	0	0.00	0	0.00
15–19	8	0.73	1	0.10
20–24	6	0.53	5	0.44
25–29	14	0.97	19	1.28
30–34	43	2.76	32	2.11
35–39	61	4.56	38	3.02
40–44	66	5.99	57	5.86
45–49	86	11.77	63	10.55
50–54	130	18.74	84	14.75
55–59	204	29.19	164	26.92
60–64	375	60.75	211	36.51
65+	1488	134.33	1394	99.22
TOTAL	2481	16.96	2068	14.78

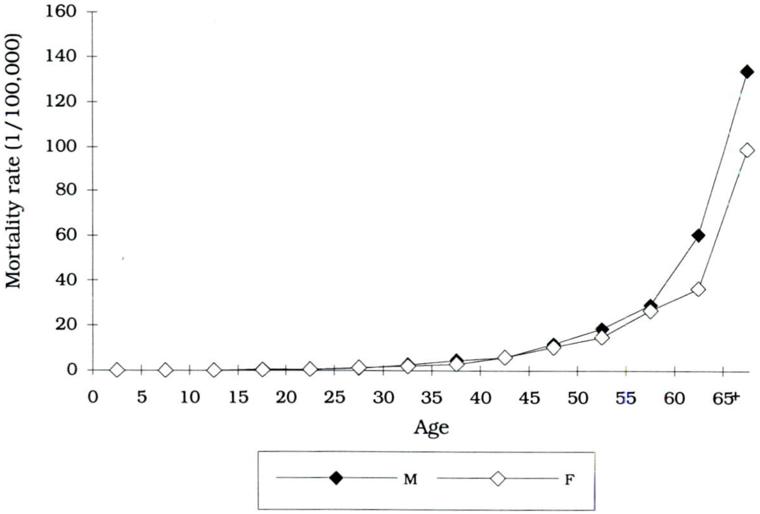

Number of communities on map by category based on standardized mortality ratio (SMR) during 1989–1993

Category	Number of communities Male	Female
SMR significantly high, in top 20%	1	2
SMR significantly high , not in top 20%	0	0
SMR not significantly high, in top 20%	12	11
SMR not significantly low, in bottom 20%	11	11
SMR significantly low, not in bottom 20%	0	1
SMR significantly low, in bottom 20%	2	2
other communities	39	38

Values of the standardized mortality ratio (SMR) which divide the 65 communities into quintile

Percentile	Male	Female
20th	84.24	81.42
40th	94.24	95.35
60th	107.24	105.45
80th	117.95	119.19
Lowest SMR	42.83	0.00
Highest SMR	190.82	205.59
No. of communities with zero cases	0	1

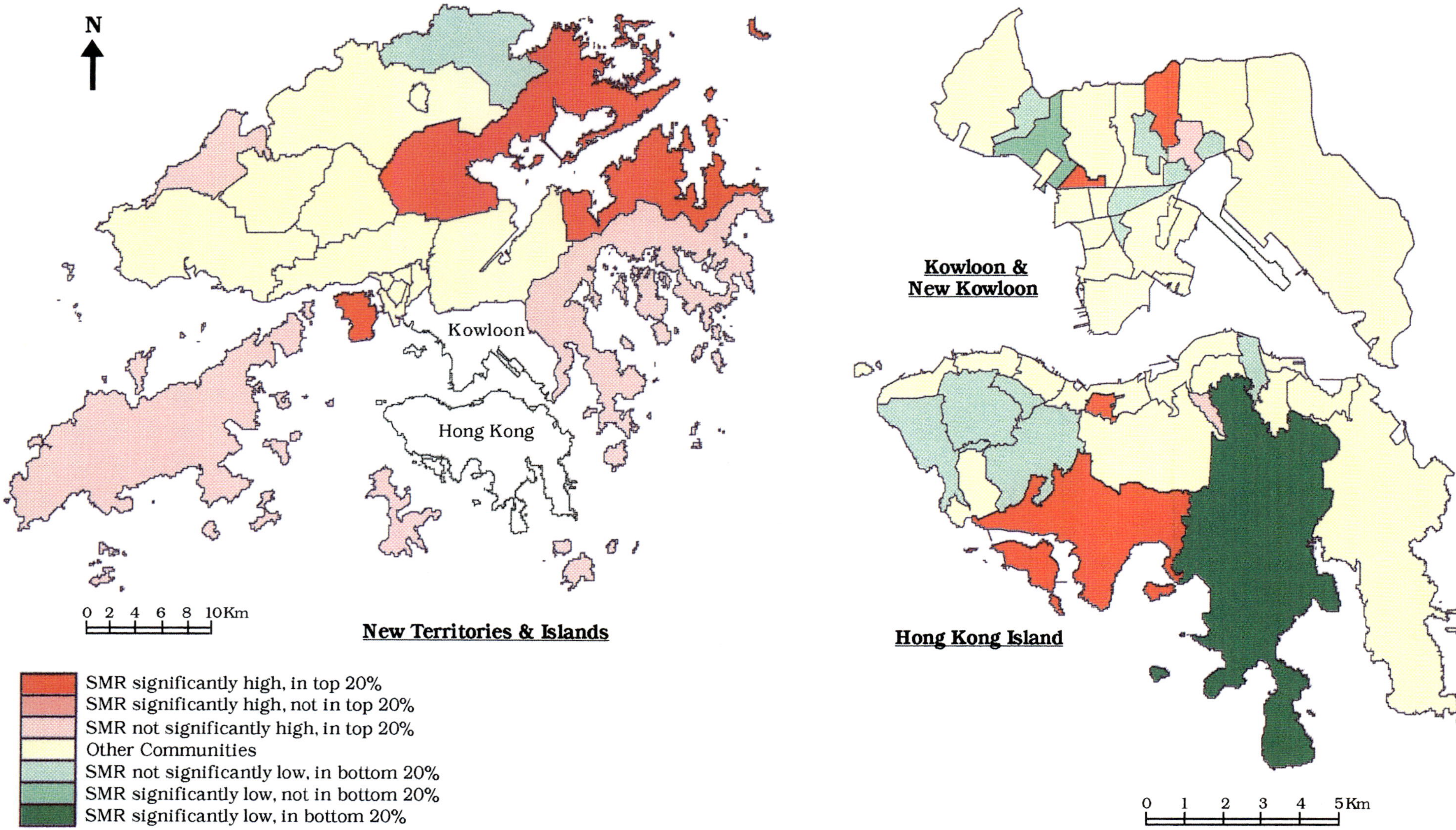

Liver Cancer (Male, 1979 – 1983)

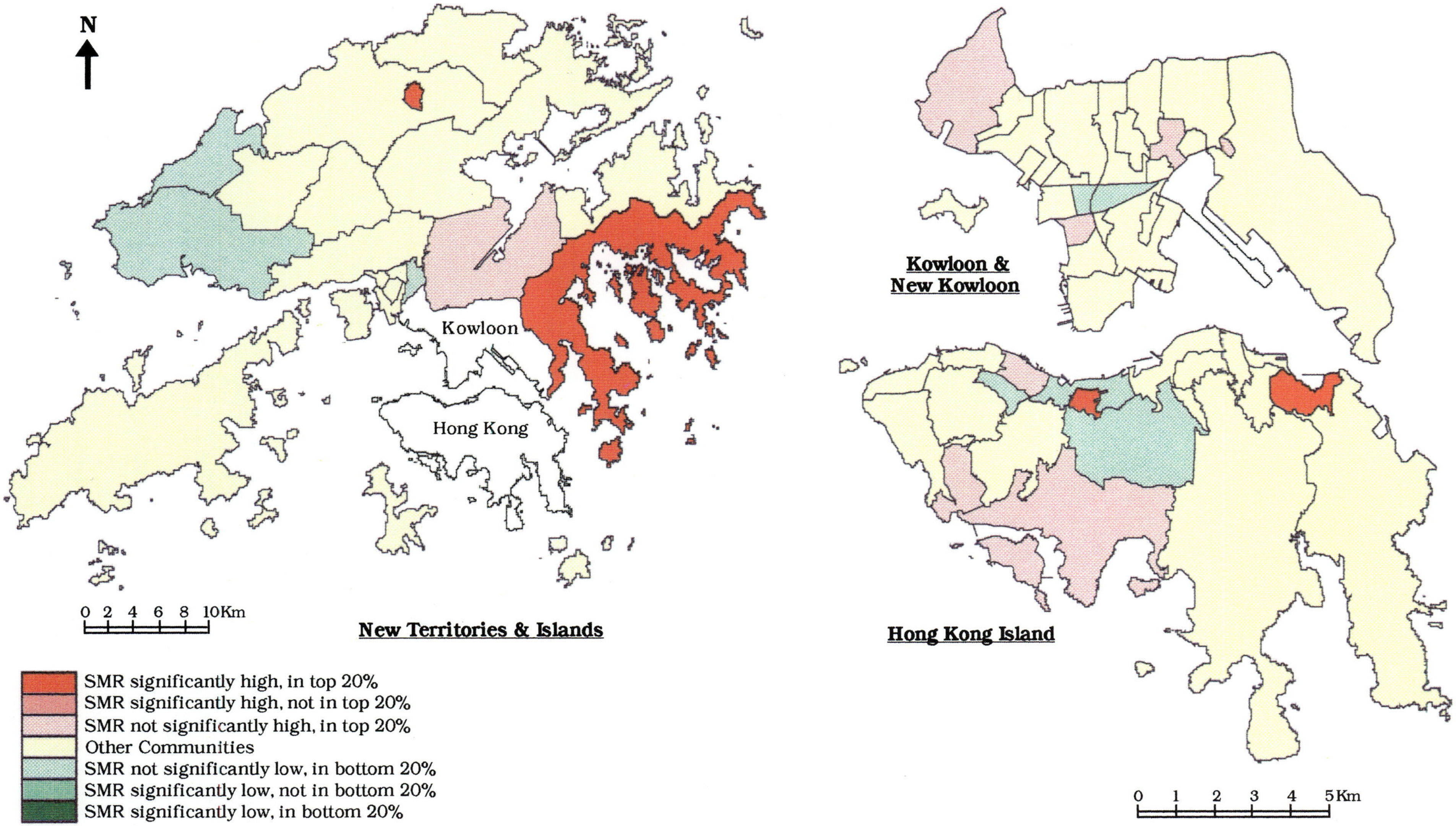

Liver Cancer (Female, 1979 – 1983)

Number of Deaths, Standardised Mortality Ratio (SMR) and 95% Confidence Interval of Liver Cancer by 65 Communities in 1979–1983

	Male			Female		
Community	Number of deaths	SMR	95% C.I.	Number of deaths	SMR	95% C.I.
HK1	60	100.4	75.0 - 125.8	20	117.5	71.6 - 181.6
HK2	99	108.1	86.8 - 129.4	25	103.4	62.9 - 143.9
HK3	41	114.1	79.2 - 149.1	13	148.0	78.7 - 253.0
HK4	49	83.4	60.0 - 106.7	11	70.4	35.2 - 125.9
HK5	84	152.1	119.6 - 184.6	24	164.2	105.3 - 244.4
HK6	43	92.3	64.7 - 119.9	12	69.0	35.6 - 120.4
HK7	5	53.3	17.2 - 124.4	3	83.8	17.3 - 245.0
HK8	10	55.0	26.5 - 101.2	2	28.1	3.4 - 101.6
HK9	4	44.4	12.1 - 113.6	2	60.6	7.3 - 219.0
HK10	117	90.7	74.3 - 107.2	49	114.2	82.2 - 146.2
HK11	15	122.8	68.6 - 202.7	3	94.0	19.4 - 274.8
HK12	9	85.6	39.3 - 162.5	3	74.0	15.2 - 216.2
HK13	9	56.4	25.9 - 107.1	6	124.2	45.5 - 270.5
HK14	41	109.5	76.0 - 143.1	10	86.9	41.8 - 159.8
HK15	18	111.8	66.2 - 176.6	4	80.0	21.8 - 204.5
HK16	79	114.2	89.0 - 139.4	30	159.3	102.3 - 216.3
HK17	83	115.5	90.7 - 140.4	20	96.9	59.1 - 149.8
HK18	5	46.0	14.9 - 107.4	2	56.8	6.9 - 204.9
HK19	39	102.6	70.4 - 134.9	15	134.9	75.4 - 222.6
HK20	101	130.2	104.8 - 155.6	28	127.8	80.4 - 175.1
HK21	4	35.0	9.5 - 89.5	2	73.1	8.8 - 263.7
KL1	44	86.0	60.6 - 111.5	12	88.4	45.6 - 154.3
KL2	106	98.6	79.8 - 117.3	26	93.5	57.6 - 129.4
KL3	34	111.7	74.1 - 149.2	5	55.2	17.9 - 129.1
KL4	89	103.1	81.7 - 124.5	28	128.3	80.8 - 175.8
KL5	75	106.5	82.4 - 130.6	19	106.5	64.2 - 166.5
KL6	12	71.8	37.0 - 125.2	2	28.8	3.5 - 104.1
KL7	9	69.1	31.7 - 131.1	5	104.0	33.7 - 243.0
KL8	41	85.4	59.3 - 111.6	12	88.7	45.7 - 154.8
KL9	172	98.3	83.6 - 113.0	57	111.9	82.9 - 141.0
KL10	14	80.0	43.7 - 134.2	5	92.2	29.8 - 215.4
KL11	38	83.7	57.1 - 110.3	19	131.5	79.2 - 205.4
KL12	10	71.6	34.4 - 131.7	2	58.9	7.1 - 212.7
KL13	149	86.1	72.3 - 100.0	36	78.5	52.9 - 104.1
KL14	91	98.6	78.3 - 118.8	23	90.1	57.0 - 135.3
KL15	7	81.8	32.9 - 168.7	3	135.9	28.0 - 397.4
KL16	60	146.8	109.7 - 184.0	8	71.2	30.7 - 140.2
KL17	11	92.1	46.1 - 164.8	4	81.2	22.1 - 207.6
KL18	6	71.3	26.1 - 155.3	0	0.0	...
KL19	158	105.1	88.7 - 121.5	48	107.2	76.9 - 137.5
KL20	67	134.6	102.3 - 166.8	18	121.0	71.6 - 191.1
KL21	97	122.9	98.4 - 147.3	33	137.7	90.7 - 184.7
KL22	9	60.8	27.9 - 115.3	2	56.1	6.8 - 202.7
KL23	34	75.8	50.3 - 101.2	14	116.7	63.7 - 195.7
KL24	41	139.3	96.6 - 181.9	14	175.1	95.7 - 293.7
KL25	402	93.4	84.3 - 102.5	99	84.1	67.6 - 100.7
NT1	20	91.4	55.8 - 141.3	5	81.0	26.2 - 189.2
NT2	25	76.4	46.5 - 106.4	8	96.0	41.4 - 188.9
NT3	64	97.3	73.5 - 121.2	12	80.5	41.5 - 140.5
NT4	38	100.2	68.3 - 132.0	9	89.0	40.8 - 168.8
NT5	127	103.5	85.5 - 121.5	34	103.4	68.6 - 138.1
NT6	53	84.9	62.1 - 107.8	12	70.4	36.3 - 122.9
NT7	33	153.9	101.4 - 206.4	6	109.9	40.2 - 239.4
NT8	55	83.7	61.6 - 105.8	11	66.1	33.1 - 118.3
NT9	24	126.5	81.1 - 188.2	3	59.2	12.2 - 173.2
NT10	72	91.3	70.2 - 112.3	17	80.9	47.1 - 129.5
NT11	14	85.7	46.8 - 143.8	5	120.6	39.0 - 281.7
NT12	77	104.2	80.9 - 127.4	16	79.0	45.1 - 128.2
NT13	13	93.5	49.7 - 159.8	9	224.1	102.8 - 425.3
NT14	8	63.9	27.5 - 125.8	5	121.9	39.4 - 284.7
NT15	68	133.7	101.9 - 165.5	12	77.5	39.9 - 135.2
NT16	59	87.5	65.1 - 109.8	27	136.5	85.0 - 188.0
NT17	37	125.6	85.1 - 166.0	16	179.9	102.8 - 292.1
NT18	18	130.6	77.3 - 206.4	4	87.1	23.7 - 222.7
NT19	29	117.1	74.5 - 159.8	6	79.3	29.0 - 172.8

LIVER CANCER

Sex-Age specific mortality rate (1/100,000) of liver cancer in Hong Kong (1979–1983)

	Male		Female	
Age	No. of deaths	Mortality rate	No. of deaths	Mortality rate
0–4	1	0.09	1	0.10
5–9	6	0.57	0	0.00
10–14	1	0.09	3	0.28
15–19	8	0.56	4	0.30
20–24	13	0.85	7	0.50
25–29	32	2.42	10	0.86
30–34	87	7.89	9	0.98
35–39	130	18.01	15	2.70
40–44	247	35.10	36	6.51
45–49	387	53.65	58	9.58
50–54	537	78.16	86	14.10
55–59	529	93.00	96	17.95
60–64	551	120.58	127	27.84
65+	996	146.09	543	53.79
TOTAL	3525	26.74	995	8.17

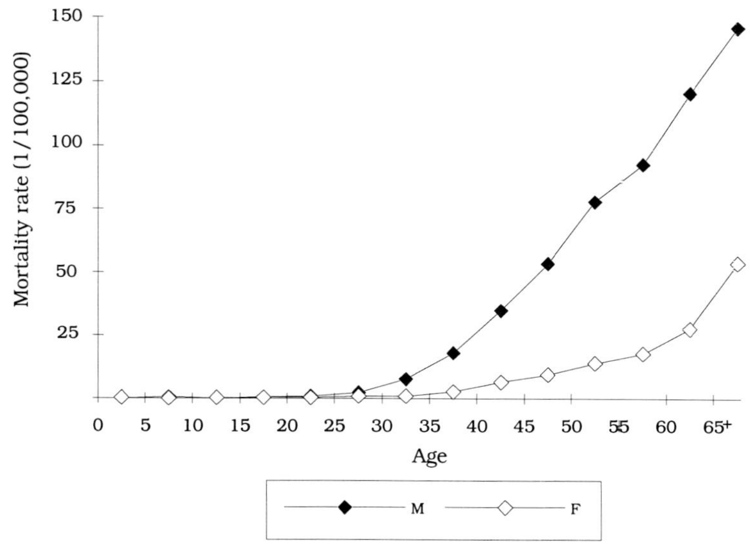

Number of communities on map by category based on standardized mortality ratio (SMR) during 1979–1983

	Number of communities	
Category	Male	Female
SMR significantly high, in top 20%	6	4
SMR significantly high , not in top 20%	0	0
SMR not significantly high, in top 20%	7	8
SMR not significantly low, in bottom 20%	12	8
SMR significantly low, not in bottom 20%	1	0
SMR significantly low, in bottom 20%	1	0
other communities	38	45

Values of the standardized mortality ratio (SMR) which divide the 65 communities into quintile

Percentile	Male	Female
20th	75.76	70.45
40th	87.47	83.79
60th	100.41	103.37
80th	115.52	124.17
Lowest SMR	35.01	0.00
Highest SMR	153.86	224.11
No. of communities with zero death	0	1

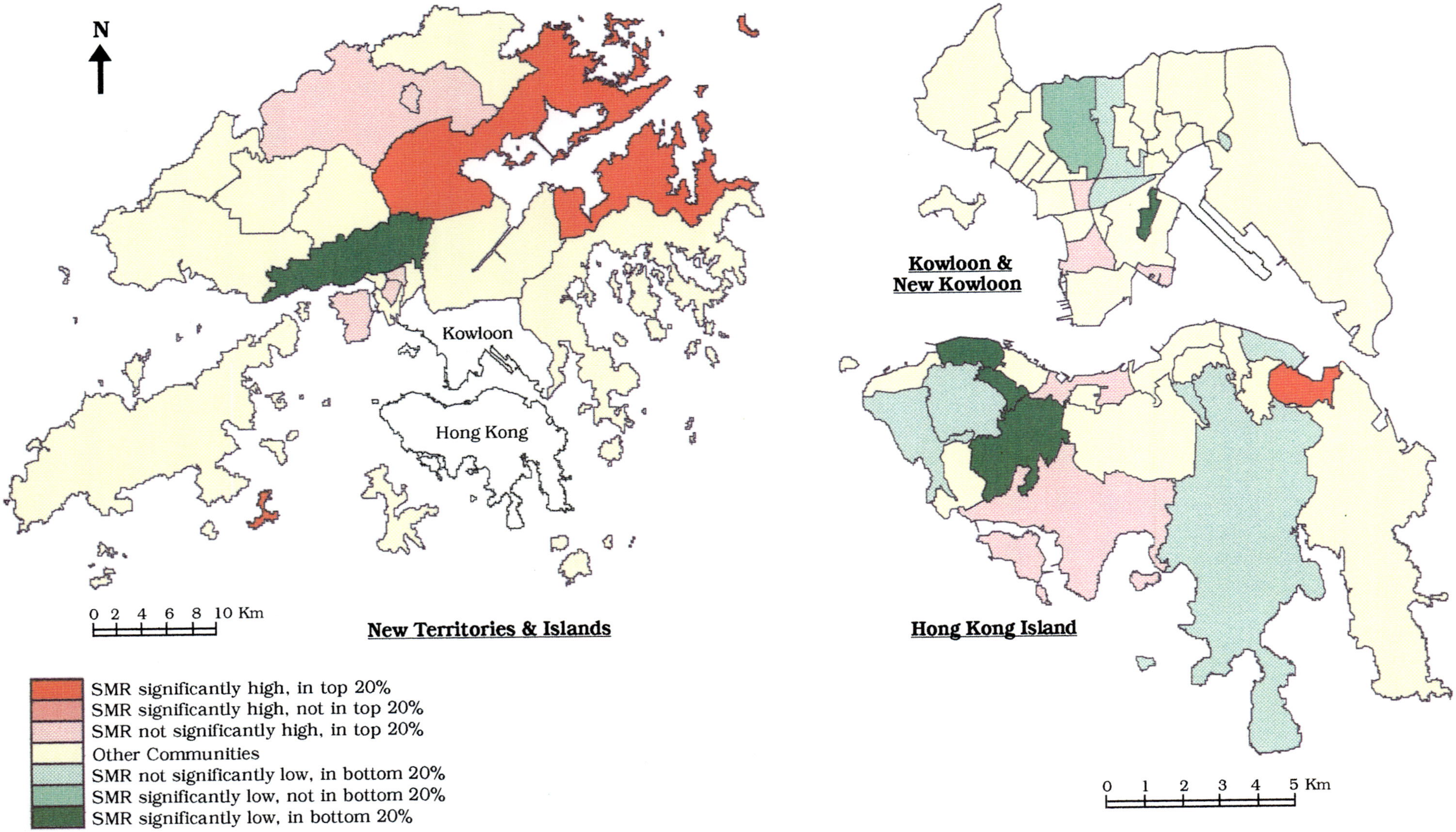

Liver Cancer (Male, 1984 -1988)

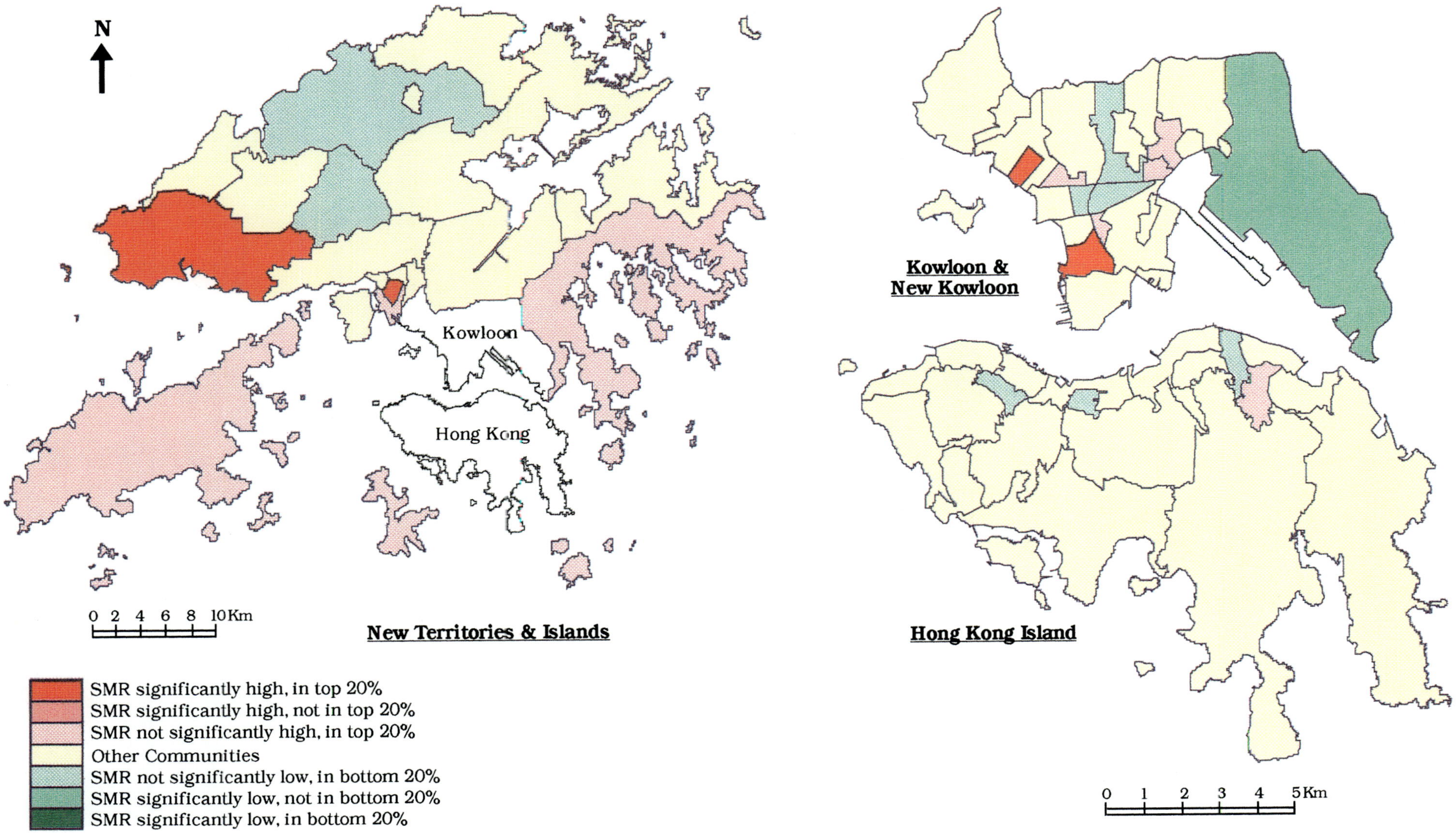

Liver Cancer (Female, 1984 – 1988)

Number of Deaths, Standardised Mortality Ratio (SMR) and 95% Confidence Interval of Liver Cancer by 65 Communities in 1984–1988

Community	Male			Female		
	Number of deaths	SMR	95% C.I.	Number of deaths	SMR	95% C.I.
HK1	68	107.1	81.6 - 132.5	13	74.1	39.4 - 126.6
HK2	61	68.5	51.3 - 85.6	24	99.1	63.5 - 147.4
HK3	29	87.2	55.5 - 118.9	6	74.5	27.3 - 162.3
HK4	62	115.3	86.6 - 144.0	13	89.0	47.3 - 152.1
HK5	41	84.1	58.3 - 109.8	8	58.5	25.2 - 115.2
HK6	41	83.8	58.2 - 109.5	15	88.2	49.0 - 145.5
HK7	4	41.0	11.2 - 104.9	2	57.8	7.0 - 208.8
HK8	5	27.6	8.9 - 64.4	4	63.9	17.4 - 163.5
HK9	1	11.4	0.3 - 63.5	1	31.3	0.8 - 174.1
HK10	125	90.1	74.3 - 106.0	39	86.5	59.3 - 113.6
HK11	10	80.3	38.6 - 147.5	4	124.3	33.9 - 317.9
HK12	10	84.7	40.7 - 155.8	2	53.0	6.4 - 191.2
HK13	15	92.0	51.4 - 151.9	1	22.8	0.6 - 126.7
HK14	40	78.5	54.2 - 102.8	16	97.7	55.8 - 158.6
HK15	17	98.8	57.4 - 158.0	8	146.4	63.1 - 288.1
HK16	89	126.8	100.5 - 153.2	19	98.5	59.3 - 153.9
HK17	96	107.7	86.2 - 129.3	21	81.7	46.8 - 116.7
HK18	8	76.6	33.0 - 150.8	1	29.3	0.7 - 162.7
HK19	46	99.2	70.5 - 127.8	11	83.4	41.7 - 149.2
HK20	106	113.1	91.6 - 134.6	28	105.1	66.1 - 144.0
HK21	10	76.8	36.9 - 141.2	0	0.0	...
KL1	52	105.1	76.5 - 133.6	15	116.2	64.9 - 191.7
KL2	104	106.4	85.9 - 126.8	27	107.3	66.8 - 147.7
KL3	31	110.5	71.6 - 149.3	5	58.6	18.9 - 136.8
KL4	90	101.7	80.7 - 122.7	20	94.9	57.9 - 146.7
KL5	80	124.3	97.1 - 151.6	27	164.1	108.0 - 238.9
KL6	11	63.5	31.7 - 113.5	4	62.9	17.1 - 160.9
KL7	13	98.4	52.3 - 168.2	8	198.9	85.7 - 391.5
KL8	34	72.1	47.9 - 96.3	15	120.2	67.1 - 198.3
KL9	181	99.8	85.3 - 114.4	45	87.9	62.2 - 113.6
KL10	22	118.6	74.1 - 179.7	4	73.4	20.0 - 187.7
KL11	50	95.3	68.9 - 121.7	11	72.0	36.0 - 128.8
KL12	13	90.0	47.9 - 153.8	3	86.5	17.8 - 253.0
KL13	169	104.9	89.1 - 120.7	47	111.2	79.4 - 143.0
KL14	84	81.5	64.1 - 98.9	32	107.4	70.2 - 144.6
KL15	20	101.3	61.8 - 156.6	12	206.2	106.3 - 359.9
KL16	43	106.0	74.3 - 137.6	15	147.4	82.4 - 243.3
KL17	10	64.1	30.8 - 117.8	3	38.6	8.0 - 112.9
KL18	7	86.8	34.9 - 179.0	2	90.4	10.9 - 326.4
KL19	156	97.5	82.2 - 112.8	39	84.7	58.1 - 111.2
KL20	37	95.3	64.6 - 126.0	11	92.8	46.4 - 166.1
KL21	63	98.9	74.5 - 123.3	26	144.5	94.5 - 211.9
KL22	16	106.6	60.9 - 173.0	4	108.4	29.5 - 277.4
KL23	38	104.1	71.0 - 137.2	14	149.1	81.5 - 250.1
KL24	24	73.0	43.8 - 102.2	6	70.7	25.9 - 153.9
KL25	529	98.3	89.9 - 106.7	113	78.5	64.0 - 92.9
NT1	18	58.0	31.2 - 84.8	8	94.0	40.5 - 185.0
NT2	37	97.6	66.1 - 129.0	16	164.7	94.1 - 267.4
NT3	74	107.0	82.6 - 131.4	19	120.8	72.8 - 188.8
NT4	70	111.8	85.6 - 138.0	21	132.2	81.6 - 202.2
NT5	136	110.6	92.0 - 129.2	46	148.4	105.5 - 191.3
NT6	73	101.1	77.9 - 124.3	19	104.2	62.7 - 162.7
NT7	43	112.0	78.6 - 145.5	10	113.7	54.7 - 209.1
NT8	131	100.1	82.9 - 117.2	53	150.8	110.2 - 191.4
NT9	23	106.0	67.1 - 159.2	5	82.4	26.7 - 192.4
NT10	89	91.2	72.3 - 110.2	28	107.2	67.5 - 146.9
NT11	19	107.2	64.6 - 167.4	2	37.6	4.5 - 135.7
NT12	98	113.4	91.0 - 135.9	17	68.0	39.5 - 108.8
NT13	31	139.5	94.8 - 198.3	4	71.8	19.6 - 183.7
NT14	14	100.0	54.6 - 167.8	3	74.1	15.3 - 216.6
NT15	107	130.6	105.9 - 155.4	32	127.3	83.2 - 171.4
NT16	211	109.0	94.3 - 123.7	60	101.9	76.1 - 127.6
NT17	35	106.2	71.0 - 141.4	16	168.1	96.1 - 272.9
NT18	33	208.9	143.4 - 293.6	7	138.9	55.8 - 286.3
NT19	21	85.6	52.8 - 130.8	11	153.3	76.7 - 274.3

LIVER CANCER

Sex-Age specific mortality rate (1/100,000) of liver cancer in Hong Kong (1984–1988)

	Male		Female	
Age	No. of deaths	Mortality rate	No of deaths	Mortality rate
0–4	0	0.00	1	0.10
5–9	4	0.36	1	0.10
10–14	9	0.79	2	0.19
15–19	7	0.58	3	0.27
20–24	18	1.25	7	0.50
25–29	41	2.61	7	0.47
30–34	89	6.58	20	1.62
35–39	146	13.16	19	1.96
40–44	203	27.69	19	3.17
45–49	345	49.01	44	7.54
50–54	463	63.17	75	11.88
55–59	656	98.77	116	19.09
60–64	651	120.53	134	25.03
65+	1420	157.27	682	55.26
TOTAL	4052	28.42	1130	8.42

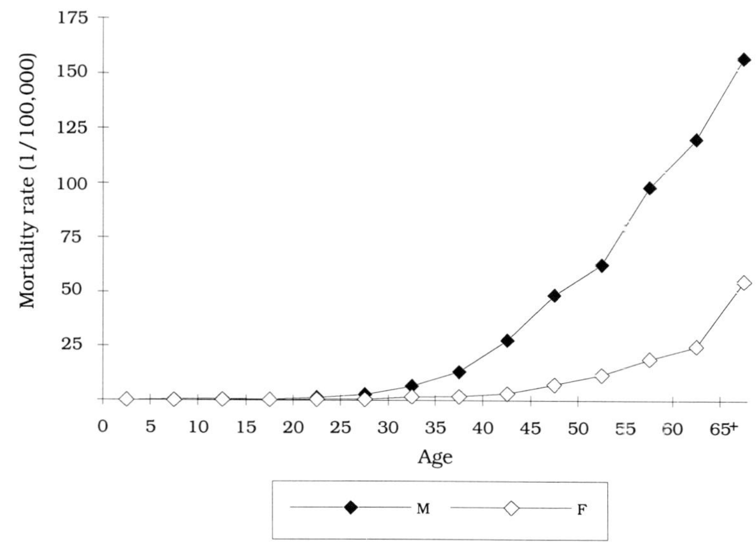

Number of communities on map by category based on standardized mortality ratio (SMR) during 1984–1988

Category	Number of communities Male	Female
SMR significantly high, in top 20%	3	4
SMR significantly high , not in top 20%	0	0
SMR not significantly high, in top 20%	10	9
SMR not significantly low, in bottom 20%	8	8
SMR significantly low, not in bottom 20%	1	1
SMR significantly low, in bottom 20%	5	0
other communities	38	43

Values of the standardized mortality ratio (SMR) which divide the 65 communities into quintile

Percentile	Male	Female
20th	80.26	68.01
40th	95.33	86.49
60th	101.73	104.15
80th	109.00	132.21
Lowest SMR	11.43	0.00
Highest SMR	208.86	206.21
No. of communities with zero death	0	1

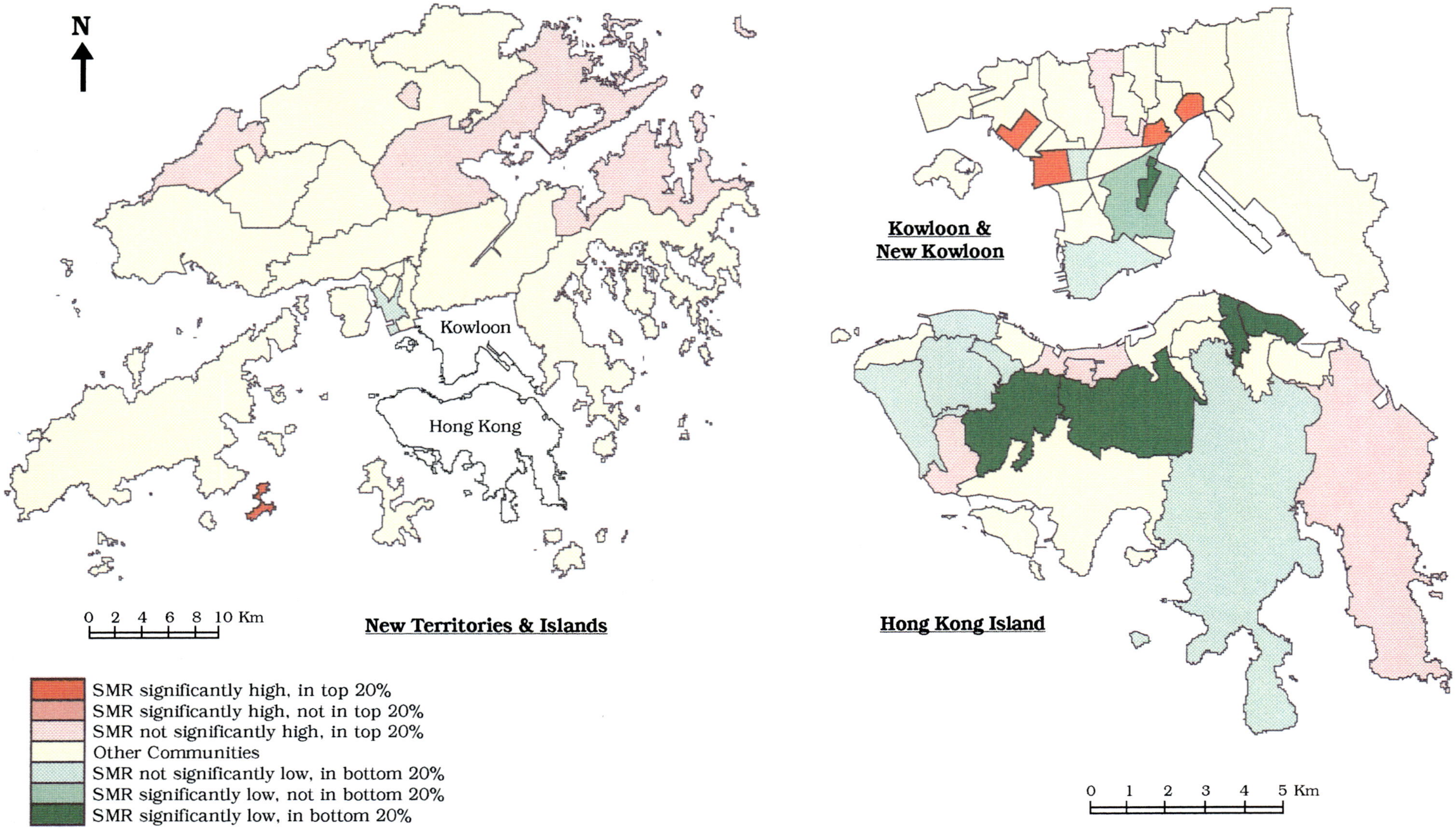

Liver Cancer (Male, 1989 -1993)

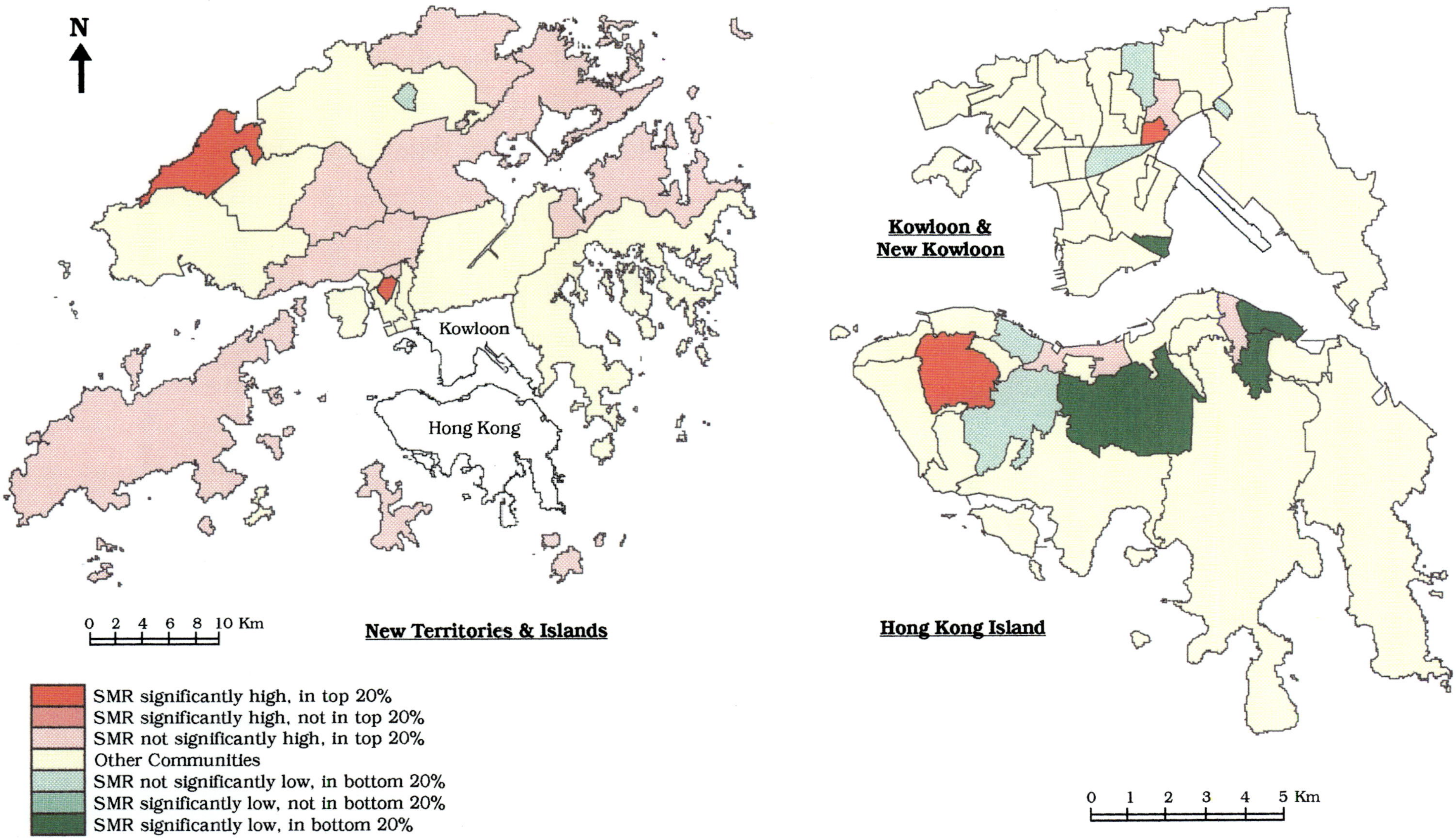

Liver Cancer (Female, 1989 -1993)

Number of Deaths, Standardised Mortality Ratio (SMR) and 95% Confidence Interval of Liver Cancer by 65 Communities in 1989–1993

Community	Male			Female		
	Number of deaths	SMR	95% C.I.	Number of deaths	SMR	95% C.I.
HK1	54	87.0	63.8 - 110.1	18	97.5	57.8 - 154.0
HK2	70	83.3	63.8 - 102.8	20	89.7	54.8 - 138.1
HK3	25	88.0	57.0 - 130.3	3	42.2	8.7 - 123.3
HK4	54	114.2	83.8 - 144.7	16	126.2	72.2 - 204.5
HK5	54	120.8	88.6 - 153.1	12	100.7	52.1 - 176.2
HK6	32	63.9	41.8 - 86.0	9	50.7	23.2 - 96.4
HK7	8	70.3	30.3 - 138.5	6	142.0	521.1 - 309.5
HK8	14	78.3	42.8 - 131.6	4	67.0	18.2 - 171.6
HK9	3	33.4	6.9 - 97.6	0	0.0	...
HK10	136	93.2	77.5 - 108.8	44	90.0	63.4 - 116.5
HK11	12	89.6	46.3 - 156.9	3	80.4	16.6 - 234.6
HK12	13	105.0	55.8 - 179.5	5	124.4	40.3 - 289.9
HK13	7	46.9	18.8 - 96.5	7	158.4	63.5 - 326.3
HK14	40	67.4	46.5 - 88.3	9	49.7	22.8 - 94.4
HK15	36	98.4	66.2 - 130.5	4	35.4	9.6 - 90.7
HK16	59	100.1	74.6 - 125.6	18	105.6	62.6 - 166.9
HK17	139	113.9	94.9 - 132.8	39	106.3	72.9 - 139.7
HK18	7	54.4	21.8 - 112.1	4	86.4	23.5 - 221.2
HK19	59	115.7	86.2 - 145.2	15	103.0	57.7 - 170.0
HK20	123	112.5	92.6 - 132.4	33	101.4	66.8 - 135.9
HK21	10	79.2	38.0 - 145.7	2	65.0	7.9 - 234.8
KL1	30	79.1	50.8 - 107.4	9	85.9	39.3 - 163.2
KL2	113	123.1	100.4 - 145.8	21	100.1	61.9 - 153.1
KL3	20	79.1	48.3 - 121.8	6	78.9	28.9 - 171.9
KL4	71	96.4	74.0 - 118.8	16	89.7	51.3 - 145.2
KL5	53	100.2	73.2 - 127.2	17	124.4	72.5 - 199.1
KL6	16	89.7	51.3 - 145.3	4	54.9	14.9 - 140.4
KL7	12	86.7	44.8 - 151.8	6	119.4	43.8 - 260.3
KL8	31	67.1	43.5 - 90.7	15	120.6	67.6 - 199.1
KL9	150	83.6	70.2 - 96.9	54	105.3	77.2 - 133.4
KL10	35	105.2	70.4 - 140.1	4	38.0	10.3 - 97.2
KL11	41	100.7	69.9 - 131.5	11	86.3	43.1 - 154.5
KL12	13	99.0	52.7 - 169.3	0	0.0	...

Community	Male			Female		
	Number of deaths	SMR	95% C.I.	Number of deaths	SIR	95% C.I.
KL13	144	89.2	74.7 - 103.8	35	82.2	55.0 - 109.5
KL14	99	106.3	85.4 - 127.3	27	89.3	55.6 - 123.0
KL15	32	159.9	104.5 - 215.3	7	118.6	47.6 - 244.3
KL16	37	99.7	67.6 - 131.9	10	104.9	50.3 - 193.0
KL17	18	127.9	75.9 - 202.1	8	126.1	54.4 - 248.4
KL18	8	104.5	45.0 - 205.9	0	0.0	...
KL19	168	105.2	89.3 - 121.1	53	102.3	74.7 - 129.8
KL20	41	109.2	75.8 - 142.6	6	52.6	19.3 - 114.7
KL21	52	93.0	67.7 - 118.3	24	130.8	83.8 - 194.8
KL22	22	173.2	108.6 - 261.5	4	116.2	31.6 - 297.5
KL23	43	170.6	119.6 - 221.5	14	198.3	108.3 - 333.2
KL24	36	111.4	75.0 - 147.8	6	65.1	23.9 - 141.9
KL25	488	93.6	85.3 - 102.0	148	97.6	81.9 - 113.4
NT1	46	98.9	70.3 - 127.4	20	151.4	92.5 - 233.2
NT2	35	80.9	54.1 - 107.8	13	104.2	55.5 - 178.2
NT3	73	87.8	67.7 - 107.9	19	93.8	56.5 - 146.3
NT4	65	112.8	85.3 - 140.2	22	138.4	86.8 - 209.0
NT5	117	102.9	84.3 - 121.6	38	239.0	163.0 - 315.0
NT6	77	98.1	76.2 - 120.0	18	84.3	50.0 - 133.2
NT7	92	110.3	87.7 - 132.8	14	67.9	37.1 - 114.1
NT8	189	99.0	84.9 - 113.1	55	108.9	80.1 - 137.6
NT9	31	153.4	99.4 - 207.4	13	204.4	108.7 - 349.5
NT10	119	112.1	91.9 - 132.2	33	110.1	72.5 - 147.6
NT11	19	104.4	62.8 - 162.9	8	138.9	59.9 - 273.7
NT12	102	102.9	82.9 - 122.8	34	117.5	78.0 - 157.0
NT13	27	127.3	79.3 - 175.3	3	46.0	9.5 - 134.4
NT14	11	104.9	52.3 - 187.8	8	224.7	96.8 - 442.6
NT15	139	119.5	99.6 - 139.3	45	126.4	89.5 - 163.4
NT16	311	103.8	92.3 - 115.4	106	113.7	92.1 - 135.4
NT17	77	104.6	81.2 - 127.9	18	80.7	47.8 - 127.5
NT18	30	176.4	113.3 - 239.5	6	107.7	39.5 - 234.8
NT19	21	96.2	59.5 - 147.1	9	131.5	60.2 - 249.9

LIVER CANCER

Sex-Age specific mortality rate (1/100,000) of liver cancer in Hong Kong (1989–1993)

	Male		Female	
Age	No. of deaths	Mortality rate	No. of deaths	Mortality rate
0–4	2	0.21	1	0.11
5–9	6	0.57	2	0.20
10–14	6	0.55	0	0.00
15–19	8	0.73	1	0.10
20–24	10	0.88	1	0.09
25–29	34	2.36	13	0.88
30–34	107	6.86	19	1.25
35–39	185	13.82	28	2.23
40–44	273	24.79	32	3.29
45–49	289	39.56	31	5.19
50–54	419	60.39	70	12.29
55–59	559	79.99	110	18.06
60–64	689	111.62	164	28.38
65+	1722	155.46	786	55.95
TOTAL	4309	29.46	1258	8.99

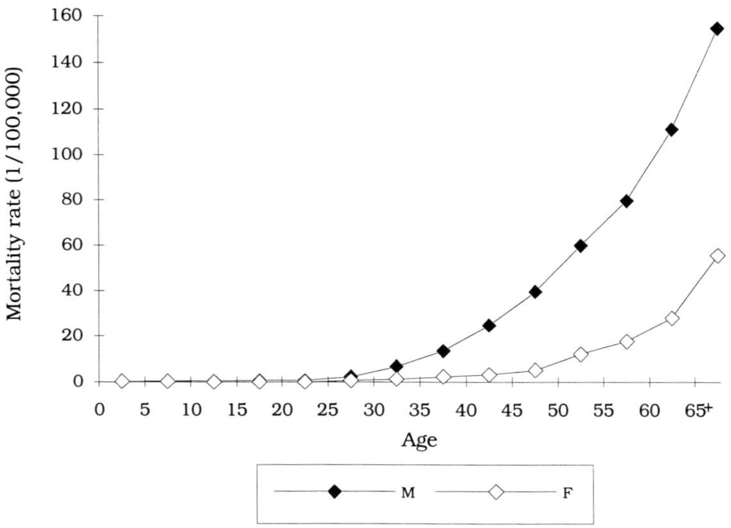

Number of communities on map by category based on standardized mortality ratio (SMR) during 1989–1993

Category	Number of communities Male	Female
SMR significantly high, in top 20%	5	4
SMR significantly high , not in top 20%	0	0
SMR not significantly high, in top 20%	8	9
SMR not significantly low, in bottom 20%	8	5
SMR significantly low, not in bottom 20%	0	4
SMR significantly low, in bottom 20%	5	4
other communities	39	39

Values of the standardized mortality ratio (SMR) which divide the 65 communities into quintile

Percentile	Male	Female
20th	83.32	65.09
40th	96.40	89.70
60th	104.39	105.65
80th	112.76	126.11
Lowest SMR	33.41	0.00
Highest SMR	176.37	239.03
No. of communities with zero cases	0	3

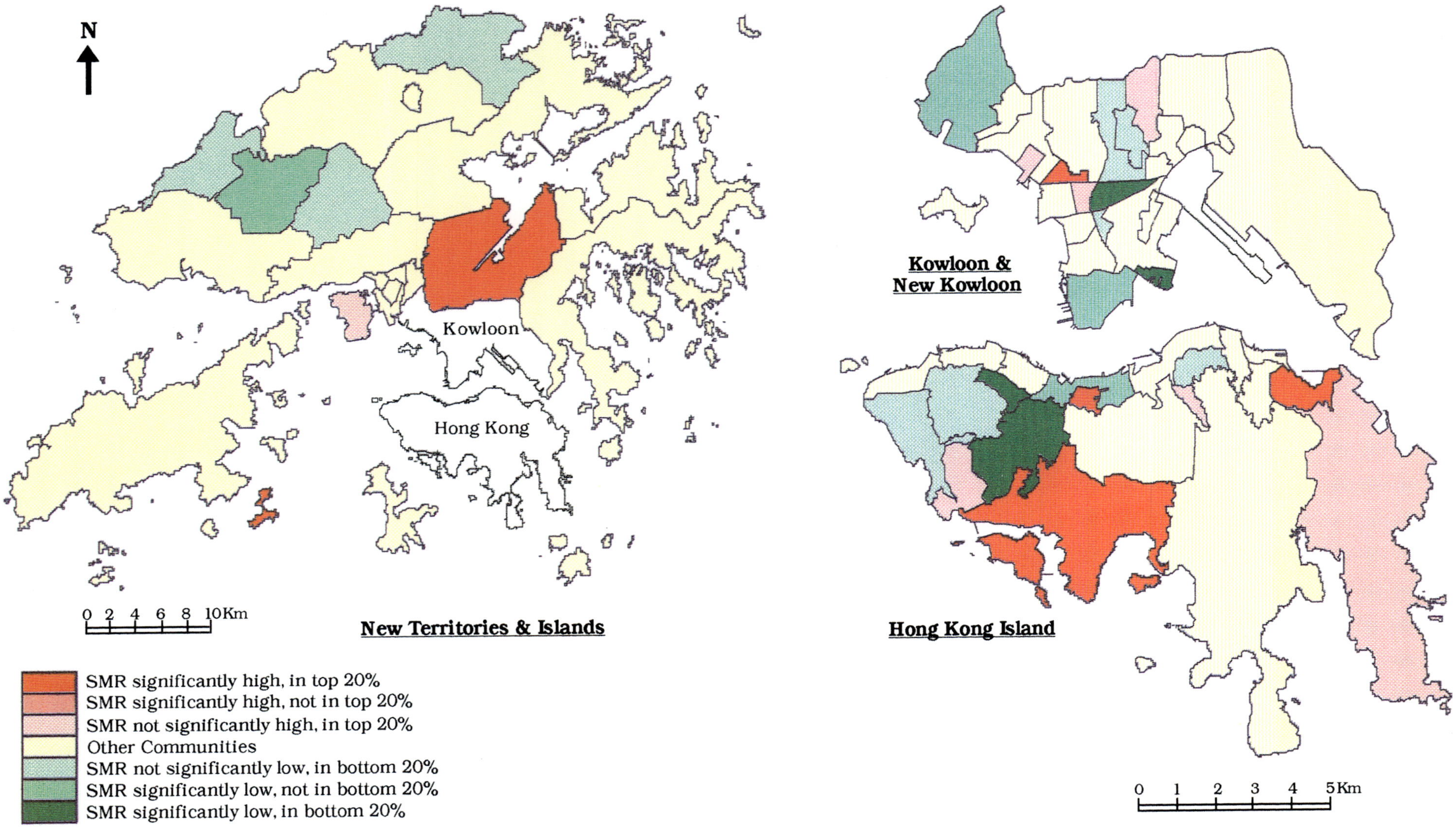

Lung Cancer (Male, 1979 - 1983)

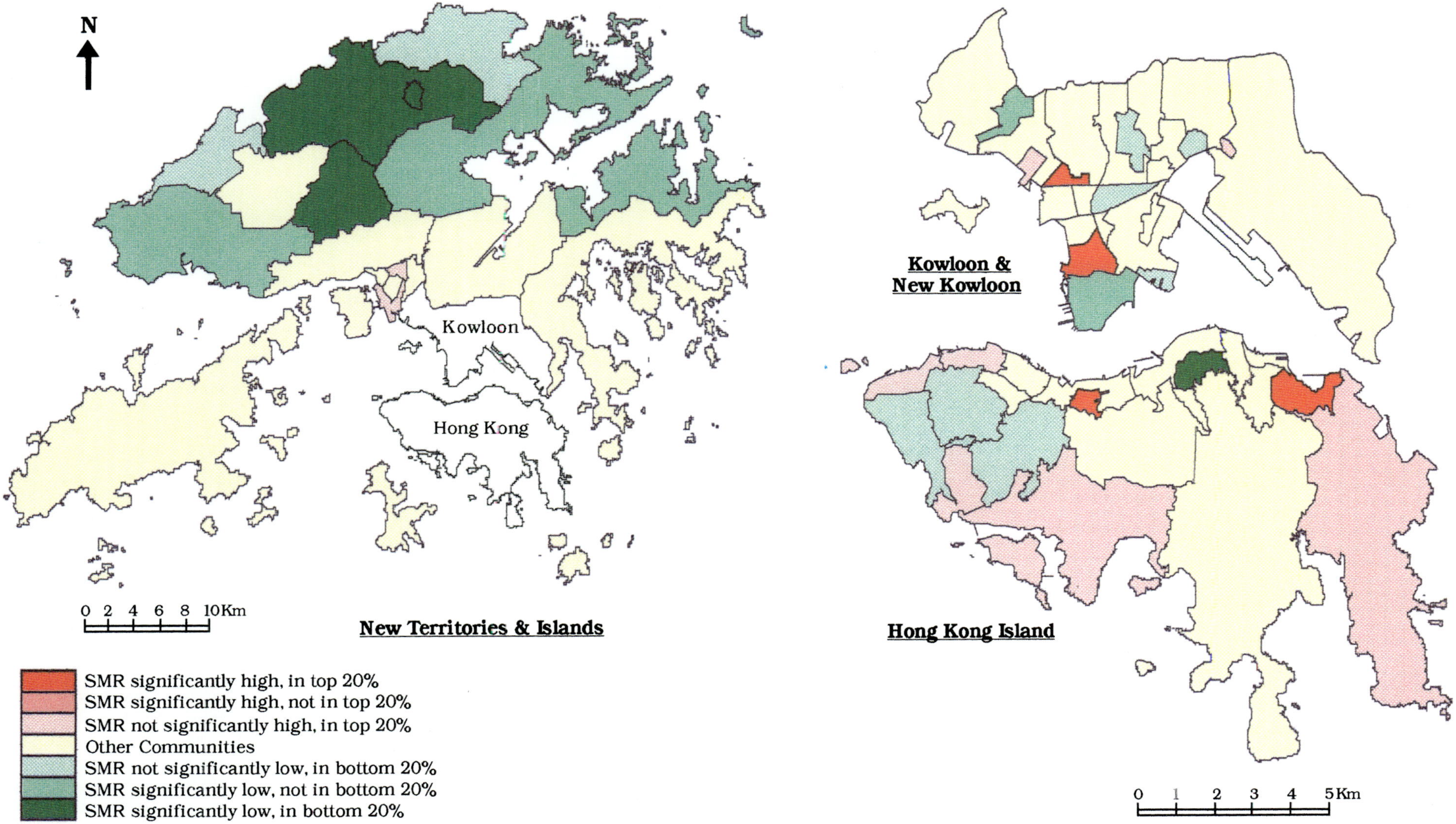

Lung Cancer (Female, 1979 - 1983)

Number of Deaths, Standardised Mortality Ratio (SMR) and 95% Confidence Interval of Lung Cancer by 65 Communities in 1979–1983

	Male			Female		
Community	Number of deaths	SMR	95% C.I.	Number of deaths	SMR	95% C.I.
HK1	115	110.4	90.2 - 130.6	67	125.6	95.5 - 155.6
HK2	185	110.7	94.7 - 126.6	94	121.6	97.0 - 146.2
HK3	65	98.6	74.6 - 122.6	30	105.6	67.8 - 143.4
HK4	82	81.0	63.4 - 98.5	50	100.6	72.7 - 128.5
HK5	144	146.2	122.3 - 170.1	72	153.3	117.9 - 188.8
HK6	66	81.4	61.8 - 101.1	53	95.6	69.8 - 121.3
HK7	9	56.3	25.8 - 106.8	7	62.1	24.9 - 128.0
HK8	17	53.6	31.1 - 85.7	23	101.1	64.0 - 151.9
HK9	4	27.5	7.5 - 70.5	4	39.3	10.7 - 100.5
HK10	226	101.9	88.6 - 115.2	127	93.2	77.0 - 109.5
HK11	26	127.6	78.6 - 176.7	7	73.0	29.3 - 150.4
HK12	10	61.2	29.4 - 112.6	5	39.3	12.7 - 91.9
HK13	25	94.3	57.4 - 131.3	12	80.6	41.6 - 140.7
HK14	61	97.1	72.8 - 121.5	28	77.8	49.0 - 106.6
HK15	24	95.1	60.9 - 141.5	14	91.0	49.7 - 152.7
HK16	167	139.3	118.2 - 160.4	78	133.0	103.5 - 162.5
HK17	149	113.8	95.6 - 132.1	76	116.2	90.1 - 142.4
HK18	11	60.8	30.4 - 108.7	7	63.5	25.5 - 130.9
HK19	71	116.1	89.1 - 143.1	46	136.5	97.0 - 175.9
HK20	170	123.9	105.3 - 142.5	79	115.9	90.3 - 141.5
HK21	15	88.1	49.2 - 145.3	8	98.9	42.6 - 194.7
KL1	70	80.1	61.3 - 98.8	31	72.7	47.1 - 98.2
KL2	160	89.2	75.3 - 103.0	97	109.4	87.6 - 131.1
KL3	60	115.0	85.9 - 144.1	31	107.1	69.4 - 144.8
KL4	144	98.4	82.4 - 114.5	80	114.8	89.6 - 139.9
KL5	122	99.2	81.6 - 116.8	76	132.7	102.8 - 162.5
KL6	17	55.2	32.1 - 88.3	14	62.1	33.9 - 104.2
KL7	14	62.7	34.3 - 105.2	12	78.3	40.4 - 136.7
KL8	71	91.3	70.1 - 112.6	42	99.7	69.5 - 129.8
KL9	281	98.1	86.6 - 109.6	180	113.9	97.3 - 130.6
KL10	14	50.3	27.5 - 84.3	9	53.3	24.5 - 101.1
KL11	59	76.7	57.1 - 96.3	44	96.4	67.9 - 124.9
KL12	19	78.2	47.1 - 122.2	8	72.1	31.1 - 142.0
KL13	280	94.1	83.1 - 105.2	167	115.4	97.9 - 132.9
KL14	194	109.3	94.0 - 124.7	71	86.8	66.6 - 107.0
KL15	21	151.3	93.4 - 231.4	12	171.4	88.4 - 299.1
KL16	90	129.9	103.1 - 156.7	58	161.5	120.0 - 203.1
KL17	13	65.2	34.7 - 111.5	15	95.4	53.3 - 157.5
KL18	9	71.3	32.7 - 135.3	4	51.9	14.1 - 132.7
KL19	253	97.9	85.9 - 110.0	147	105.2	88.2 - 122.2
KL20	105	114.9	92.9 - 136.9	45	95.3	67.5 - 123.2
KL21	147	99.3	83.2 - 115.3	63	82.1	61.8 - 102.3
KL22	20	80.6	49.2 - 124.6	8	71.3	30.7 - 140.4
KL23	62	80.8	60.7 - 101.0	32	84.4	55.2 - 113.7
KL24	47	95.5	68.2 - 122.8	34	143.5	95.3 - 191.7
KL25	724	102.2	94.7 - 109.6	344	95.1	85.1 - 105.2
NT1	35	99.4	66.5 - 132.4	19	98.8	59.5 - 154.4
NT2	54	105.2	77.2 - 133.3	34	134.9	89.6 - 180.3
NT3	89	84.9	67.2 - 102.5	44	97.8	68.9 - 126.6
NT4	50	90.5	65.4 - 115.6	36	119.8	80.7 - 159.0
NT5	204	101.9	87.9 - 115.9	95	94.6	75.6 - 113.6
NT6	110	112.6	91.6 - 133.6	41	79.4	55.1 - 103.7
NT7	40	122.7	84.7 - 160.7	15	92.1	51.4 - 151.9
NT8	106	99.0	80.1 - 117.8	38	73.9	50.4 - 97.4
NT9	26	75.6	46.6 - 104.7	10	62.4	30.0 - 114.7
NT10	118	83.2	68.2 - 98.2	53	80.4	58.7 - 102.0
NT11	19	64.5	38.9 - 100.8	5	38.4	12.4 - 89.7
NT12	117	86.3	70.6 - 101.9	46	71.4	50.8 - 92.1
NT13	20	79.2	48.3 - 122.4	4	31.2	8.5 - 79.8
NT14	18	76.4	45.2 - 120.7	7	52.5	21.1 - 108.3
NT15	93	100.1	79.7 - 120.4	37	74.7	50.6 - 98.7
NT16	147	131.0	109.9 - 152.2	66	107.6	81.6 - 133.5
NT17	60	109.5	81.8 - 137.3	21	73.6	45.4 - 112.6
NT18	46	170.2	121.0 - 219.3	13	87.4	46.5 - 149.4
NT19	38	81.6	55.7 - 107.6	22	88.1	55.1 - 133.5

LUNG CANCER

Sex-Age specific mortality rate (1/100,000) of lung cancer in Hong Kong (1979–1983)

	Male		Female	
Age	No. of deaths	Mortality rate	No. of deaths	Mortality rate
0–4	1	0.09	0	0.00
5–9	0	0.00	1	0.10
10–14	2	0.17	1	0.09
15–19	3	0.21	0	0.00
20–24	7	0.46	4	0.29
25–29	11	0.83	10	0.86
30–34	23	2.09	10	1.09
35–39	46	6.37	17	3.06
40–44	109	15.49	60	10.85
45–49	309	42.84	100	16.52
50–54	599	87.19	180	29.52
55–59	921	161.91	340	63.58
60–64	1132	247.73	475	104.13
65+	2865	420.23	1921	190.30
TOTAL	6028	45.72	3119	25.62

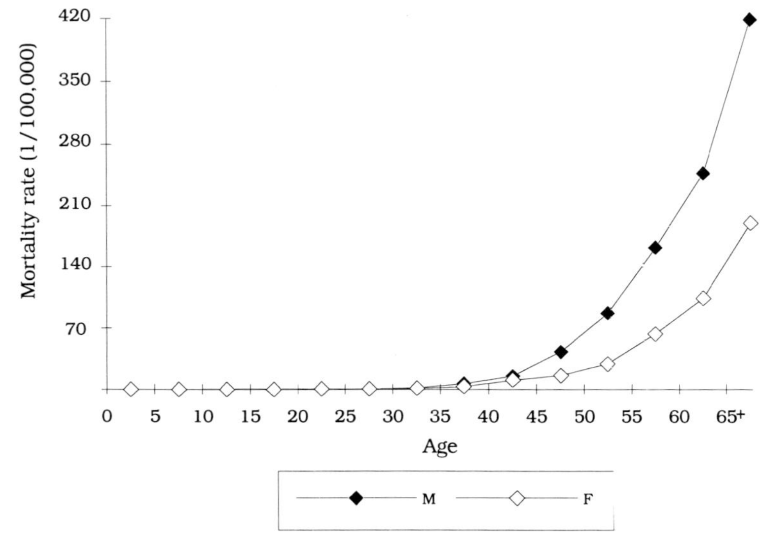

Number of communities on map by category based on standardized mortality ratio (SMR) during 1979–1983

Category	Number of communities Male	Number of communities Female
SMR significantly high, in top 20%	6	4
SMR significantly high , not in top 20%	0	0
SMR not significantly high, in top 20%	7	9
SMR not significantly low, in bottom 20%	9	9
SMR significantly low, not in bottom 20%	4	4
SMR significantly low, in bottom 20%	4	4
other communities	35	35

Values of the standardized mortality ratio (SMR) which divide the 65 communities into quintile

Percentile	Male	Female
20th	76.39	71.42
40th	88.07	84.42
60th	98.99	97.76
80th	112.59	115.44
Lowest SMR	27.55	31.20
Highest SMR	170.17	171.41
No. of communities with zero death	0	0

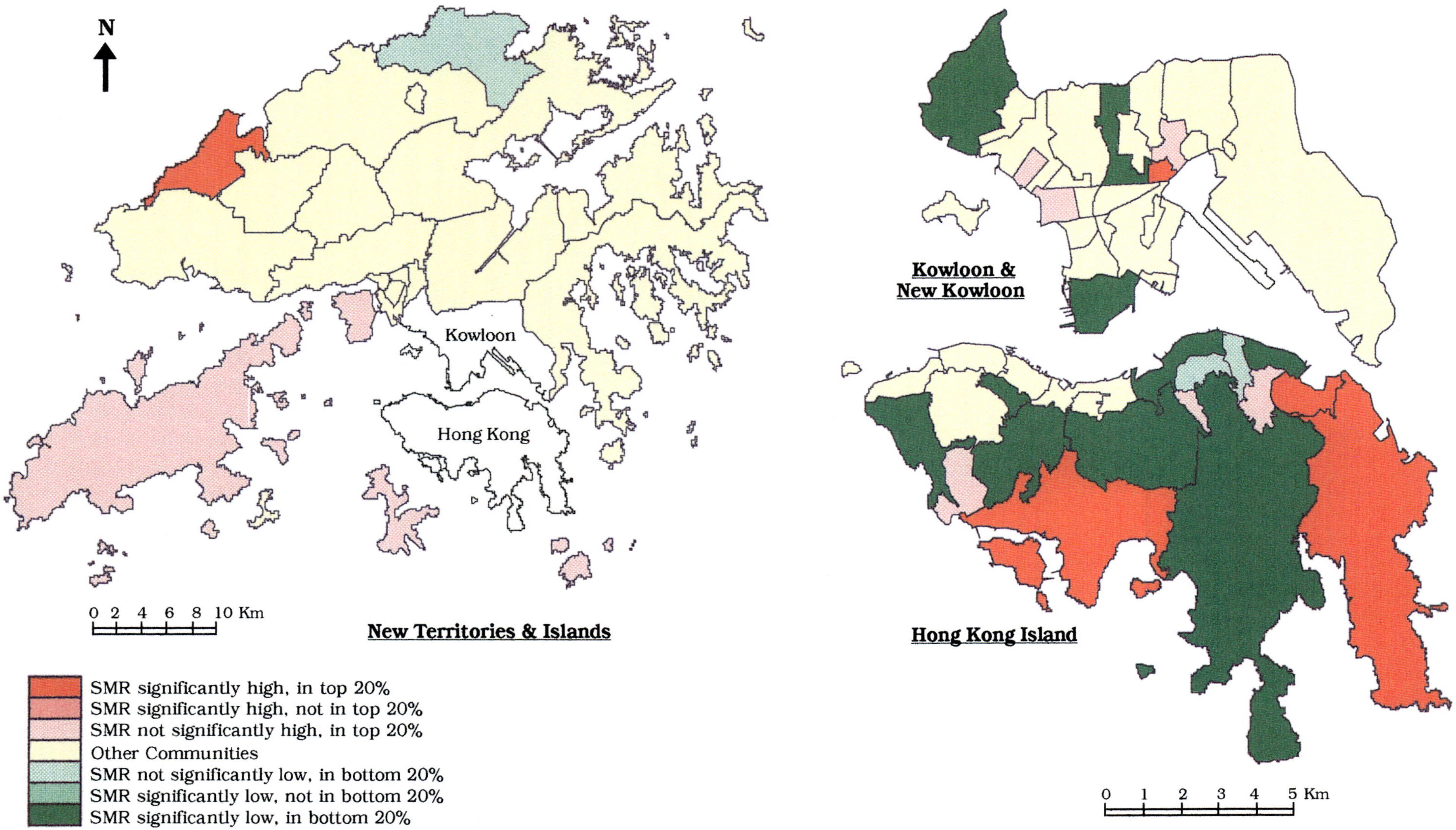

Lung Cancer (Male, 1984 -1988)

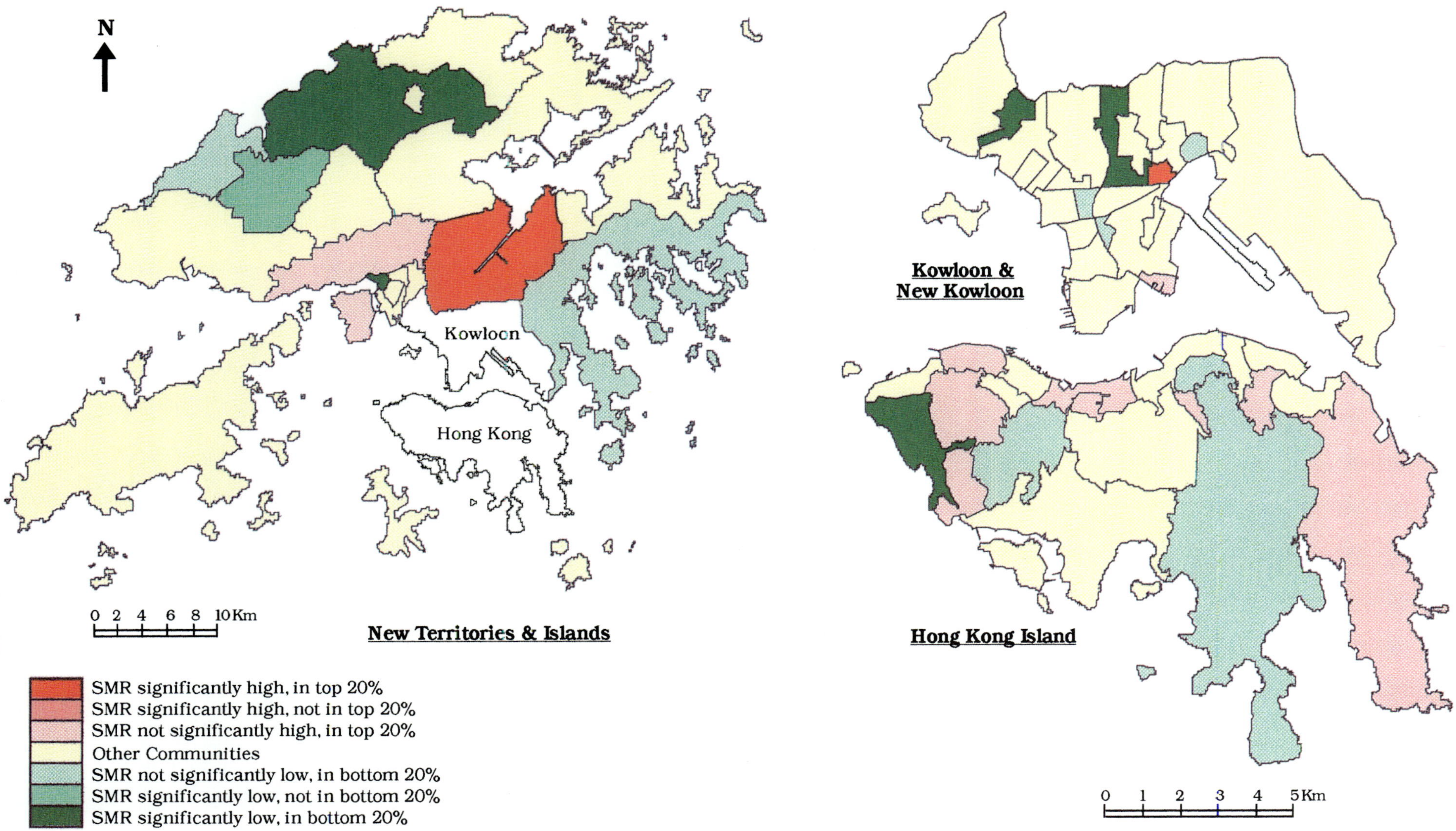

Lung Cancer (Female, 1984 – 1988)

Number of Deaths, Standardised Mortality Ratio (SMR) and 95% Confidence Interval of Lung Cancer by 65 Communities in 1984–1988

	Male			Female		
Community	Number of deaths	SMR	95% C.I.	Number of deaths	SMR	95% C.I.
HK1	119	98.7	81.0 - 116.5	62	98.3	73.8 - 122.7
HK2	157	92.0	77.6 - 106.4	107	120.9	98.0 - 143.9
HK3	68	105.4	80.3 - 130.5	31	104.8	67.9 - 141.6
HK4	100	98.2	79.0 - 117.5	64	119.9	90.5 - 149.3
HK5	100	108.2	87.0 - 129.4	65	129.1	97.7 - 160.5
HK6	64	69.7	52.7 - 86.8	54	87.4	64.1 - 110.7
HK7	17	92.4	53.7 - 147.8	15	121.1	67.7 - 199.8
HK8	17	49.4	25.9 - 72.9	25	111.6	72.0 - 164.7
HK9	2	13.4	1.6 - 48.5	7	63.1	25.3 - 130.0
HK10	190	74.9	64.3 - 85.6	160	98.3	83.1 - 113.6
HK11	26	111.4	72.8 - 163.4	17	154.0	89.6 - 246.5
HK12	13	62.4	33.2 - 106.6	9	67.5	31.0 - 128.1
HK13	23	74.1	43.8 - 104.4	16	103.1	58.9 - 167.4
HK14	64	69.0	52.1 - 85.9	54	92.0	67.4 - 116.5
HK15	39	132.2	90.7 - 173.7	25	129.0	83.3 - 190.3
HK16	157	120.3	101.5 - 139.1	70	101.0	77.4 - 124.7
HK17	229	132.2	115.1 - 149.3	109	117.4	95.3 - 139.4
HK18	9	48.4	22.2 - 91.8	4	32.7	8.9 - 83.7
HK19	94	114.7	91.5 - 137.9	53	115.4	84.4 - 146.5
HK20	256	143.1	125.6 - 160.7	96	100.9	80.7 - 121.1
HK21	12	56.0	28.9 - 97.8	9	72.0	33.0 - 136.5
KL1	69	75.2	57.5 - 92.9	53	113.8	83.2 - 144.5
KL2	197	111.6	96.0 - 127.1	102	111.5	89.8 - 133.1
KL3	55	103.0	75.8 - 130.3	23	73.2	43.3 - 103.1
KL4	149	89.8	75.4 - 104.3	78	101.0	78.6 - 123.4
KL5	113	92.3	75.3 - 109.4	54	89.7	65.8 - 113.6
KL6	35	101.3	67.8 - 134.9	25	107.2	69.2 - 158.2
KL7	21	86.5	53.4 - 132.2	10	70.0	33.6 - 128.7
KL8	78	91.8	71.5 - 112.2	43	96.7	67.8 - 125.7
KL9	334	100.9	90.1 - 111.7	181	99.3	84.9 - 113.8
KL10	35	109.1	73.0 - 145.2	22	115.0	71.9 - 174.2
KL11	73	76.2	58.7 - 93.7	47	85.9	61.3 - 110.4
KL12	26	96.2	59.2 - 133.1	3	23.1	4.8 - 67.6
KL13	301	100.3	89.0 - 111.7	156	101.6	85.7 - 117.6
KL14	233	107.7	93.8 - 121.5	118	106.9	87.6 - 126.2
KL15	45	123.0	87.1 - 159.0	22	105.5	65.9 - 159.8
KL16	65	87.4	66.1 - 108.6	42	114.0	79.5 - 148.4
KL17	17	51.7	27.1 - 76.2	20	67.4	37.9 - 96.9
KL18	14	101.2	55.3 - 169.8	6	78.7	28.8 - 171.4
KL19	322	104.5	93.1 - 115.9	172	103.8	88.3 - 119.3
KL20	75	98.9	76.5 - 121.3	39	90.9	62.4 - 119.5
KL21	152	116.3	97.8 - 134.8	64	97.8	73.9 - 121.8
KL22	27	100.3	62.5 - 138.1	9	67.5	31.0 - 128.0
KL23	98	148.3	119.0 - 177.7	51	152.0	110.3 - 193.7
KL24	54	83.5	61.2 - 105.8	26	88.4	54.4 - 122.3
KL25	965	99.4	93.2 - 105.7	471	92.9	84.5 - 101.3
NT1	43	81.6	57.2 - 106.0	37	124.7	84.5 - 164.9
NT2	57	85.7	63.4 - 107.9	36	105.6	71.1 - 140.1
NT3	118	97.8	80.2 - 115.5	39	72.7	49.9 - 95.5
NT4	104	101.2	81.7 - 120.6	59	108.2	80.6 - 135.8
NT5	215	98.0	84.9 - 111.1	124	114.8	94.6 - 135.0
NT6	111	86.3	70.3 - 102.4	70	110.0	84.2 - 135.7
NT7	74	118.5	91.5 - 145.6	39	132.0	90.6 - 173.5
NT8	207	97.4	84.2 - 110.7	107	88.0	71.3 - 104.7
NT9	60	149.2	111.4 - 186.9	14	63.6	34.8 - 106.8
NT10	190	100.9	86.5 - 115.2	75	79.5	61.5 - 97.5
NT11	26	77.3	47.6 - 107.0	21	108.7	67.1 - 166.2
NT12	172	104.5	88.9 - 120.2	54	59.2	43.4 - 75.0
NT13	47	110.6	79.0 - 142.2	16	81.1	46.3 - 131.6
NT14	21	75.8	43.4 - 108.2	12	79.7	41.1 - 139.0
NT15	159	106.1	89.6 - 122.6	98	108.1	86.7 - 129.5
NT16	336	103.2	92.1 - 114.2	250	120.6	105.7 - 135.6
NT17	65	100.3	75.9 - 124.7	26	74.8	46.0 - 103.5
NT18	35	108.1	72.3 - 144.0	21	112.2	69.3 - 171.6
NT19	57	115.7	85.6 - 145.7	23	85.6	50.6 - 120.6

LUNG CANCER

Sex-Age specific mortality rate (1/100,000) of lung cancer in Hong Kong (1984–1988)

	Male		Female	
Age	No. of deaths	Mortality rate	No. of deaths	Mortality rate
0–4	1	0.09	0	0.00
5–9	0	0.00	0	0.00
10–14	0	0.00	0	0.00
15–19	3	0.25	0	0.00
20–24	3	0.21	2	0.14
25–29	8	0.51	7	0.47
30–34	33	2.44	18	1.45
35–39	63	5.68	43	4.43
40–44	116	15.83	48	8.01
45–49	242	34.38	80	13.71
50–54	641	87.46	186	29.45
55–59	988	148.75	312	51.36
60–64	1330	246.25	521	97.33
65+	4059	449.55	2812	227.84
TOTAL	7487	52.51	4029	30.02

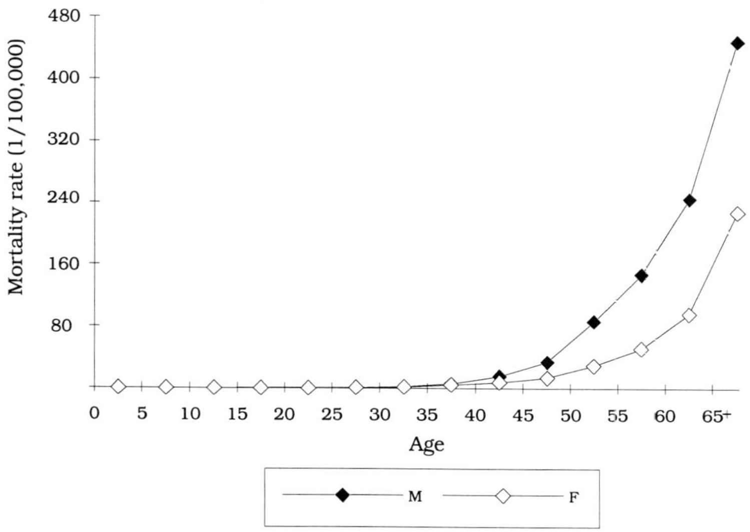

Number of communities on map by category based on standardized mortality ratio (SMR) during 1984–1988

Category	Number of communities Male	Female
SMR significantly high, in top 20%	5	2
SMR significantly high , not in top 20%	0	0
SMR not significantly high, in top 20%	8	11
SMR not significantly low, in bottom 20%	3	8
SMR significantly low, not in bottom 20%	0	1
SMR significantly low, in bottom 20%	10	5
other communities	39	38

Values of the standardized mortality ratio (SMR) which divide the 65 communities into quintile

Percentile	Male	Female
20th	76.21	74.77
40th	96.17	92.93
60th	101.17	105.45
80th	110.59	114.75
Lowest SMR	13.44	23.11
Highest SMR	149.15	154.04
No. of communities with zero death	0	0

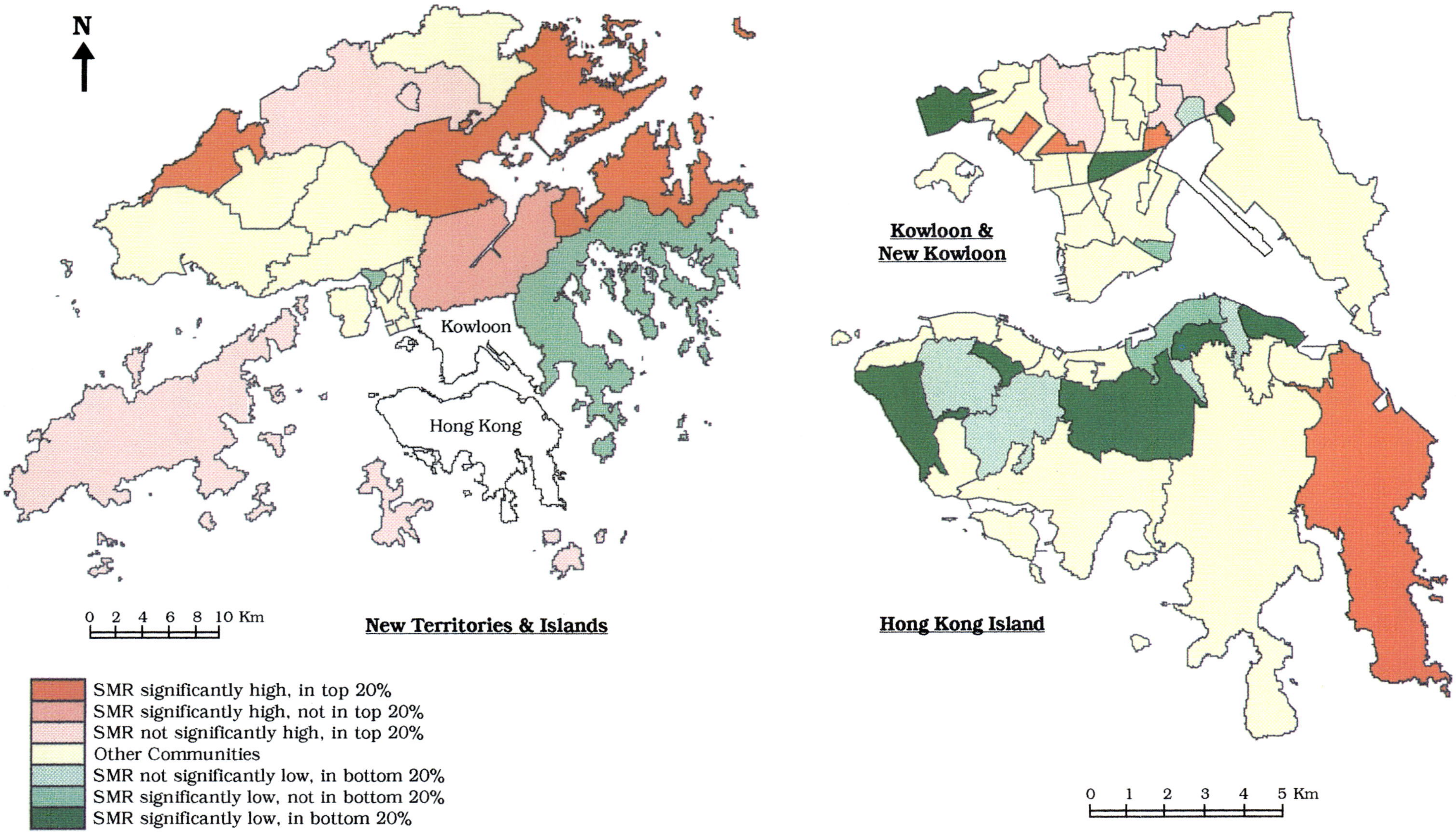

Lung Cancer (Male, 1989 -1993)

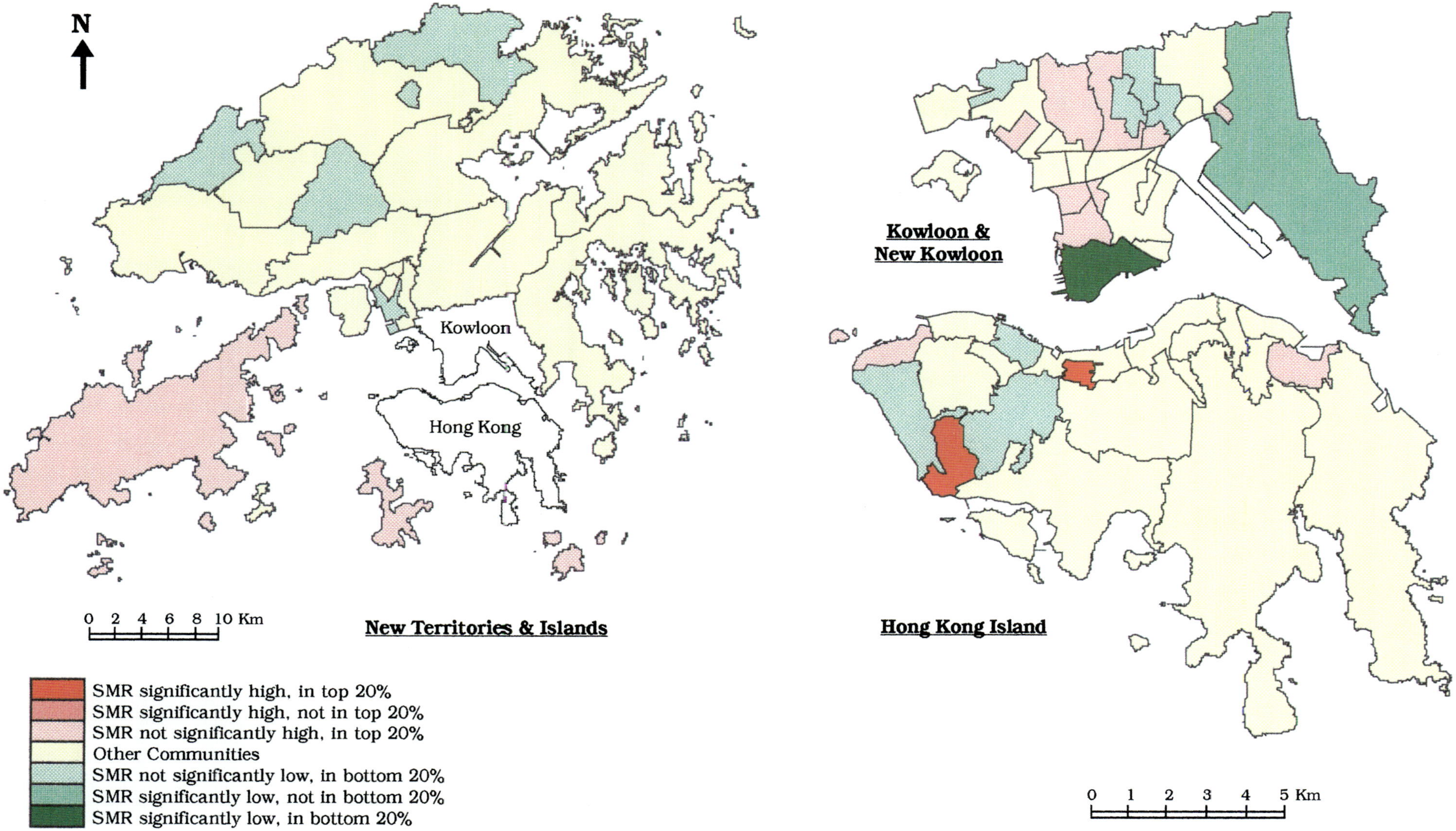

Lung Cancer (Female, 1989 -1993)

Number of Deaths, Standardised Mortality Ratio (SMR) and 95% Confidence Interval of Lung Cancer by 65 Communities in 1989–1993

Community	Male			Female		
	Number of deaths	SMR	95% C.I.	Number of deaths	SMR	95% C.I.
HK1	128	97.6	80.7 - 114.5	78	118.5	92.2 - 144.8
HK2	164	92.4	78.3 - 106.6	86	107.7	84.9 - 130.4
HK3	57	92.7	68.6 - 116.7	17	65.6	38.3 - 105.0
HK4	85	84.6	66.6 - 102.6	43	93.4	65.5 - 121.3
HK5	104	108.5	87.6 - 129.3	63	144.9	109.1 - 180.6
HK6	61	58.2	43.6 - 72.7	56	87.8	64.8 - 110.8
HK7	14	61.4	33.5 - 103.1	16	106.2	60.8 - 172.1
HK8	22	59.4	37.2 - 89.7	20	95.5	58.3 - 147.1
HK9	12	72.3	37.4 - 126.6	7	69.1	27.7 - 142.4
HK10	237	79.4	69.3 - 89.6	165	93.8	79.5 - 108.1
HK11	21	73.1	45.2 - 111.8	14	108.9	59.5 - 183.0
HK12	8	33.5	14.4 - 65.9	14	100.0	54.6 - 168.0
HK13	23	69.8	44.3 - 104.7	18	113.7	67.4 - 179.7
HK14	72	61.7	47.4 - 75.9	73	115.9	89.3 - 142.4
HK15	68	98.9	75.4 - 122.4	42	109.3	76.2 - 142.3
HK16	134	108.2	89.9 - 126.5	77	127.3	98.9 - 155.7
HK17	307	120.1	106.7 - 133.6	126	96.4	79.5 - 113.2
HK18	10	37.5	18.0 - 69.0	13	75.8	40.3 - 129.6
HK19	116	110.1	90.1 - 130.1	67	132.3	100.6 - 164.0
HK20	244	106.2	92.9 - 119.5	135	115.4	96.0 - 134.9
HK21	21	97.9	60.6 - 149.9	9	88.0	40.3 - 167.2
KL1	64	81.0	61.2 - 100.9	24	64.1	41.1 - 95.5
KL2	204	109.5	94.5 - 124.5	93	111.2	88.6 - 133.8
KL3	49	91.0	65.5 - 116.4	25	89.6	58.0 - 132.7
KL4	160	103.3	87.3 - 119.3	78	120.8	94.0 - 147.6
KL5	111	98.2	79.9 - 116.4	65	129.6	98.1 - 161.2
KL6	23	55.7	35.3 - 83.6	28	101.3	63.8 - 138.8
KL7	23	80.0	50.7 - 120.0	22	120.2	75.4 - 181.5
KL8	94	99.6	79.5 - 119.7	44	99.9	70.4 - 129.4
KL9	352	94.4	84.6 - 104.3	176	97.0	82.7 - 111.3
KL10	56	75.9	54.0 - 97.9	32	88.1	57.6 - 118.7
KL11	63	75.9	57.2 - 94.7	40	88.0	60.7 - 115.2
KL12	18	98.9	58.6 - 156.2	10	80.6	38.7 - 148.3

Community	Male			Female		
	Number of deaths	SMR	95% C.I.	Number of deaths	SMR	95% C.I.
KL13	341	98.9	88.4 - 109.4	147	95.5	80.0 - 110.9
KL14	246	112.3	98.3 - 126.4	133	118.4	98.3 - 138.6
KL15	65	154.6	117.0 - 192.2	25	117.2	75.8 - 173.5
KL16	101	132.7	106.8 - 158.5	38	110.3	75.2 - 145.3
KL17	30	93.7	60.2 - 127.3	31	128.4	83.2 - 173.6
KL18	13	85.2	45.3 - 145.8	5	55.3	17.9 - 128.9
KL19	394	110.6	99.6 - 121.5	200	105.4	90.8 - 120.0
KL20	69	84.9	64.9 - 104.9	30	74.9	48.1 - 101.6
KL21	143	110.6	92.5 - 128.7	57	85.0	62.9 - 107.0
KL22	19	72.6	43.7 - 113.2	13	104.2	55.4 - 178.2
KL23	81	152.0	118.9 - 185.1	37	144.0	97.6 - 190.3
KL24	55	72.8	53.6 - 92.1	42	131.2	91.5 - 170.9
KL25	1118	103.4	97.3 - 109.4	493	91.3	83.3 - 99.4
NT1	74	90.0	69.5 - 110.5	51	113.2	82.1 - 144.3
NT2	74	83.9	64.8 - 103.1	37	82.3	55.8 - 108.8
NT3	126	78.1	64.5 - 91.8	59	85.6	63.7 - 107.4
NT4	116	103.1	84.3 - 121.8	51	91.5	66.4 - 116.6
NT5	258	108.9	95.6 - 122.2	105	94.3	76.3 - 112.4
NT6	165	104.9	88.9 - 120.9	76	101.0	78.3 - 123.7
NT7	151	104.9	88.1 - 121.6	59	85.4	63.6 - 107.2
NT8	333	99.6	88.9 - 110.3	177	101.8	86.8 - 116.8
NT9	66	144.3	109.5 - 179.2	20	83.2	50.8 - 128.1
NT10	211	95.0	82.1 - 107.8	115	106.6	87.2 - 126.1
NT11	34	82.3	54.6 - 110.0	16	73.8	42.2 - 119.6
NT12	228	111.3	96.8 - 125.7	98	93.8	75.2 - 112.3
NT13	48	112.5	80.7 - 144.3	19	80.9	48.7 - 126.1
NT14	23	95.3	60.4 - 142.9	9	66.7	30.5 - 126.6
NT15	273	120.4	106.1 - 134.7	128	100.6	83.2 - 118.1
NT16	620	110.2	101.5 - 118.9	321	97.3	86.6 - 107.9
NT17	116	82.6	67.5 - 97.6	68	86.7	66.1 - 107.4
NT18	48	122.3	87.7 - 156.9	24	116.0	74.3 - 172.8
NT19	57	120.3	89.1 - 151.6	30	116.5	74.8 - 158.1

LUNG CANCER

Sex-Age specific mortality rate (1/100,000) of lung cancer in Hong Kong (1989–1993)

	Male		Female	
Age	No. of deaths	Mortality rate	No. of deaths	Mortality rate
0–4	0	0.00	0	0.00
5–9	0	0.00	0	0.00
10–14	0	0.00	0	0.00
15–19	0	0.00	1	0.10
20–24	3	0.26	4	0.35
25–29	8	0.55	9	0.61
30–34	35	2.24	21	1.38
35–39	69	5.15	52	4.13
40–44	160	14.53	85	8.74
45–49	231	31.62	78	13.06
50–54	488	70.34	147	25.82
55–59	983	140.67	300	49.25
60–64	1435	232.46	465	80.46
65+	5410	488.40	3328	236.89
TOTAL	8822	0.06	4490	32.09

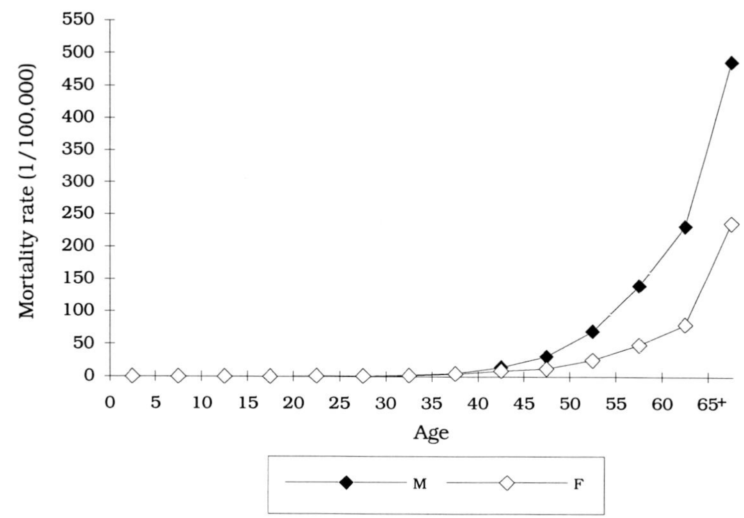

Number of communities on map by category based on standardized mortality ratio (SMR) during 1989–1993

Category	Number of communities Male	Female
SMR significantly high, in top 20%	6	2
SMR significantly high , not in top 20%	1	0
SMR not significantly high, in top 20%	7	11
SMR not significantly low, in bottom 20%	5	12
SMR significantly low, not in bottom 20%	4	1
SMR significantly low, in bottom 20%	8	1
other communities	34	38

Values of the standardized mortality ratio (SMR) which divide the 65 communities into quintile

Percentile	Male	Female
20th	75.94	84.98
40th	90.96	93.80
60th	99.57	104.23
80th	110.21	115.98
Lowest SMR	33.46	55.33
Highest SMR	154.64	144.87
No. of communities with zero cases	0	0

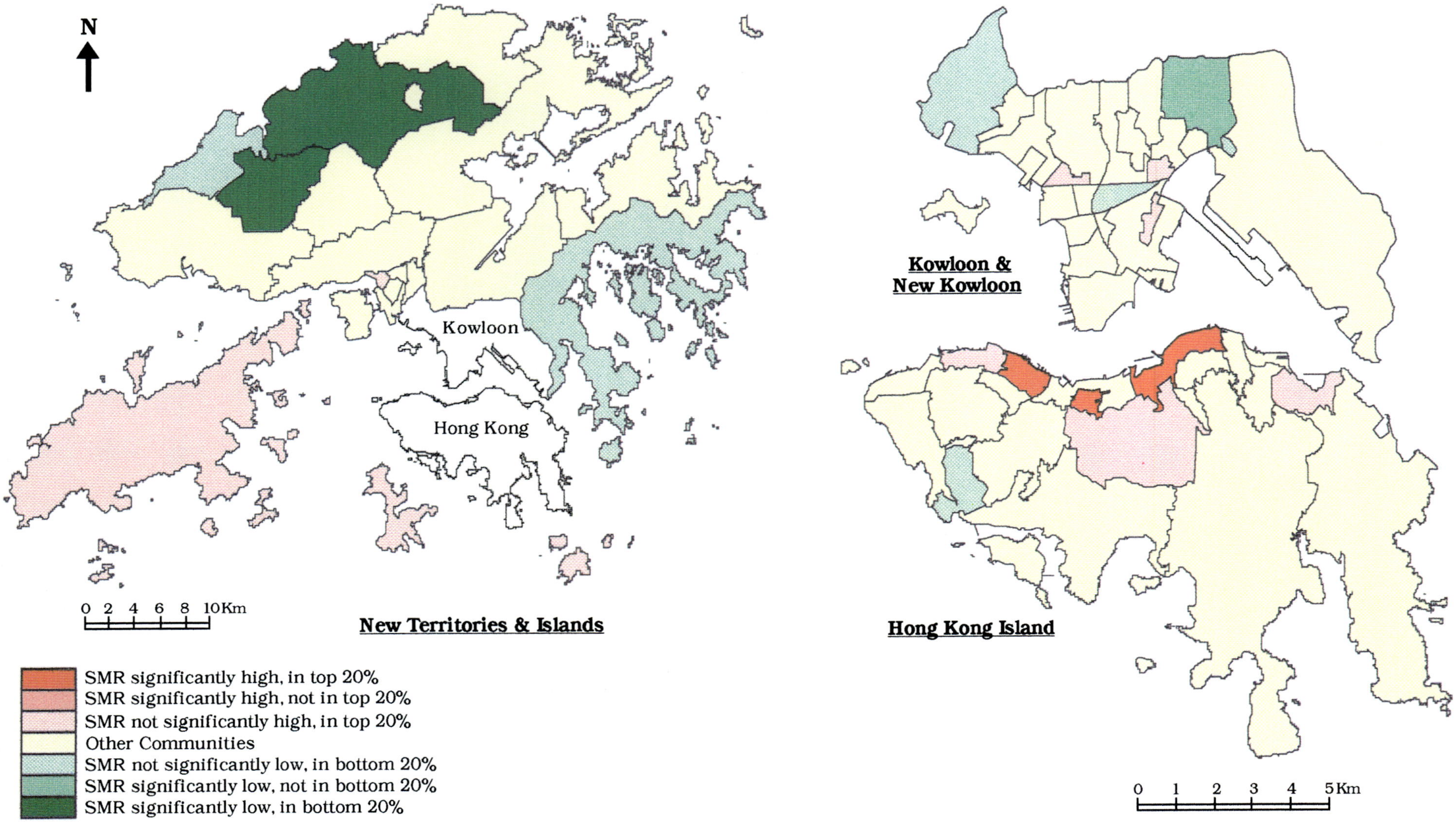

Breast Cancer (Female, 1979 – 1983)

Number of Deaths, Standardised Mortality Ratio (SMR) and 95% Confidence Interval of Breast Cancer by 65 Communities in 1979–1983

Community	Female			Community	Female			Community	Female		
	Number of deaths	SMR	95% C.I.		Number of deaths	SMR	95% C.I.		Number of deaths	SMR	95% C.I.
HK1	20	112.5	68.6 - 173.9	KL1	15	105.2	58.8 - 173.6	NT1	6	96.0	35.2 - 209.2
HK2	32	130.7	85.4 - 176.0	KL2	31	111.0	71.9 - 150.0	NT2	7	77.2	31.0 - 159.2
HK3	18	206.9	122.4 - 326.9	KL3	9	99.1	45.5 - 188.0	NT3	23	142.5	90.2 - 213.9
HK4	12	74.5	38.4 - 129.9	KL4	22	100.1	62.5 - 151.6	NT4	14	127.5	69.7 - 213.9
HK5	26	177.2	109.1 - 245.3	KL5	15	83.7	46.8 - 138.1	NT5	27	77.2	48.1 - 106.3
HK6	25	138.0	83.9 - 192.1	KL6	4	57.5	15.7 - 147.0	NT6	13	71.5	38.0 - 122.2
HK7	2	52.4	6.3 - 189.3	KL7	4	80.8	22.0 - 206.8	NT7	6	100.6	36.8 - 219.1
HK8	8	108.7	46.8 - 213.9	KL8	20	142.2	86.7 - 219.7	NT8	20	115.8	70.6 - 178.9
HK9	3	82.0	16.9 - 239.7	KL9	70	130.1	99.6 - 160.6	NT9	2	39.1	4.7 - 141.3
HK10	71	158.4	121.6 - 195.2	KL10	4	69.2	18.9 - 177.0	NT10	11	51.4	25.7 - 91.9
HK11	2	56.2	6.8 - 202.8	KL11	10	66.3	31.9 - 122.0	NT11	4	94.9	25.9 - 242.7
HK12	4	91.6	25.0 - 234.2	KL12	1	30.9	0.8 - 171.6	NT12	10	49.5	23.8 - 91.0
HK13	6	116.9	42.8 - 254.7	KL13	37	79.2	53.7 - 104.8	NT13	4	100.1	27.3 - 256.1
HK14	12	97.6	50.3 - 170.3	KL14	23	88.0	55.7 - 132.2	NT14	0	0.0	...
HK15	6	108.8	39.9 - 237.1	KL15	2	90.6	11.0 - 327.0	NT15	11	71.5	35.8 - 127.9
HK16	29	147.3	93.7 - 201.0	KL16	16	142.7	81.5 - 231.7	NT16	23	112.3	71.0 - 168.5
HK17	15	70.7	39.5 - 116.7	KL17	6	117.5	43.1 - 256.1	NT17	6	67.8	24.9 - 147.8
HK18	3	80.9	16.7 - 236.5	KL18	4	147.3	40.1 - 376.7	NT18	6	133.6	48.9 - 291.0
HK19	8	66.3	28.6 - 130.5	KL19	32	69.2	45.3 - 93.2	NT19	11	154.1	77.0 - 275.6
HK20	23	100.8	63.8 - 151.3	KL20	12	79.1	40.8 - 138.0				
HK21	4	126.7	34.5 - 324.1	KL21	18	74.4	44.0 - 117.5				
				KL22	2	54.5	6.6 - 196.8				
				KL23	17	137.2	79.8 - 219.5				
				KL24	5	56.9	18.4 - 133.0				
				KL25	119	95.8	78.6 - 113.0				

BREAST CANCER

Sex-Age specific mortality rate (1/100,000) of breast cancer in Hong Kong (1979–1983)

	Male		Female	
Age	No. of deaths	Mortality rate	No. of deaths	Mortality rate
0–4	-	-	0	0.00
5–9	-	-	0	0.00
10–14	-	-	0	0.00
15–19	-	-	0	0.00
20–24	-	-	3	0.22
25–29	-	-	7	0.60
30–34	-	-	28	3.05
35–39	-	-	35	6.29
40–44	-	-	56	10.12
45–49	-	-	95	15.70
50–54	-	-	130	21.32
55–59	-	-	128	23.93
60–64	-	-	150	32.88
65+	-	-	399	39.53
TOTAL	-	-	1031	8.47

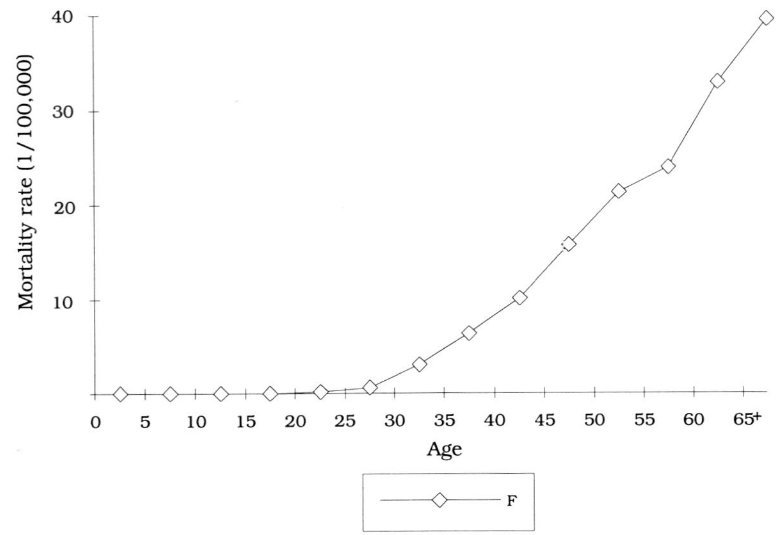

Number of communities on map by category based on standardized mortality ratio (SMR) during 1979–1983

	Number of communities	
Category	Male	Female
SMR significantly high, in top 20%	-	3
SMR significantly high , not in top 20%	-	0
SMR not significantly high, in top 20%	-	9
SMR not significantly low, in bottom 20%	-	6
SMR significantly low, not in bottom 20%	-	1
SMR significantly low, in bottom 20%	-	2
other communities	-	44

Values of the standardized mortality ratio (SMR) which divide the 65 communities into quintile

Percentile	Male	Female
20th	-	67.84
40th	-	80.87
60th	-	100.57
80th	-	130.08
Lowest SMR	-	0.00
Highest SMR	-	206.91
No. of communities with zero death	-	1

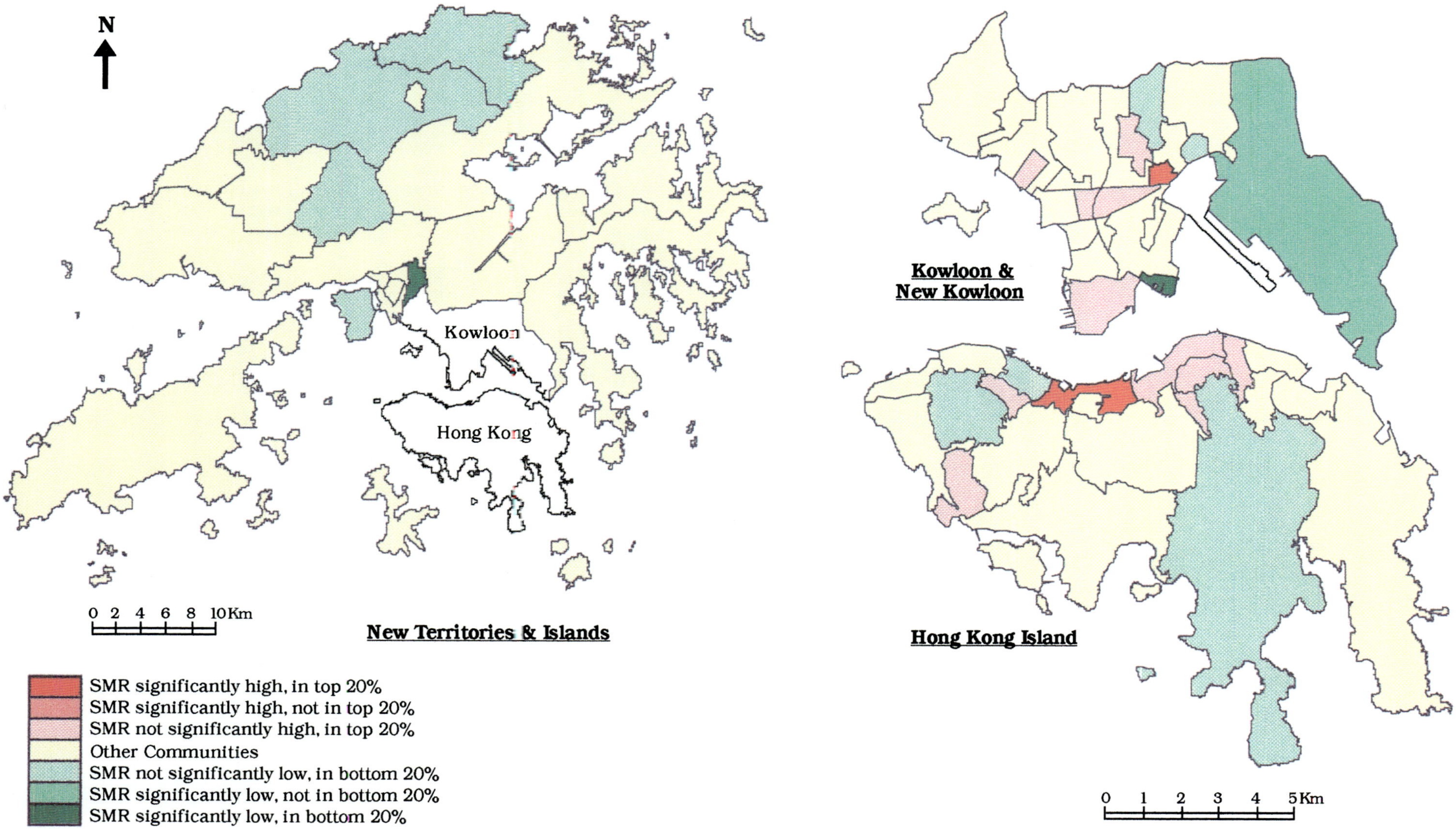

Breast Cancer (Female, 1984 - 1988)

Number of Deaths, Standardised Mortality Ratio (SMR) and 95% Confidence Interval of Breast Cancer by 65 Communities in 1984–1988

Community	Female			Community	Female			Community	Female		
	Number of deaths	SMR	95% C.I.		Number of deaths	SMR	95% C.I.		Number of deaths	SMR	95% C.I.
HK1	24	121.1	77.6 - 180.3	KL1	20	135.7	82.8 - 209.8	NT1	11	110.4	55.2 - 197.4
HK2	28	105.4	66.4 - 144.5	KL2	30	107.4	69.0 - 145.8	NT2	11	95.4	47.7 - 170.6
HK3	5	56.7	18.4 - 132.5	KL3	16	171.2	97.8 - 278.0	NT3	18	93.1	55.1 - 147.0
HK4	26	160.8	105.1 - 235.8	KL4	27	117.0	77.0 - 170.3	NT4	19	96.5	58.1 - 150.8
HK5	18	120.6	71.3 - 190.5	KL5	18	99.7	59.0 - 157.5	NT5	41	111.0	77.1 - 145.0
HK6	21	109.1	67.3 - 166.7	KL6	9	128.0	58.7 - 242.8	NT6	9	41.2	18.9 - 78.2
HK7	3	74.6	15.4 - 218.3	KL7	6	125.7	46.0 - 273.8	NT7	8	72.5	31.3 - 142.8
HK8	13	179.3	95.4 - 306.5	KL8	14	96.8	52.9 - 162.4	NT8	42	103.7	72.3 - 135.0
HK9	5	123.8	40.1 - 289.4	KL9	68	114.9	87.6 - 142.2	NT9	5	75.2	24.3 - 175.7
HK10	65	126.7	95.9 - 157.5	KL10	1	15.5	0.4 - 86.1	NT10	22	76.4	44.5 - 108.3
HK11	6	149.8	54.9 - 326.4	KL11	21	117.8	72.7 - 180.2	NT11	2	34.4	4.2 - 124.1
HK12	7	156.0	62.6 - 321.6	KL12	2	55.2	6.7 - 199.2	NT12	20	74.2	41.7 - 106.7
HK13	7	136.8	54.9 - 282.0	KL13	45	96.1	68.0 - 124.2	NT13	5	80.6	26.1 - 188.3
HK14	20	105.9	64.6 - 163.7	KL14	25	79.4	48.3 - 110.6	NT14	1	23.2	0.6 - 128.9
HK15	6	92.8	34.0 - 202.1	KL15	11	168.3	84.1 - 301.0	NT15	22	79.9	46.5 - 113.3
HK16	25	114.7	74.0 - 169.2	KL16	9	79.6	36.5 - 151.0	NT16	75	110.0	85.1 - 134.9
HK17	24	84.7	50.8 - 118.6	KL17	10	126.0	60.6 - 231.6	NT17	13	125.6	66.8 - 214.6
HK18	2	51.1	6.2 - 184.4	KL18	5	183.5	59.4 - 428.8	NT18	6	113.3	41.5 - 246.9
HK19	24	150.9	96.7 - 224.6	KL19	53	103.1	75.4 - 130.9	NT19	6	80.7	29.5 - 175.7
HK20	23	76.4	45.2 - 107.6	KL20	8	61.7	26.6 - 121.5				
HK21	3	68.9	14.2 - 201.5	KL21	20	101.7	62.0 - 157.2				
				KL22	2	48.2	5.8 - 174.0				
				KL23	22	206.2	128.9 - 312.5				
				KL24	8	79.0	34.0 - 155.4				
				KL25	133	79.3	65.8 - 92.7				

BREAST CANCER

Sex-Age specific mortality rate (1/100,000) of breast cancer in Hong Kong (1984–1988)

	Male		Female	
Age	No. of deaths	Mortality rate	No. of deaths	Mortality rate
0–4	–	–	0	0.00
5–9	–	–	0	0.00
10–14	–	–	0	0.00
15–19	–	–	0	0.00
20–24	–	–	0	0.00
25–29	–	–	7	0.47
30–34	–	–	23	1.86
35–39	–	–	60	6.19
40–44	–	–	52	8.67
45–49	–	–	123	21.08
50–54	–	–	138	21.85
55–59	–	–	163	26.83
60–64	–	–	152	28.40
65+	–	–	561	45.45
TOTAL	–	–	1279	9.53

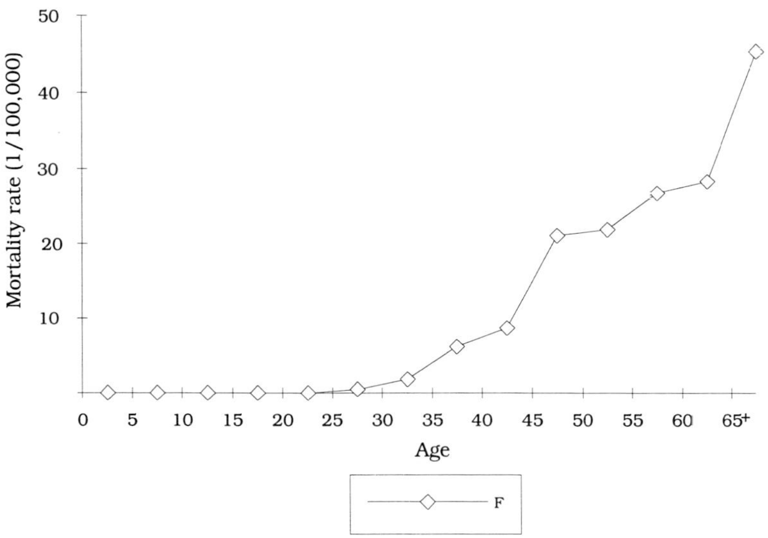

Number of communities on map by category based on standardized mortality ratio (SMR) during 1984–1988

Category	Number of communities Male	Female
SMR significantly high, in top 20%	–	2
SMR significantly high , not in top 20%	–	0
SMR not significantly high, in top 20%	–	11
SMR not significantly low, in bottom 20%	–	9
SMR significantly low, not in bottom 20%	–	1
SMR significantly low, in bottom 20%	–	2
other communities	–	40

Values of the standardized mortality ratio (SMR) which divide the 65 communities into quintile

Percentile	Male	Female
20th	–	74.64
40th	–	93.07
60th	–	109.99
80th	–	125.97
Lowest SMR	–	15.50
Highest SMR	–	206.23
No. of communities with zero death	–	0

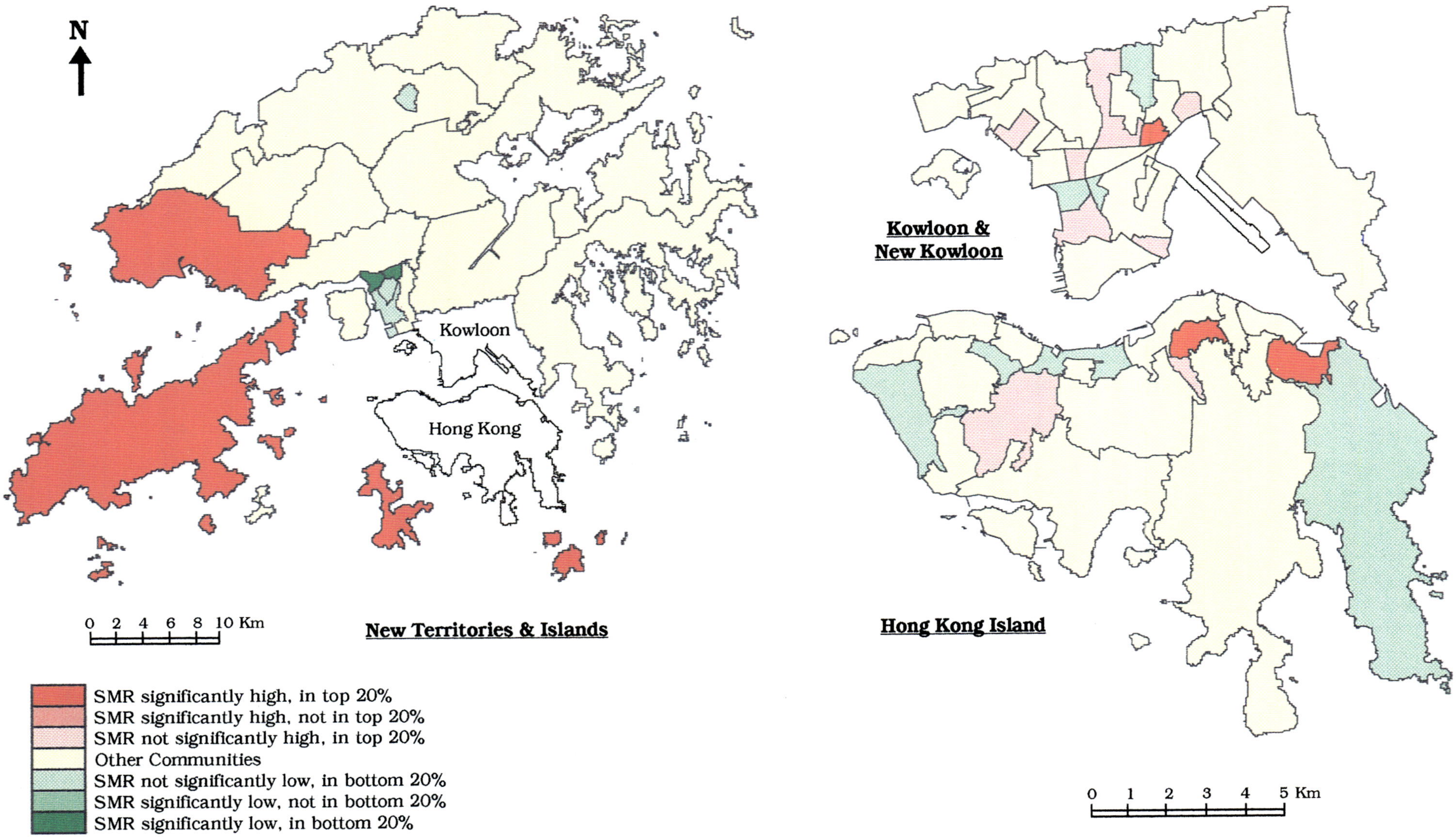

Breast Cancer (Female, 1989 -1993)

Number of Deaths, Standardised Mortality Ratio (SMR) and 95% Confidence Interval of Breast Cancer by 65 Communities in 1989–1993

Community	Female			Community	Female			Community	Female		
	Number of deaths	SMR	95% C.I.		Number of deaths	SMR	95% C.I.		Number of deaths	SMR	95% C.I.
HK1	24	108.0	69.2 - 160.9	KL1	11	85.1	42.4 - 152.3	NT1	18	102.0	60.5 - 161.1
HK2	28	104.0	65.5 - 142.5	KL2	29	106.2	67.6 - 144.9	NT2	9	58.3	26.7 - 105.0
HK3	8	95.8	41.3 - 188.8	KL3	13	146.2	77.8 - 249.9	NT3	12	45.5	23.5 - 79.6
HK4	11	73.5	36.7 - 131.5	KL4	16	76.0	43.4 - 123.0	NT4	11	53.5	26.7 - 95.8
HK5	16	114.9	65.7 - 186.2	KL5	19	119.9	72.2 - 187.0	NT5	29	76.0	48.3 - 103.7
HK6	21	94.5	58.5 - 144.6	KL6	9	109.6	50.2 - 208.3	NT6	24	90.5	58.0 - 134.9
HK7	5	92.4	29.9 - 215.4	KL7	4	64.9	17.6 - 166.1	NT7	28	97.9	61.2 - 134.5
HK8	5	64.8	21.0 - 150.9	KL8	15	98.6	55.2 - 162.7	NT8	86	126.4	102.6 - 150.1
HK9	7	155.3	62.3 - 319.9	KL9	67	107.0	81.4 - 132.6	NT9	7	102.3	41.0 - 210.8
HK10	71	118.5	91.0 - 146.1	KL10	17	122.3	71.3 - 195.7	NT10	33	93.3	60.4 - 126.3
HK11	7	149.6	64.5 - 308.3	KL11	15	93.4	52.3 - 154.2	NT11	6	95.8	35.2 - 208.9
HK12	14	260.6	142.3 - 437.8	KL12	2	53.9	6.5 - 194.7	NT12	32	94.3	60.7 - 128.0
HK13	6	114.2	41.9 - 249.0	KL13	47	95.8	68.4 - 123.2	NT13	4	51.7	14.1 - 132.4
HK14	23	97.3	61.7 - 145.9	KL14	29	88.2	56.1 - 120.3	NT14	4	105.1	28.6 - 268.9
HK15	16	106.5	60.9 - 172.6	KL15	10	146.2	70.2 - 268.9	NT15	40	91.7	62.0 - 121.4
HK16	33	161.0	106.0 - 215.9	KL16	11	97.1	48.5 - 173.8	NT16	133	112.4	94.3 - 130.4
HK17	34	77.5	51.5 - 103.6	KL17	9	124.2	56.9 - 236.0	NT17	25	89.3	57.8 - 132.1
HK18	2	34.9	4.2 - 126.1	KL18	3	94.3	19.4 - 275.4	NT18	7	114.1	45.7 - 235.0
HK19	21	113.3	70.2 - 173.4	KL19	62	107.7	80.9 - 134.5	NT19	17	225.6	131.5 - 361.0
HK20	40	102.6	70.8 - 134.4	KL20	11	82.0	40.9 - 146.9				
HK21	4	87.4	23.8 - 223.8	KL21	20	99.4	60.7 - 153.0				
				KL22	6	146.8	53.9 - 320.1				
				KL23	16	194.6	111.3 - 315.2				
				KL24	10	94.8	45.5 - 174.5				
				KL25	158	86.6	73.1 - 100.1				

BREAST CANCER

Sex-Age specific mortality rate (1/100,000) of breast cancer in Hong Kong (1989–1993)

	Male		Female	
Age	No. of deaths	Mortality rate	No. of deaths	Mortality rate
0–4	–	–	0	0.00
5–9	–	–	0	0.00
10–14	–	–	0	0.00
15–19	–	–	0	0.00
20–24	–	–	0	0.00
25–29	–	–	16	1.08
30–34	–	–	41	2.70
35–39	–	–	93	7.39
40–44	–	–	137	14.09
45–49	–	–	104	17.42
50–54	–	–	140	24.59
55–59	–	–	157	25.78
60–64	–	–	162	28.03
65+	–	–	680	48.40
TOTAL	–	–	1530	10.93

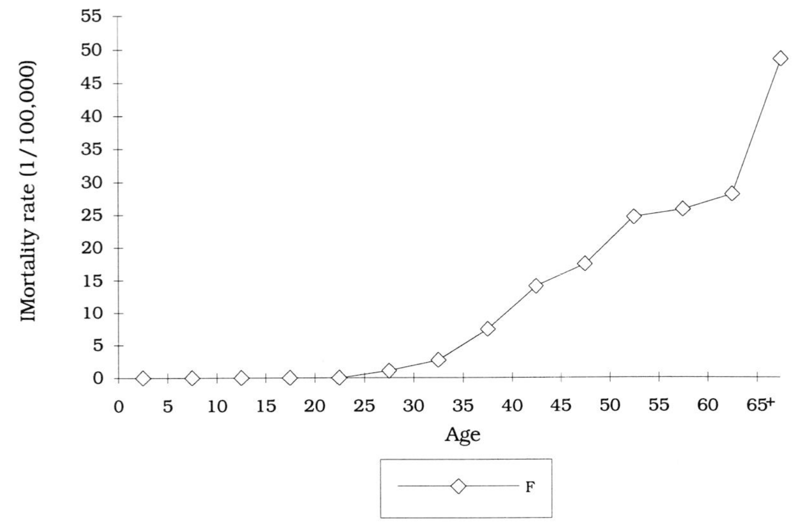

Number of communities on map by category based on standardized mortality ratio (SMR) during 1989–1993

Category	Number of communities Male	Number of communities Female
SMR significantly high, in top 20%	–	5
SMR significantly high , not in top 20%	–	0
SMR not significantly high, in top 20%	–	8
SMR not significantly low, in bottom 20%	–	10
SMR significantly low, not in bottom 20%	–	0
SMR significantly low, in bottom 20%	–	2
other communities	–	40

Values of the standardized mortality ratio (SMR) which divide the 65 communities into quintile

Percentile	Male	Female
20th	–	82.04
40th	–	94.54
60th	–	103.97
80th	–	118.53
Lowest SMR	–	34.94
Highest SMR	–	260.57
No. of communities with zero cases	–	0

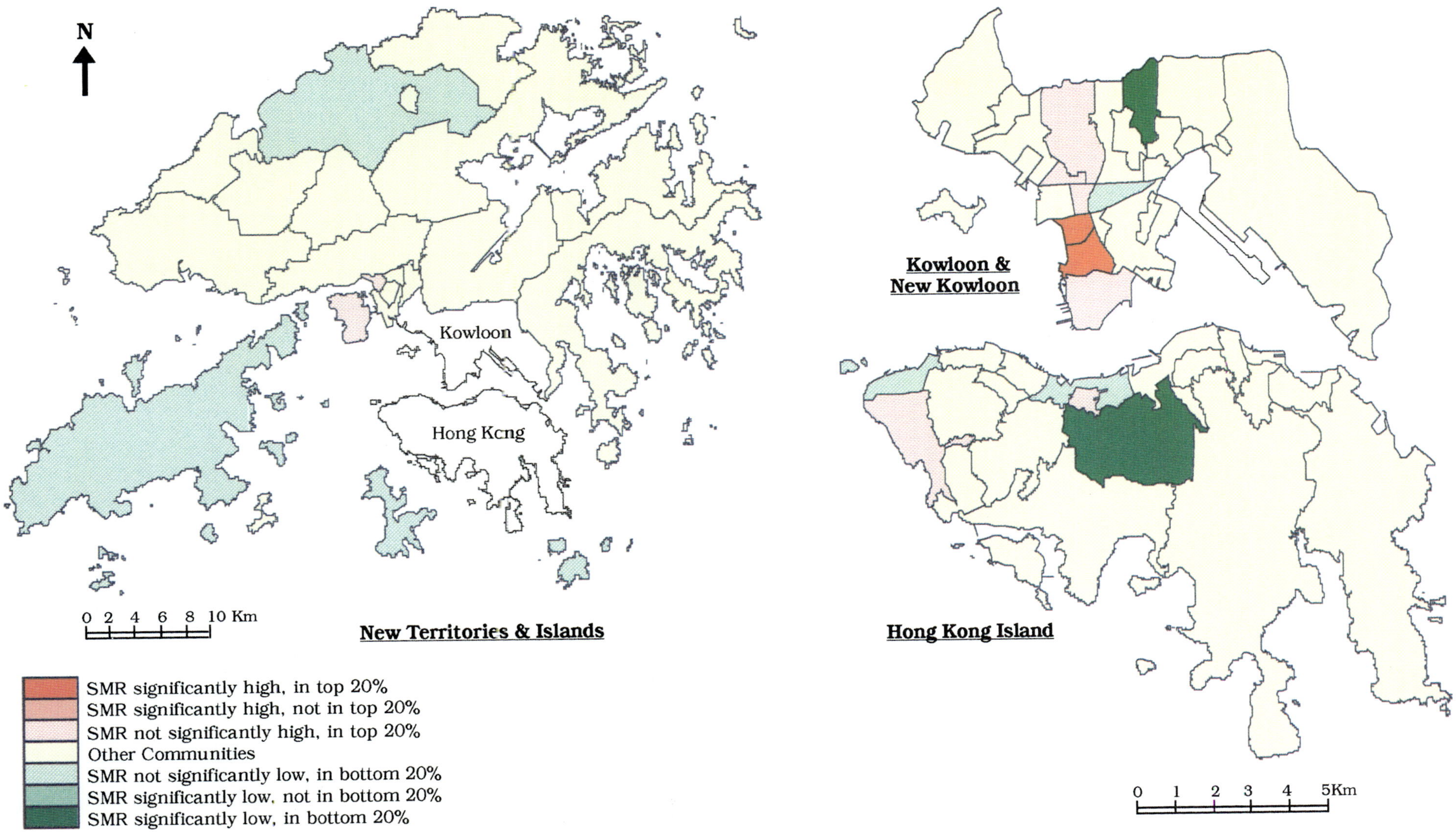

Cervical Cancer (Female, 1979 -1983)

Number of Deaths, Standardised Mortality Ratio (SMR) and 95% Confidence Interval
of Cervical Cancer by 65 Communities in 1979–1983

Community	Female			Community	Female			Community	Female		
	Number of deaths	SMR	95% C.I.		Number of deaths	SMR	95% C.I.		Number of deaths	SMR	95% C.I.
HK1	6	50.7	18.6 - 110.5	KL1	14	147.6	80.7 - 247.7	NT1	3	74.5	15.4 - 217.8
HK2	10	61.4	29.5 - 112.9	KL2	13	70.8	37.7 - 121.0	NT2	7	118.3	47.5 - 243.9
HK3	4	69.9	19.0 - 178.8	KL3	9	151.3	69.4 - 287.1	NT3	14	132.1	72.2 - 221.6
HK4	6	56.1	20.5 - 122.1	KL4	23	158.1	100.1 - 237.4	NT4	8	114.5	49.3 - 225.4
HK5	16	164.7	94.1 - 267.4	KL5	23	194.0	122.8 - 291.2	NT5	27	117.5	73.2 - 161.8
HK6	4	33.2	9.1 - 85.0	KL6	1	21.6	0.5 - 120.1	NT6	15	126.4	70.6 - 208.6
HK7	3	118.3	24.4 - 345.8	KL7	4	123.1	33.5 - 314.9	NT7	7	181.5	72.9 - 374.1
HK8	4	82.0	22.3 - 209.7	KL8	11	119.1	59.5 - 213.0	NT8	13	115.6	61.5 - 197.6
HK9	0	0.0	...	KL9	38	106.6	72.7 - 140.5	NT9	3	87.6	18.1 - 256.1
HK10	25	83.3	50.6 - 115.9	KL10	4	103.7	28.3 - 265.3	NT10	12	84.5	43.5 - 147.4
HK11	0	0.0	...	KL11	11	110.6	55.3 - 197.8	NT11	2	71.3	8.6 - 257.4
HK12	2	69.3	8.4 - 250.3	KL12	2	94.5	11.4 - 341.2	NT12	8	59.6	25.7 - 117.3
HK13	4	118.4	32.3 - 302.8	KL13	32	103.7	67.8 - 139.7	NT13	2	75.5	9.1 - 272.5
HK14	6	73.4	26.9 - 159.9	KL14	25	139.7	84.9 - 194.4	NT14	1	37.7	1.0 - 209.4
HK15	2	54.4	6.6 - 196.3	KL15	2	139.1	16.8 - 502.0	NT15	8	78.5	33.8 - 154.5
HK16	16	121.9	69.6 - 197.8	KL16	10	135.8	65.3 - 249.7	NT16	13	96.6	51.4 - 165.2
HK17	11	76.8	38.4 - 137.3	KL17	4	118.5	32.3 - 303.0	NT17	6	102.4	37.5 - 223.1
HK18	5	207.0	67.0 - 483.7	KL18	1	57.0	1.4 - 316.7	NT18	4	134.0	36.5 - 342.6
HK19	10	126.8	60.9 - 233.0	KL19	29	94.3	60.0 - 128.6	NT19	1	21.2	0.5 - 117.8
HK20	19	125.4	75.5 - 195.9	KL20	4	38.3	19.6 - 99.3				
HK21	2	96.6	11.7 - 348.6	KL21	20	121.8	74.3 - 188.2				
				KL22	0	0.0	...				
				KL23	9	109.0	50.0 - 206.9				
				KL24	5	85.9	27.8 - 200.8				
				KL25	80	97.6	76.2 - 119.0				

CERVICAL CANCER

Sex-Age specific mortality rate (1/100,000) of cervical cancer in Hong Kong (1979–1983)

	Male		Female	
Age	No. of deaths	Mortality rate	No. of deaths	Mortality rate
0–4	–	–	0	0.00
5–9	–	–	0	0.00
10–14	–	–	0	0.00
15–19	–	–	0	0.00
20–24	–	–	0	0.00
25–29	–	–	4	0.34
30–34	–	–	13	1.42
35–39	–	–	19	3.42
40–44	–	–	30	5.42
45–49	–	–	45	7.44
50–54	–	–	97	15.91
55–59	–	–	138	25.80
60–64	–	–	97	21.26
65+	–	–	240	23.78
TOTAL	–	–	683	5.61

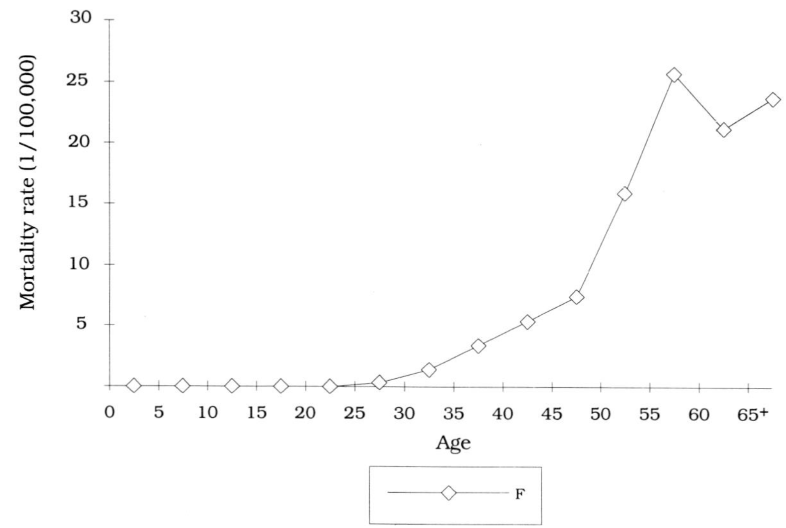

Number of communities on map by category based on standardized mortality ratio (SMR) during 1979–1983

	Number of communities	
Category	Male	Female
SMR significantly high, in top 20%	–	2
SMR significantly high , not in top 20%	–	0
SMR not significantly high, in top 20%	–	8
SMR not significantly low, in bottom 20%	–	5
SMR significantly low, not in bottom 20%	–	0
SMR significantly low, in bottom 20%	–	2
other communities	–	48

Values of the standardized mortality ratio (SMR) which divide the 65 communities into quintile

Percentile	Male	Female
20th	–	59.57
40th	–	84.46
60th	–	110.56
80th	–	126.42
Lowest SMR	–	0.00
Highest SMR	–	207.04
No. of communities with zero death	–	3

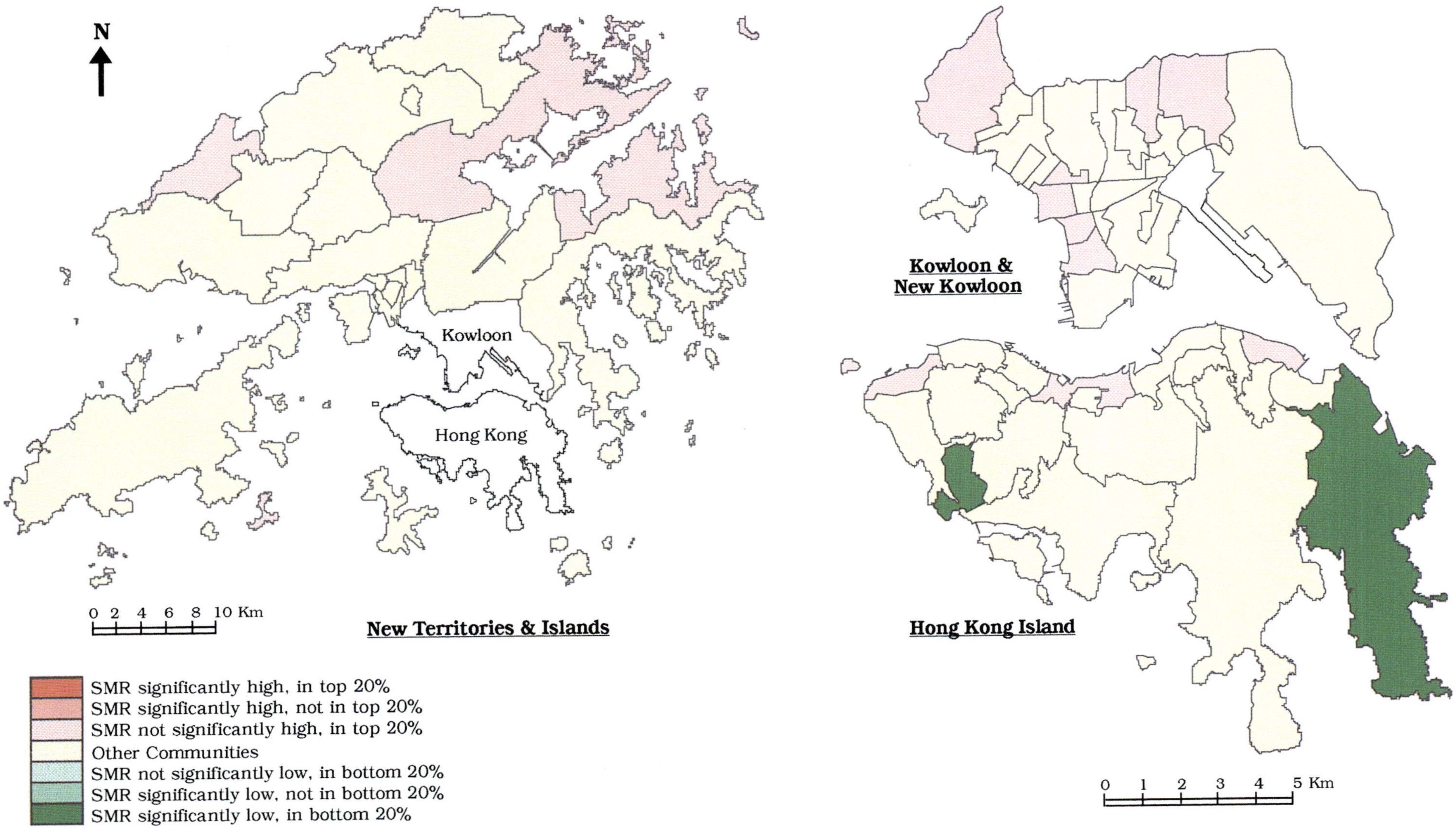

Cervical Cancer (Female, 1984 -1988)

Number of Deaths, Standardised Mortality Ratio (SMR) and 95% Confidence Interval of Cervical Cancer by 65 Communities in 1984–1988

	Female		
Community	Number of deaths	SMR	95% C.I.
HK1	15	144.2	80.6 - 237.9
HK2	12	86.9	44.8 - 151.7
HK3	3	65.3	13.5 - 190.9
HK4	12	142.8	73.6 - 249.2
HK5	9	115.1	52.8 - 218.4
HK6	7	70.5	28.3 - 145.3
HK7	1	48.2	1.2 - 267.8
HK8	3	79.5	16.4 - 232.4
HK9	1	48.9	1.2 - 271.6
HK10	24	89.9	54.0 - 125.9
HK11	1	46.1	1.2 - 256.4
HK12	1	42.7	1.1 - 237.0
HK13	0	0.0	...
HK14	15	152.1	85.0 - 251.1
HK15	3	89.8	18.5 - 262.6
HK16	10	87.7	42.2 - 161.2
HK17	7	46.8	18.8 - 96.5
HK18	0	0.0	...
HK19	2	24.4	3.0 - 88.3
HK20	16	102.2	58.4 - 165.9
HK21	0	0.0	...

	Female		
Community	Number of deaths	SMR	95% C.I.
KL1	5	65.1	21.1 - 152.0
KL2	17	116.8	67.9 - 187.0
KL3	5	104.2	33.7 - 243.4
KL4	17	141.8	82.5 - 226.9
KL5	14	148.5	81.1 - 249.1
KL6	3	82.5	17.0 - 241.3
KL7	0	0.0	...
KL8	8	106.8	46.0 - 210.3
KL9	31	100.1	64.8 - 135.3
KL10	3	89.3	18.4 - 261.1
KL11	15	163.1	91.1 - 269.2
KL12	1	53.1	1.3 - 295.1
KL13	20	81.5	49.7 - 125.9
KL14	17	101.2	58.8 - 161.9
KL15	1	29.5	0.7 - 163.7
KL16	8	135.2	58.3 - 266.2
KL17	3	74.9	15.4 - 218.9
KL18	0	0.0	...
KL19	33	121.0	79.7 - 162.3
KL20	10	145.1	69.8 - 266.7
KL21	8	75.9	32.7 - 149.4
KL22	0	0.0	...
KL23	6	107.5	39.4 - 234.3
KL24	5	91.5	29.6 - 213.7
KL25	101	114.6	92.3 - 137.0

	Female		
Community	Number of deaths	SMR	95% C.I.
NT1	5	96.2	31.1 - 224.9
NT2	4	66.8	18.2 - 170.8
NT3	11	108.4	54.2 - 193.9
NT4	7	69.7	28.0 - 143.7
NT5	20	103.5	63.1 - 159.9
NT6	12	105.3	54.3 - 183.7
NT7	5	87.0	28.2 - 203.2
NT8	24	113.3	72.6 - 168.6
NT9	4	115.5	31.5 - 295.4
NT10	15	99.0	55.3 - 163.4
NT11	3	97.9	20.2 - 286.3
NT12	14	99.3	54.3 - 166.7
NT13	2	60.5	7.3 - 218.5
NT14	0	0.0	...
NT15	20	138.9	84.7 - 214.7
NT16	36	101.8	68.6 - 135.1
NT17	3	55.6	11.5 - 162.7
NT18	5	180.5	58.4 - 421.7
NT19	3	77.7	16.0 - 227.2

CERVICAL CANCER

Sex-Age specific mortality rate (1/100,000) of cervical cancer in Hong Kong (1984–1988)

	Male		Female	
Age	No. of deaths	Mortality rate	No. of deaths	Mortality rate
0–4	–	–	0	0.00
5–9	–	–	0	0.00
10–14	–	–	0	0.00
15–19	–	–	0	0.00
20–24	–	–	0	0.00
25–29	–	–	5	0.34
30–34	–	–	18	1.45
35–39	–	–	24	2.47
40–44	–	–	20	3.34
45–49	–	–	52	8.91
50–54	–	–	85	13.46
55–59	–	–	95	15.64
60–64	–	–	110	20.55
65+	–	–	263	21.31
TOTAL	–	–	672	5.01

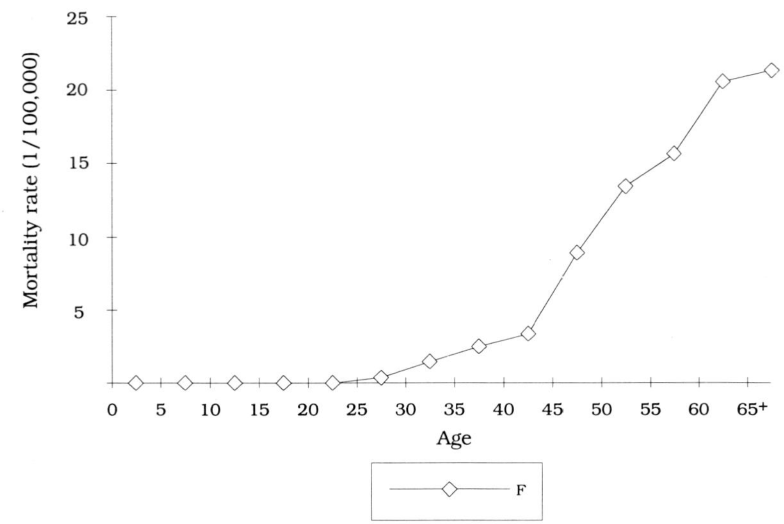

Number of communities on map by category based on standardized mortality ratio (SMR) during 1984–1988

Category	Number of communities Male	Female
SMR significantly high, in top 20%	–	0
SMR significantly high , not in top 20%	–	0
SMR not significantly high, in top 20%	–	13
SMR not significantly low, in bottom 20%	–	0
SMR significantly low, not in bottom 20%	–	0
SMR significantly low, in bottom 20%	–	2
other communities	–	50

Values of the standardized mortality ratio (SMR) which divide the 65 communities into quintile

Percentile	Male	Female
20th	–	48.20
40th	–	79.48
60th	–	99.34
80th	–	115.08
Lowest SMR	–	0.00
Highest SMR	–	180.47
No. of communities with zero death	–	7

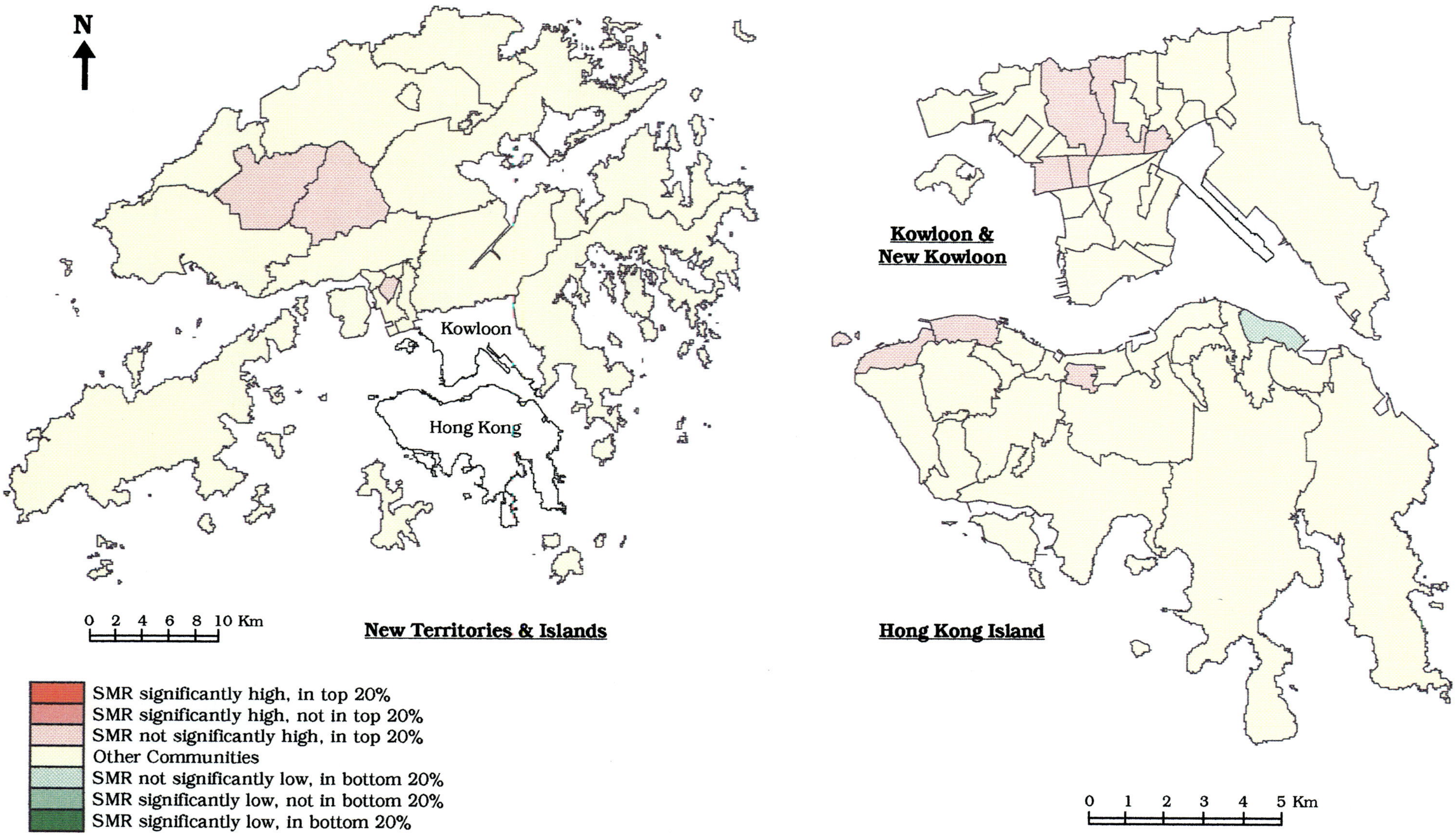

Cervical Cancer (Female, 1989 -1993)

Number of Deaths, Standardised Mortality Ratio (SMR) and 95% Confidence Interval of Cervical Cancer by 65 Communities in 1989–1993

Community	Female			Community	Female			Community	Female		
	Number of deaths	SMR	95% C.I.		Number of deaths	SMR	95% C.I.		Number of deaths	SMR	95% C.I.
HK1	15	151.1	84.6 - 249.3	KL1	6	105.5	38.7 - 230.1	NT1	8	109.6	47.2 - 216.0
HK2	16	133.6	76.4 - 216.4	KL2	17	139.0	81.0 - 222.4	NT2	7	103.6	41.5 - 213.4
HK3	1	26.7	0.7 - 148.7	KL3	8	200.1	86.2 - 394.1	NT3	7	61.5	24.7 - 126.6
HK4	5	74.3	24.1 - 173.1	KL4	8	84.4	36.4 - 166.3	NT4	9	101.0	46.2 - 191.8
HK5	9	143.1	65.6 - 271.9	KL5	6	83.8	30.7 - 182.6	NT5	23	134.3	85.2 - 201.5
HK6	6	62.9	23.1 - 137.1	KL6	4	109.0	29.7 - 279.2	NT6	11	94.0	46.9 - 168.2
HK7	0	0.0	...	KL7	1	37.5	0.9 - 208.7	NT7	12	102.6	53.0 - 179.5
HK8	2	60.7	7.3 - 219.3	KL8	7	103.5	41.5 - 213.2	NT8	28	101.2	63.7 - 138.7
HK9	0	0.0	...	KL9	33	117.6	77.5 - 157.8	NT9	1	31.7	0.8 - 176.4
HK10	21	79.3	49.1 - 121.4	KL10	5	85.2	27.6 - 198.6	NT10	22	140.4	88.0 - 212.0
HK11	1	47.3	1.2 - 263.2	KL11	6	86.3	31.7 - 188.2	NT11	4	139.9	38.0 - 358.1
HK12	3	133.9	27.6 - 390.9	KL12	0	0.0	...	NT12	18	119.9	71.1 - 189.4
HK13	4	167.5	45.6 - 428.9	KL13	19	84.7	51.0 - 132.1	NT13	1	29.4	0.7 - 163.6
HK14	4	39.6	10.8 - 101.3	KL14	21	135.2	83.7 - 206.9	NT14	2	112.6	13.6 - 406.4
HK15	5	78.3	25.4 - 182.4	KL15	1	32.1	0.8 - 178.8	NT15	18	96.1	57.0 - 151.9
HK16	6	65.4	24.0 - 142.5	KL16	4	79.1	21.5 - 202.4	NT16	62	123.3	92.6 - 154.0
HK17	13	66.2	35.2 - 113.2	KL17	6	189.5	69.6 - 413.2	NT17	12	100.4	51.9 - 175.7
HK18	1	41.8	1.1 - 232.9	KL18	1	74.8	1.9 - 416.9	NT18	3	106.0	21.8 - 309.5
HK19	6	73.8	27.1 - 160.9	KL19	26	97.0	59.7 - 134.3	NT19	1	29.2	0.7 - 162.4
HK20	16	92.7	53.0 - 150.2	KL20	7	113.9	45.7 - 234.7				
HK21	0	0.0	...	KL21	7	73.3	29.4 - 151.0				
				KL22	2	109.5	13.2 - 395.1				
				KL23	8	216.5	93.3 - 426.5				
				KL24	3	59.4	12.2 - 173.4				
				KL25	86	105.2	82.9 - 127.4				

CERVICAL CANCER

Sex-Age specific mortality rate (1/100,000) of cervical cancer in Hong Kong (1989–1993)

	Male		Female	
Age	No. of deaths	Mortality rate	No. of deaths	Mortality rate
0–4	–	–	0	0.00
5–9	–	–	0	0.00
10–14	–	–	0	0.00
15–19	–	–	0	0.00
20–24	–	–	0	0.00
25–29	–	–	3	0.20
30–34	–	–	9	0.59
35–39	–	–	21	1.67
40–44	–	–	34	3.50
45–49	–	–	41	6.87
50–54	–	–	44	7.73
55–59	–	–	80	13.13
60–64	–	–	96	16.61
65+	–	–	347	24.70
TOTAL	–	–	675	4.82

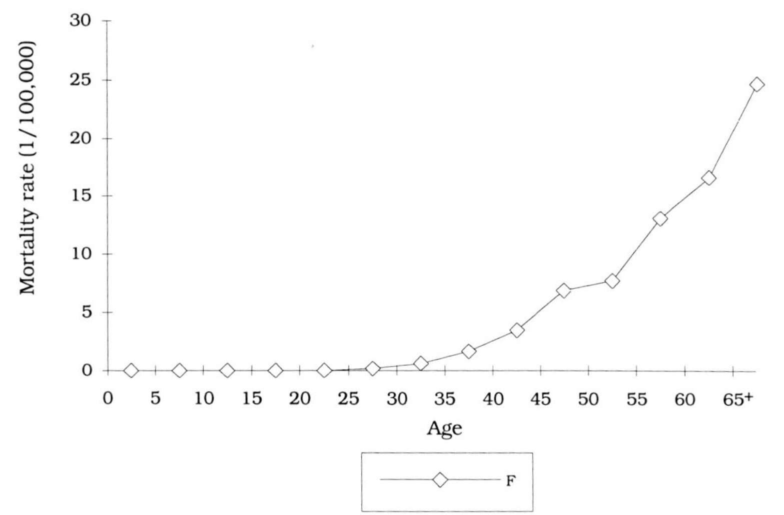

Number of communities on map by category based on standardized mortality ratio (SMR) during 1989–1993

	Number of communities	
Category	Male	Female
SMR significantly high, in top 20%	–	2
SMR significantly high , not in top 20%	–	0
SMR not significantly high, in top 20%	–	11
SMR not significantly low, in bottom 20%	–	1
SMR significantly low, not in bottom 20%	–	0
SMR significantly low, in bottom 20%	–	0
other communities	–	51

Values of the standardized mortality ratio (SMR) which divide the 65 communities into quintile

Percentile	Male	Female
20th	–	47.25
40th	–	79.34
60th	–	102.55
80th	–	123.33
Lowest SMR	–	0.00
Highest SMR	–	216.48
No. of communities with zero cases	–	0

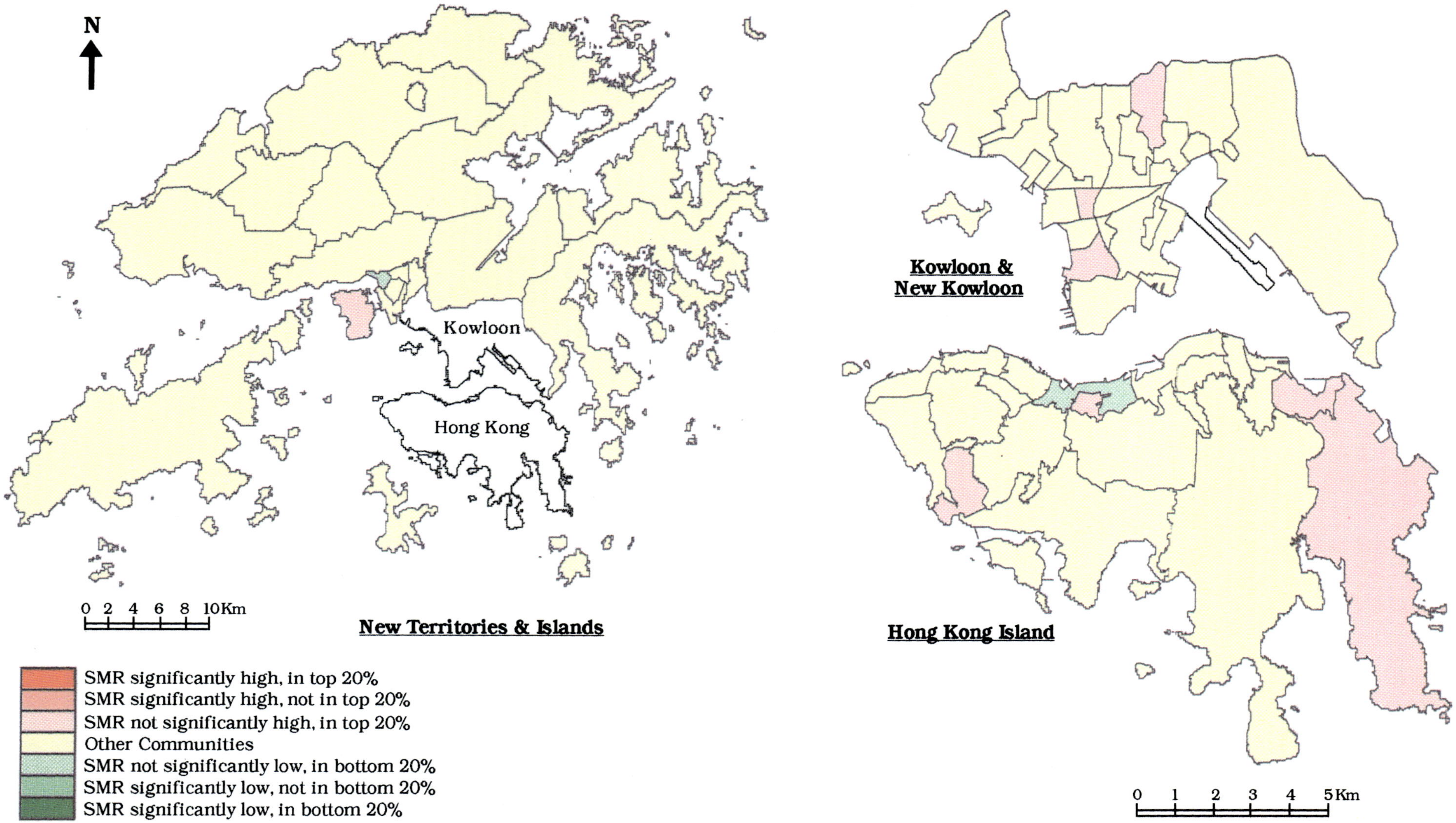

Leukaemia (Male, 1979 – 1983)

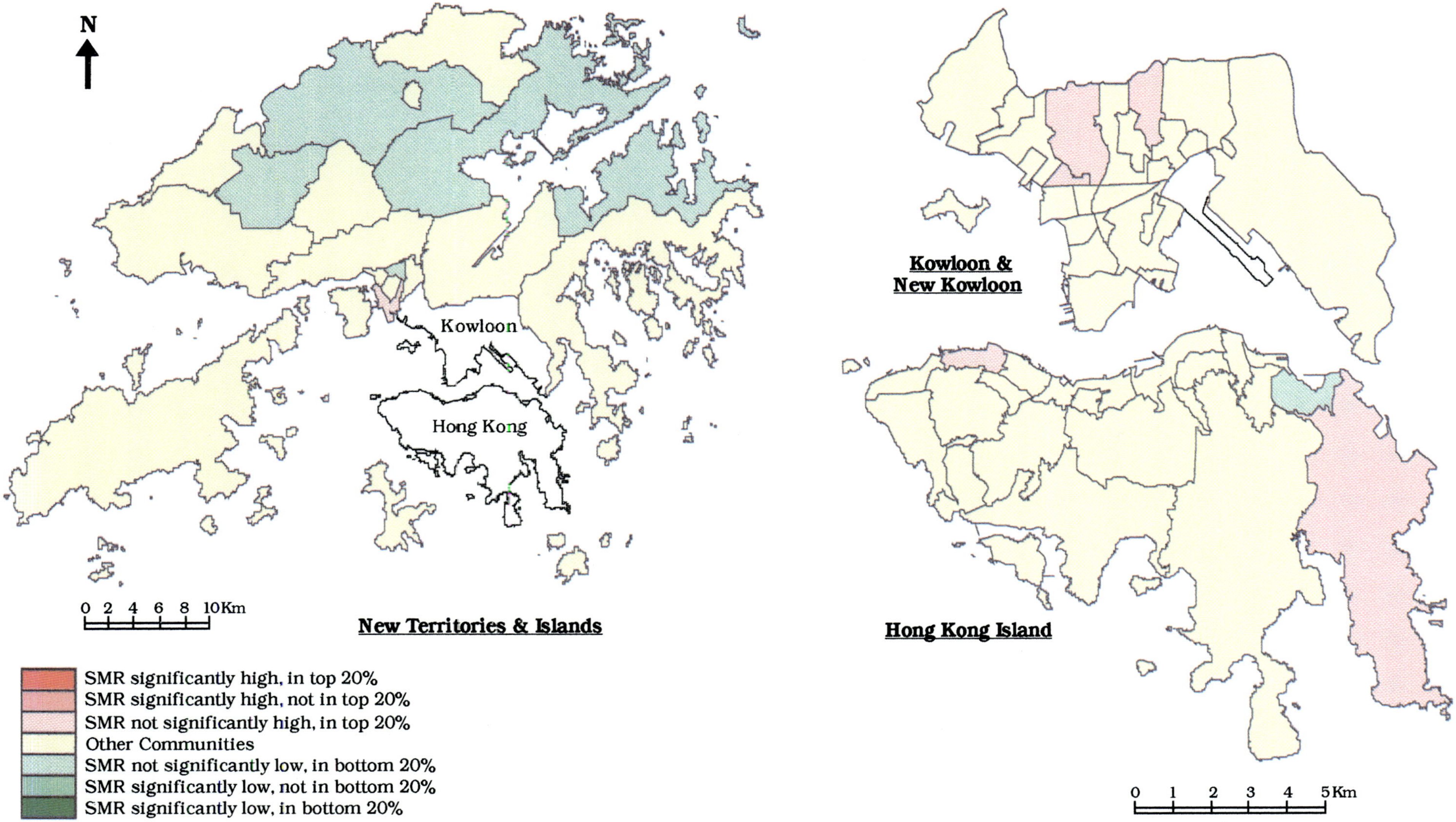

Leukaemia (Female, 1979 – 1983)

Number of Deaths, Standardised Mortality Ratio (SMR) and 95% Confidence Interval of Leukaemia by 65 Communities in 1979–1983

	Male			Female				Male			Female		
Community	Number of deaths	SMR	95% C.I.	Number of deaths	SMR	95% C.I.	Community	Number of deaths	SMR	95% C.I.	Number of deaths	SMR	95% C.I.
HK1	11	143.3	71.7 - 256.4	4	64.1	17.5 - 163.9	KL13	17	80.8	47.0 - 129.3	23	142.7	90.3 - 214.3
HK2	16	146.5	83.7 - 237.8	13	156.5	83.3 - 267.6	KL14	11	97.2	48.6 - 173.9	14	158.8	86.8 - 266.4
HK3	2	50.1	6.1 - 180.8	3	106.2	21.9 - 310.6	KL15	1	91.0	2.3 - 505.3	1	126.1	3.2 - 700.6
HK4	4	57.2	15.6 - 146.4	5	93.1	30.1 - 217.6	KL16	5	99.3	32.1 - 231.9	6	156.1	57.2 - 340.1
HK5	11	173.3	86.6 - 310.0	5	104.0	33.7 - 243.1	KL17	1	71.9	1.8 - 399.5	3	188.1	38.8 - 549.9
HK6	6	112.8	41.3 - 245.8	4	70.7	19.3 - 180.8	KL18	0	0.0	...	3	292.2	60.2 - 854.3
HK7	0	0.0	...	1	81.6	2.1 - 453.2	KL19	18	90.2	53.4 - 142.5	22	131.5	82.2 - 199.3
HK8	2	97.3	11.8 - 351.2	4	175.7	47.9 - 449.5	KL20	10	160.1	77.0 - 294.3	9	172.4	79.1 - 327.2
HK9	1	104.1	2.6 - 578.4	1	91.3	2.3 - 507.2	KL21	7	72.2	29.0 - 149.0	10	122.9	59.1 - 226.0
HK10	13	82.6	43.9 - 141.1	14	97.4	53.2 - 163.4	KL22	3	162.1	33.4 - 474.1	1	75.2	1.9 - 418.0
HK11	2	130.5	15.8 - 471.0	2	158.9	19.2 - 573.7	KL23	5	84.4	27.3 - 197.3	6	135.0	49.5 - 294.2
HK12	1	75.5	1.9 - 419.4	3	208.0	42.9 - 608.2	KL24	5	141.6	45.8 - 330.9	2	66.0	8.0 - 238.4
HK13	1	51.1	1.3 - 283.8	0	0.0	...	KL25	57	96.9	71.7 - 122.1	38	80.2	54.7 - 105.7
HK14	4	80.9	22.0 - 207.0	6	140.2	51.4 - 305.6	NT1	2	61.4	7.4 - 221.5	1	40.0	1.0 - 222.1
HK15	0	0.0	...	0	0.0	...	NT2	5	102.7	33.2 - 239.9	6	160.7	58.9 - 350.1
HK16	13	146.8	78.1 - 250.9	4	57.0	15.5 - 145.7	NT3	5	56.7	18.4 - 132.5	8	130.0	56.0 - 255.9
HK17	14	148.7	81.2 - 249.4	11	145.4	72.7 - 260.1	NT4	6	104.8	38.4 - 228.3	2	41.6	5.0 - 150.2
HK18	1	72.8	1.8 - 404.5	1	77.8	2.0 - 432.3	NT5	17	99.6	57.9 - 159.4	20	144.6	88.1 - 223.4
HK19	8	149.4	64.4 - 294.1	3	63.8	13.2 - 186.5	NT6	7	79.0	31.7 - 162.8	8	110.0	47.4 - 216.6
HK20	7	65.3	26.2 - 134.6	7	80.4	32.3 - 165.8	NT7	6	174.9	64.1 - 381.0	2	74.7	9.0 - 269.7
HK21	1	63.2	1.6 - 350.9	0	0.0	...	NT8	8	80.0	34.5 - 157.5	6	80.1	29.3 - 174.6
KL1	5	82.9	26.8 - 193.7	6	126.6	46.4 - 275.8	NT9	4	160.4	43.7 - 410.3	0	0.0	...
KL2	14	105.8	57.8 - 177.5	6	61.6	22.6 - 134.3	NT10	14	132.4	72.4 - 222.2	4	48.6	13.2 - 124.2
KL3	7	190.9	76.7 - 393.6	2	65.6	7.9 - 237.0	NT11	0	0.0	...	1	60.1	1.5 - 333.8
KL4	7	67.2	27.0 - 138.6	8	106.2	45.8 - 209.0	NT12	8	83.3	35.9 - 163.9	4	53.3	14.5 - 136.2
KL5	13	157.5	83.8 - 269.3	6	99.7	36.5 - 217.2	NT13	4	222.7	60.7 - 569.6	3	205.7	42.4 - 601.3
KL6	3	166.2	34.3 - 485.9	2	95.3	11.5 - 344.1	NT14	0	0.0	...	1	70.4	1.8 - 391.1
KL7	0	0.0	...	2	124.2	15.0 - 448.2	NT15	7	101.6	40.8 - 209.5	2	34.7	4.2 - 125.4
KL8	6	99.9	36.6 - 217.6	4	80.4	21.9 - 205.5	NT16	10	101.6	48.9 - 186.8	8	98.7	42.5 - 194.3
KL9	23	100.5	63.6 - 151.0	17	88.3	51.3 - 141.2	NT17	4	102.8	28.0 - 262.8	3	92.2	19.0 - 269.5
KL10	4	162.8	44.3 - 416.3	4	191.7	52.2 - 490.3	NT18	2	114.7	13.9 - 414.1	0	0.0	...
KL11	5	86.3	43.2 - 154.4	3	57.6	11.9 - 168.3	NT19	1	33.1	0.8 - 184.0	2	83.6	10.1 - 301.9
KL12	2	127.8	15.5 - 461.5	1	92.3	2.3 - 512.7							

LEUKAEMIA

Sex-Age specific mortality rate (1/100,000) of leukaemia in Hong Kong (1979–1983)

	Male		Female	
Age	No. of deaths	Mortality rate	No. of deaths	Mortality rate
0–4	18	1.71	12	1.21
5–9	24	2.26	17	1.72
10–14	28	2.45	29	2.71
15–19	33	2.31	22	1.65
20–24	36	2.35	26	1.87
25–29	32	2.42	13	1.12
30–34	18	1.63	14	1.53
35–39	26	3.60	12	2.16
40–44	24	3.41	18	3.25
45–49	28	3.88	20	3.30
50–54	27	3.93	23	3.77
55–59	35	6.15	24	4.49
60–64	40	8.75	24	5.26
65+	88	12.91	117	11.59
TOTAL	457	3.47	371	3.05

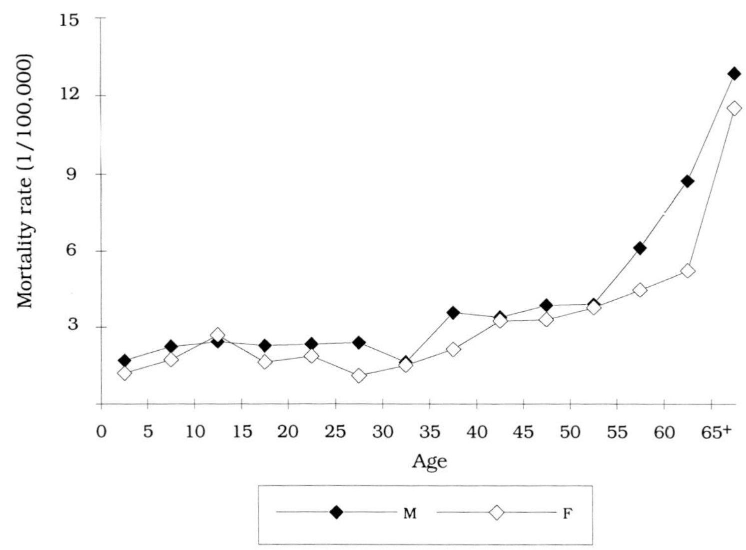

Number of communities on map by category based on standardized mortality ratio (SMR) during 1979–1983

Category	Number of communities Male	Female
SMR significantly high, in top 20%	0	0
SMR significantly high , not in top 20%	0	0
SMR not significantly high, in top 20%	8	6
SMR not significantly low, in bottom 20%	2	5
SMR significantly low, not in bottom 20%	0	0
SMR significantly low, in bottom 20%	0	0
other communities	55	54

Values of the standardized mortality ratio (SMR) which divide the 65 communities into quintile

Percentile	Male	Female
20th	63.17	60.08
40th	83.28	80.35
60th	101.63	104.03
80th	146.47	144.56
Lowest SMR	0.00	0.00
Highest SMR	222.70	292.17
No. of communities with zero death	6	5

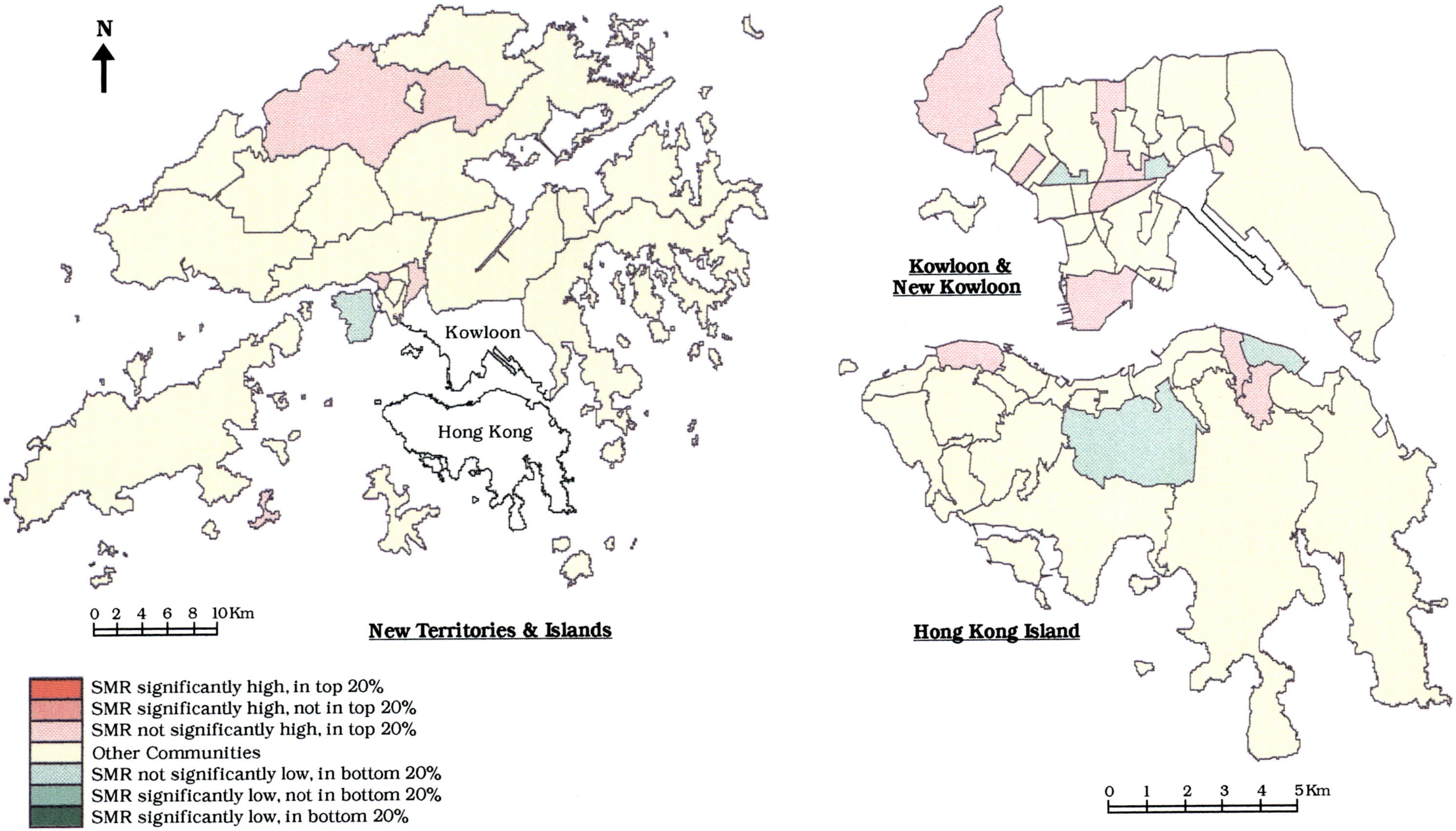

Leukaemia (Male, 1984 - 1988)

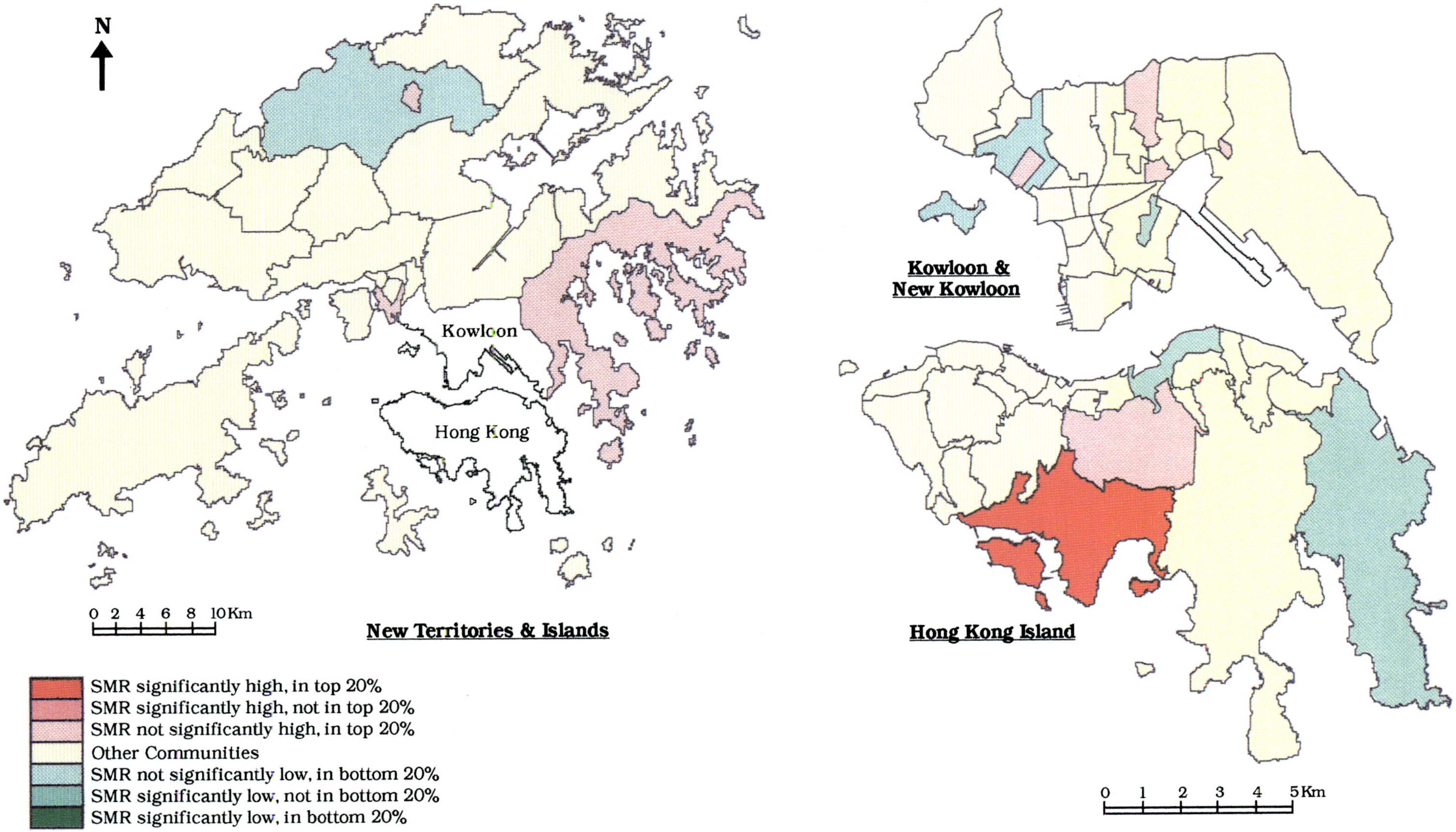

Leukaemia (Female, 1984 – 1988)

Number of Deaths, Standardised Mortality Ratio (SMR) and 95% Confidence Interval of Leukaemia by 65 Communities in 1984–1988

Community	Male			Female		
	Number of deaths	SMR	95% C.I.	Number of deaths	SMR	95% C.I.
HK1	9	111.2	51.0 - 211.1	6	96.4	35.3 - 210.1
HK2	15	135.8	75.8 - 224.0	11	132.3	66.1 - 236.6
HK3	4	105.3	28.7 - 269.3	1	38.7	1.0 - 215.1
HK4	4	61.7	16.8 - 157.9	6	123.6	45.3 - 269.3
HK5	7	125.5	50.4 - 258.8	6	135.6	49.7 - 295.5
HK6	2	34.0	4.1 - 122.7	8	137.8	59.4 - 271.4
HK7	0	0.0	...	1	81.0	2.0 - 450.1
HK8	2	96.0	11.6 - 346.4	3	143.5	29.6 - 419.6
HK9	0	0.0	...	2	176.3	21.3 - 636.3
HK10	21	118.4	73.1 - 181.0	8	51.2	22.1 - 100.9
HK11	0	0.0	...	2	167.2	20.2 - 603.8
HK12	2	128.9	15.6 - 465.4	3	203.0	41.9 - 593.6
HK13	3	145.8	30.1 - 426.4	1	63.4	1.6 - 352.1
HK14	2	29.4	3.6 - 106.3	5	82.6	26.7 - 193.1
HK15	4	168.5	45.9 - 431.0	2	97.0	11.7 - 350.3
HK16	7	74.8	30.0 - 154.1	6	86.1	31.5 - 187.6
HK17	13	107.2	57.0 - 183.2	6	65.1	23.8 - 141.8
HK18	0	0.0	...	0	0.0	...
HK19	8	123.0	53.0 - 242.1	4	76.7	20.9 - 196.2
HK20	12	90.9	46.8 - 158.6	18	176.4	104.4 - 278.7
HK21	1	49.7	1.3 - 275.9	1	68.8	1.7 - 382.3
KL1	10	168.4	81.0 - 309.6	3	67.2	13.9 - 196.6
KL2	15	122.4	68.4 - 201.9	9	104.0	47.7 - 197.4
KL3	2	57.0	6.9 - 205.9	2	71.7	8.7 - 258.7
KL4	8	75.1	32.4 - 147.9	6	84.2	30.9 - 183.5
KL5	7	91.9	36.9 - 189.4	7	128.4	51.5 - 264.6
KL6	5	257.3	83.3 - 601.1	0	0.0	...
KL7	2	114.9	13.9 - 414.7	1	65.6	1.7 - 364.5
KL8	4	66.6	18.2 - 170.4	2	44.6	5.4 - 161.0
KL9	22	93.3	58.3 - 141.4	22	119.1	74.5 - 180.5
KL10	1	38.4	1.0 - 213.6	2	93.6	11.3 - 337.8
KL11	10	149.7	72.0 - 275.3	5	88.4	28.6 - 206.5
KL12	2	117.7	14.3 - 425.1	1	88.3	2.2 - 490.5
KL13	25	124.5	80.3 - 183.6	7	49.0	19.7 - 101.0
KL14	14	108.1	59.1 - 181.3	10	101.5	48.8 - 186.5
KL15	4	157.0	42.8 - 401.6	5	249.1	80.6 - 582.0
KL16	2	38.3	4.6 - 138.3	1	28.2	0.7 - 156.9
KL17	5	269.9	87.3 - 630.6	2	88.1	10.7 - 317.9
KL18	1	88.0	2.2 - 489.1	1	109.3	2.8 - 607.1
KL19	21	99.4	61.4 - 152.0	15	92.8	51.8 - 153.1
KL20	6	118.1	43.3 - 257.4	8	197.3	85.0 - 388.4
KL21	5	63.4	20.5 - 148.2	5	83.0	26.9 - 193.9
KL22	0	0.0	...	1	77.1	1.9 - 428.1
KL23	1	20.1	0.5 - 111.5	8	225.3	97.1 - 443.5
KL24	6	159.0	58.2 - 346.4	4	138.6	37.8 - 354.6
KL25	75	100.7	77.9 - 123.4	49	87.2	62.8 - 111.7
NT1	4	81.7	22.3 - 209.0	4	109.8	29.9 - 280.9
NT2	6	110.3	40.4 - 240.3	8	200.8	86.6 - 395.3
NT3	15	155.3	86.8 - 256.3	5	77.6	25.1 - 181.3
NT4	9	96.8	44.4 - 183.7	9	130.0	59.6 - 246.6
NT5	13	76.4	40.6 - 130.6	17	136.9	79.6 - 219.0
NT6	14	138.8	75.8 - 232.9	9	123.4	56.6 - 234.2
NT7	3	48.3	10.0 - 141.2	6	136.4	49.9 - 297.1
NT8	24	103.2	66.1 - 153.5	21	118.8	73.3 - 181.6
NT9	3	99.3	20.5 - 290.4	2	87.1	10.5 - 314.4
NT10	8	60.0	25.8 - 118.0	9	91.5	42.0 - 173.6
NT11	1	38.7	1.0 - 215.1	1	49.7	1.3 - 276.2
NT12	16	129.9	74.2 - 210.9	6	64.2	23.5 - 140.0
NT13	1	29.7	0.8 - 164.7	4	171.4	46.7 - 438.5
NT14	1	55.6	1.4 - 308.8	1	72.2	1.8 - 400.9
NT15	8	62.7	27.0 - 123.5	12	117.6	60.6 - 205.2
NT16	40	129.7	89.5 - 169.8	20	79.1	44.4 - 113.8
NT17	4	87.7	23.9 - 224.4	7	198.1	79.6 - 408.4
NT18	4	188.7	51.4 - 482.6	2	114.1	13.8 - 412.0
NT19	2	61.6	7.5 - 222.4	0	0.0	...

LEUKAEMIA

Sex-Age specific mortality rate (1/100,000) of leukaemia in Hong Kong (1984–1988)

	Male		Female	
Age	No. of deaths	Mortality rate	No. of deaths	Mortality rate
0–4	20	1.87	16	1.61
5–9	23	2.10	17	1.67
10–14	18	1.58	19	1.82
15–19	46	3.84	22	2.00
20–24	31	2.15	19	1.37
25–29	41	2.61	18	1.22
30–34	33	2.44	25	2.02
35–39	33	2.97	15	1.55
40–44	24	3.27	14	2.33
45–49	32	4.55	16	2.74
50–54	42	5.73	20	3.17
55–59	35	5.27	41	6.75
60–64	45	8.33	38	7.10
65+	131	14.51	139	11.26
TOTAL	554	3.89	419	3.12

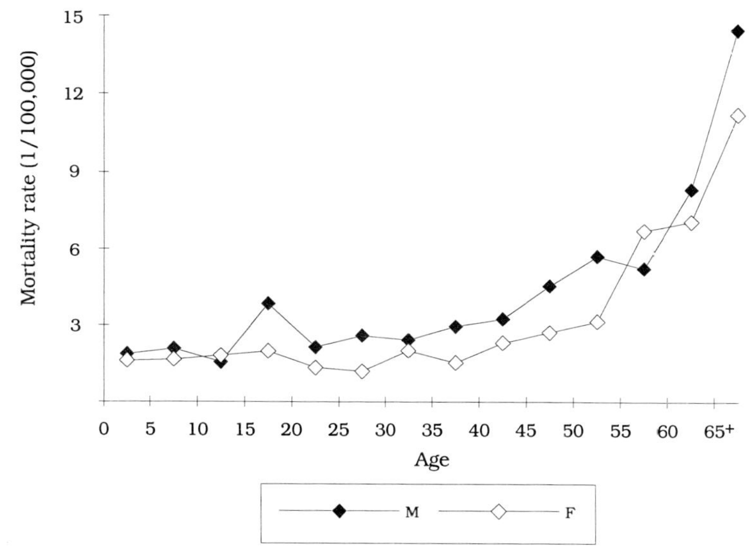

Number of communities on map by category based on standardized mortality ratio (SMR) during 1984–1988

Category	Number of communities Male	Number of communities Female
SMR significantly high, in top 20%	0	1
SMR significantly high , not in top 20%	0	0
SMR not significantly high, in top 20%	13	8
SMR not significantly low, in bottom 20%	5	5
SMR significantly low, not in bottom 20%	0	0
SMR significantly low, in bottom 20%	0	0
other communities	47	51

Values of the standardized mortality ratio (SMR) which divide the 65 communities into quintile

Percentile	Male	Female
20th	48.29	65.62
40th	81.70	86.12
60th	107.18	109.28
80th	129.67	136.90
Lowest SMR	0.00	0.00
Highest SMR	269.91	249.11
No. of communities with zero death	5	3

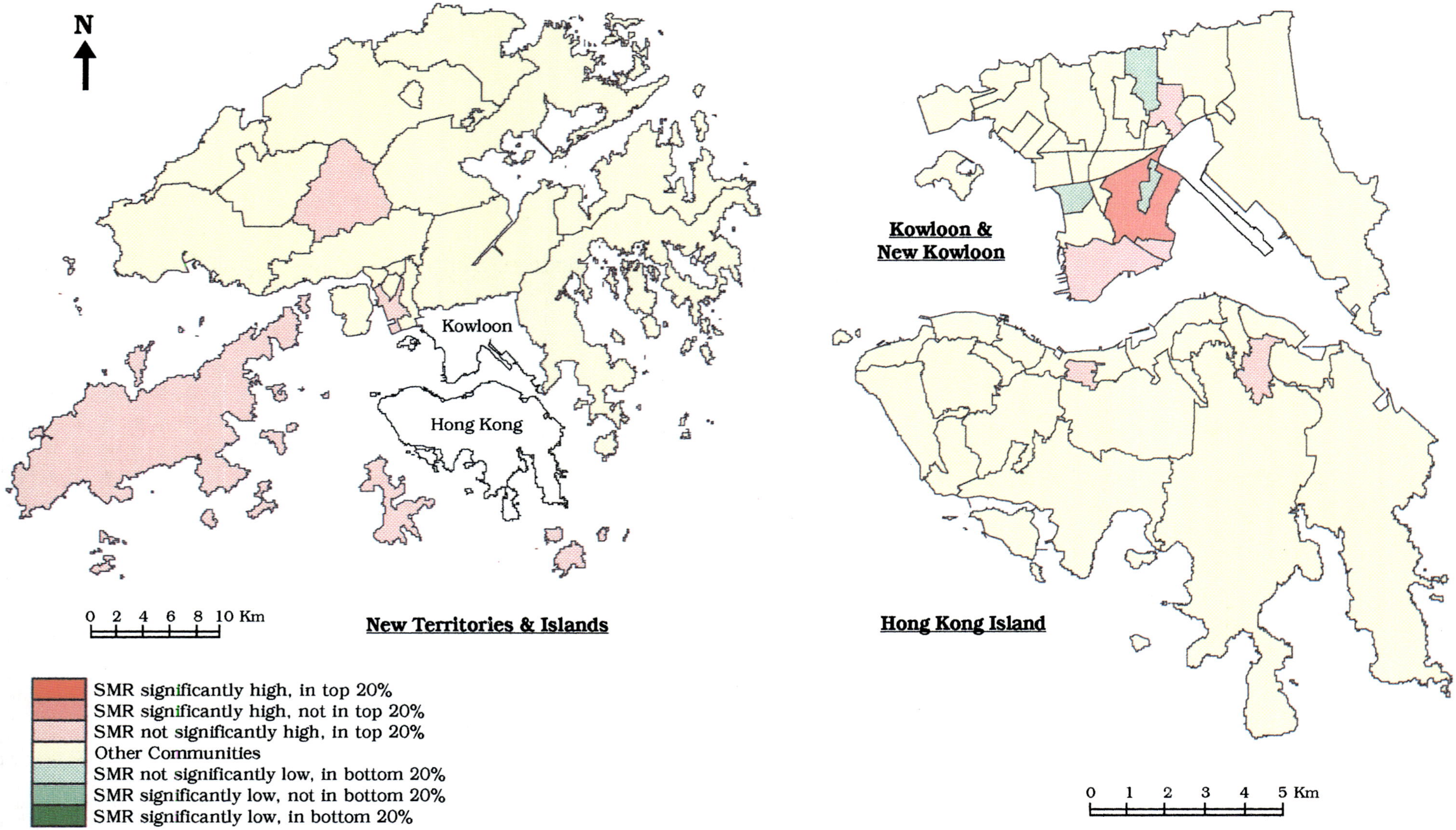

Leukaemia (Male, 1989 -1993)

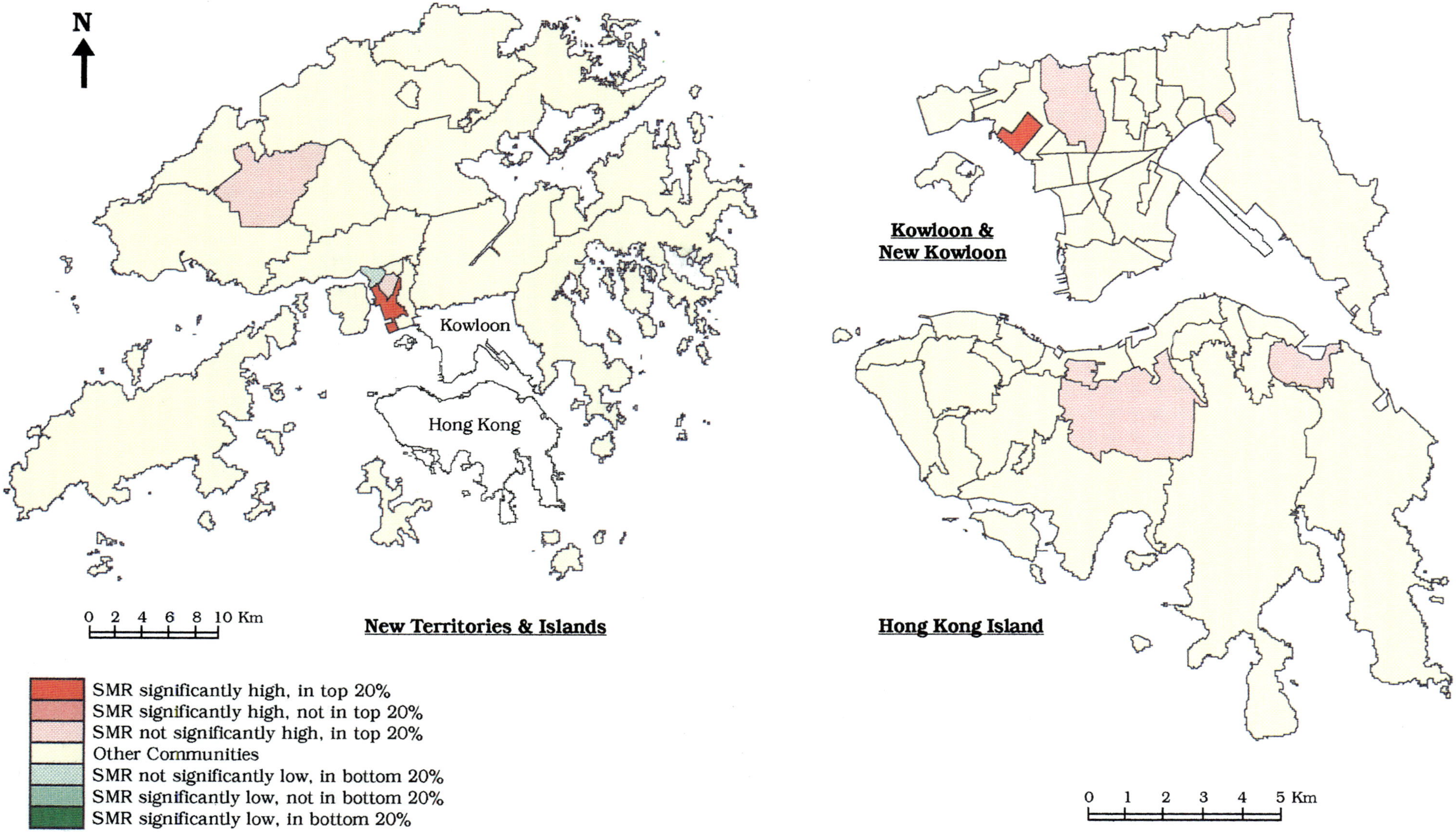

Leukaemia (Female, 1989 -1993)

Number of Deaths, Standardised Mortality Ratio (SMR) and 95% Confidence Interval of Leukaemia by 65 Communities in 1989–1993

Community	Male			Female		
	Number of deaths	SMR	95% C.I.	Number of deaths	SMR	95% C.I.
HK1	5	65.4	21.2 - 152.3	8	134.1	57.8 - 264.2
HK2	12	119.3	61.7 - 208.8	4	55.6	15.1 - 142.3
HK3	1	30.9	0.8 - 172.2	3	137.4	28.3 - 401.3
HK4	4	74.9	20.4 - 191.8	3	78.3	16.1 - 228.5
HK5	7	138.9	55.7 - 286.1	6	167.7	61.6 - 365.6
HK6	6	102.2	37.5 - 222.7	9	155.9	71.4 - 296.3
HK7	0	0.0	...	0	0.0	...
HK8	1	46.6	1.2 - 259.4	0	0.0	...
HK9	3	288.3	59.4 - 841.9	0	0.0	...
HK10	14	80.8	44.1 - 135.7	20	129.7	79.2 - 199.7
HK11	3	196.7	40.5 - 574.3	2	169.8	20.5 - 613.0
HK12	2	134.7	16.3 - 486.3	2	139.2	16.8 - 502.7
HK13	3	171.7	35.4 - 501.4	0	0.0	...
HK14	5	67.6	21.9 - 157.6	5	78.6	25.5 - 183.1
HK15	7	145.6	58.4 - 299.9	2	48.4	5.9 - 174.6
HK16	7	97.9	39.3 - 201.7	9	164.8	75.5 - 313.2
HK17	19	121.4	73.1 - 189.3	8	65.7	30.1 - 129.4
HK18	0	0.0	...	1	64.9	1.6 - 361.5
HK19	7	112.8	45.2 - 232.4	5	102.0	33.0 - 237.7
HK20	12	84.7	43.8 - 148.1	9	81.3	37.2 - 154.5
HK21	1	54.0	1.4 - 300.8	1	76.4	1.9 - 425.6
KL1	6	137.3	50.4 - 299.3	4	120.0	32.6 - 307.2
KL2	7	65.8	26.4 - 135.6	5	69.4	22.5 - 161.6
KL3	1	34.3	0.9 - 191.1	2	87.4	10.6 - 315.5
KL4	4	47.2	12.8 - 120.7	6	108.3	39.7 - 236.1
KL5	5	83.8	27.2 - 195.4	2	48.8	5.9 - 176.0
KL6	0	0.0	...	1	47.4	1.2 - 264.2
KL7	3	183.0	37.7 - 534.3	0	0.0	...
KL8	3	55.3	11.4 - 161.4	4	100.8	27.4 - 258.1
KL9	26	122.3	169.4 - 169.4	19	116.6	70.2 - 181.8
KL10	6	136.7	50.2 - 297.9	1	25.3	0.6 - 141.1
KL11	5	102.0	33.0 - 237.5	1	23.7	0.6 - 132.1
KL12	2	130.9	15.8 - 472.7	1	99.2	2.5 - 552.4
KL13	15	79.8	44.7 - 131.7	11	86.2	43.0 - 154.2
KL14	11	98.5	49.2 - 176.4	12	138.2	71.4 - 241.8
KL15	0	0.0	...	7	386.7	155.1 - 796.6
KL16	3	68.7	14.1 - 200.6	4	134.4	36.6 - 344.1
KL17	2	120.1	14.5 - 433.6	1	53.0	1.3 - 295.2
KL18	0	0.0	...	1	115.0	2.9 - 640.7
KL19	18	92.4	54.8 - 146.0	20	131.3	80.2 - 202.3
KL20	2	41.7	5.0 - 150.6	3	82.1	16.9 - 239.8
KL21	11	164.5	82.1 - 294.4	9	82.1	37.6 - 156.0
KL22	2	132.7	16.1 - 479.0	0	0.0	...
KL23	4	131.9	35.9 - 337.6	3	136.2	28.1 - 397.6
KL24	3	85.9	17.7 - 250.9	5	198.1	64.2 - 461.5
KL25	62	96.5	72.5 - 120.6	51	103.6	75.2 - 132.1
NT1	5	74.4	24.1 - 173.4	5	94.5	30.6 - 220.2
NT2	9	169.8	77.8 - 322.7	10	236.5	113.5 - 435.1
NT3	11	104.6	52.2 - 187.2	3	41.4	8.5 - 120.8
NT4	5	69.9	22.6 - 162.9	5	89.6	29.0 - 208.7
NT5	8	57.4	24.7 - 113.0	16	155.7	89.1 - 252.3
NT6	6	62.1	22.8 - 135.5	4	56.5	15.4 - 144.7
NT7	11	90.9	45.4 - 162.8	6	67.2	24.6 - 146.4
NT8	35	122.7	82.1 - 163.4	14	63.0	34.4 - 105.9
NT9	2	80.5	9.7 - 290.7	2	105.9	12.8 - 382.4
NT10	19	132.6	79.8 - 206.8	15	142.8	80.0 - 235.6
NT11	4	167.1	45.5 - 427.9	0	0.0	...
NT12	17	125.8	73.4 - 201.3	8	79.1	34.1 - 155.9
NT13	0	0.0	...	1	43.3	1.1 - 241.2
NT14	1	78.1	2.0 - 435.2	0	0.0	...
NT15	14	84.4	46.1 - 141.8	12	90.4	46.7 - 158.2
NT16	59	84.4	56.3 - 112.4	42	120.6	84.1 - 157.1
NT17	9	85.1	39.0 - 161.8	5	59.7	19.3 - 139.1
NT18	4	183.2	49.8 - 469.0	2	112.9	13.7 - 407.4
NT19	4	137.4	37.4 - 351.7	2	98.4	11.9 - 355.1

LEUKAEMIA

Sex-Age specific mortality rate (1/100,000) of leukaemia in Hong Kong (1989–1993)

	Male		Female	
Age	No. of deaths	Mortality rate	No. of deaths	Mortality rate
0–4	12	1.26	10	1.13
5–9	14	1.32	8	0.82
10–14	14	1.28	16	1.59
15–19	15	1.37	17	1.70
20–24	23	2.01	14	1.23
25–29	35	2.43	17	1.15
30–34	35	2.24	21	1.38
35–39	36	2.69	24	1.91
40–44	27	2.45	32	3.29
45–49	26	3.56	17	2.85
50–54	41	5.91	17	2.99
55–59	39	5.58	25	4.10
60–64	50	8.10	37	6.40
65+	176	15.89	167	11.89
TOTAL	543	3.71	422	3.02

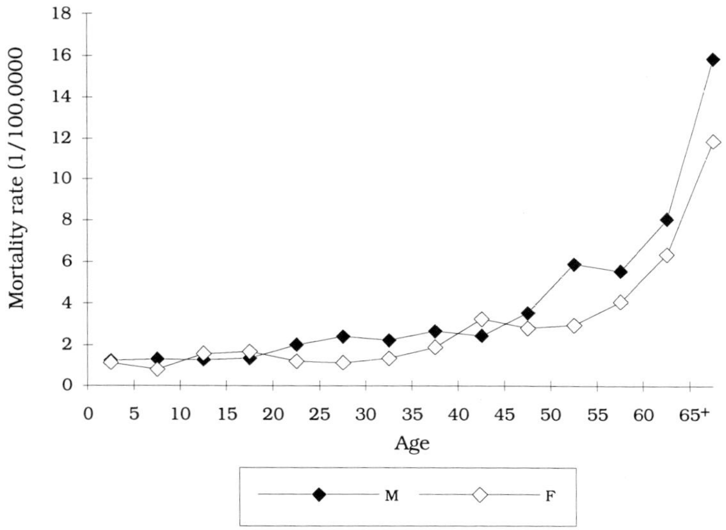

Number of communities on map by category based on standardized mortality ratio (SMR) during 1989–1993

Category	Number of communities Male	Number of communities Female
SMR significantly high, in top 20%	0	2
SMR significantly high , not in top 20%	1	0
SMR not significantly high, in top 20%	9	7
SMR not significantly low, in bottom 20%	3	1
SMR significantly low, not in bottom 20%	0	0
SMR significantly low, in bottom 20%	0	0
other communities	52	55

Values of the standardized mortality ratio (SMR) which divide the 65 communities into quintile

Percentile	Male	Female
20th	55.28	47.43
40th	80.77	78.27
60th	102.17	100.83
80th	134.72	134.42
Lowest SMR	0.00	0.00
Highest SMR	288.31	386.71
No. of communities with zero cases	6	8

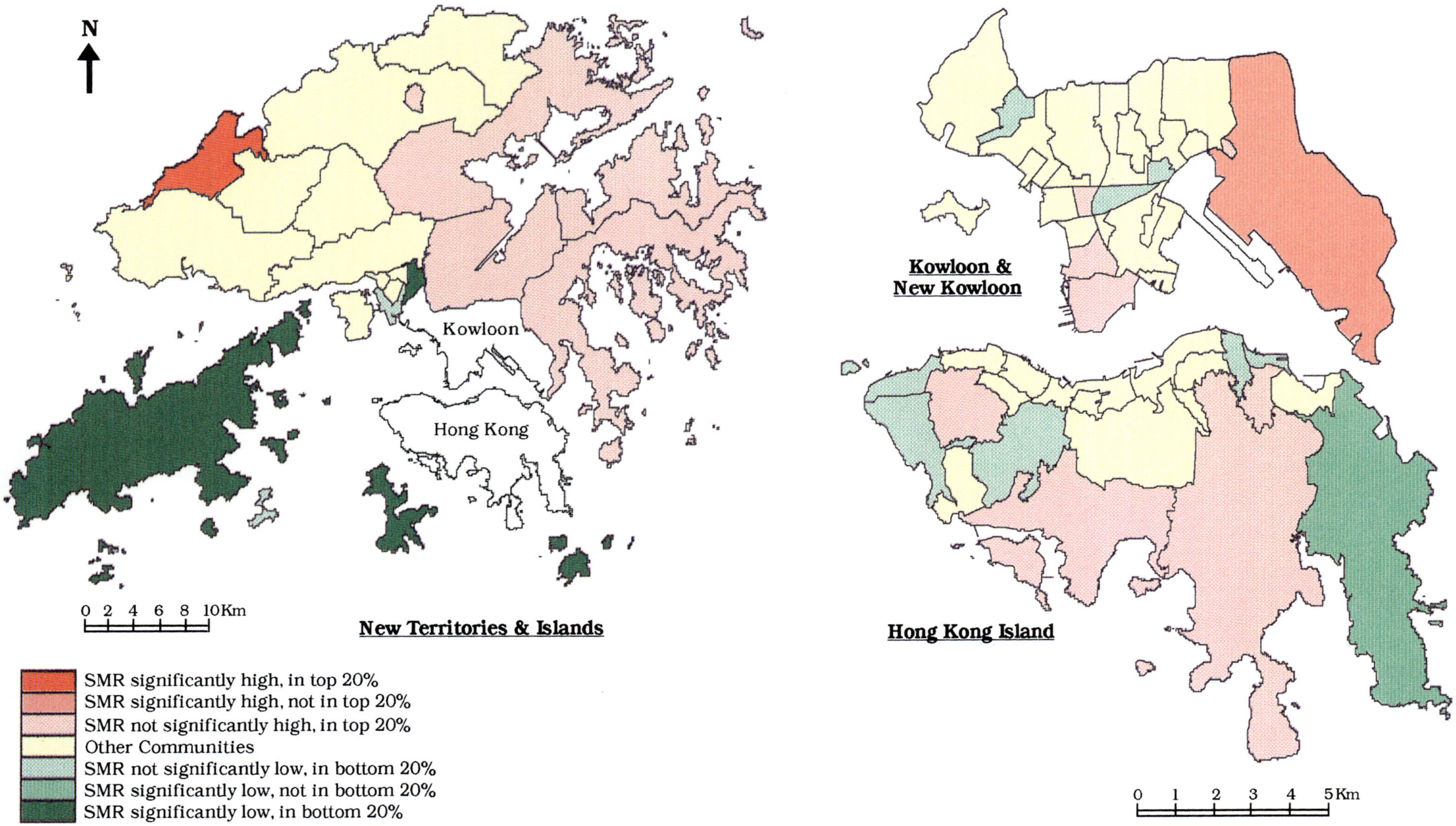

HBP (Male, 1979 – 1983)

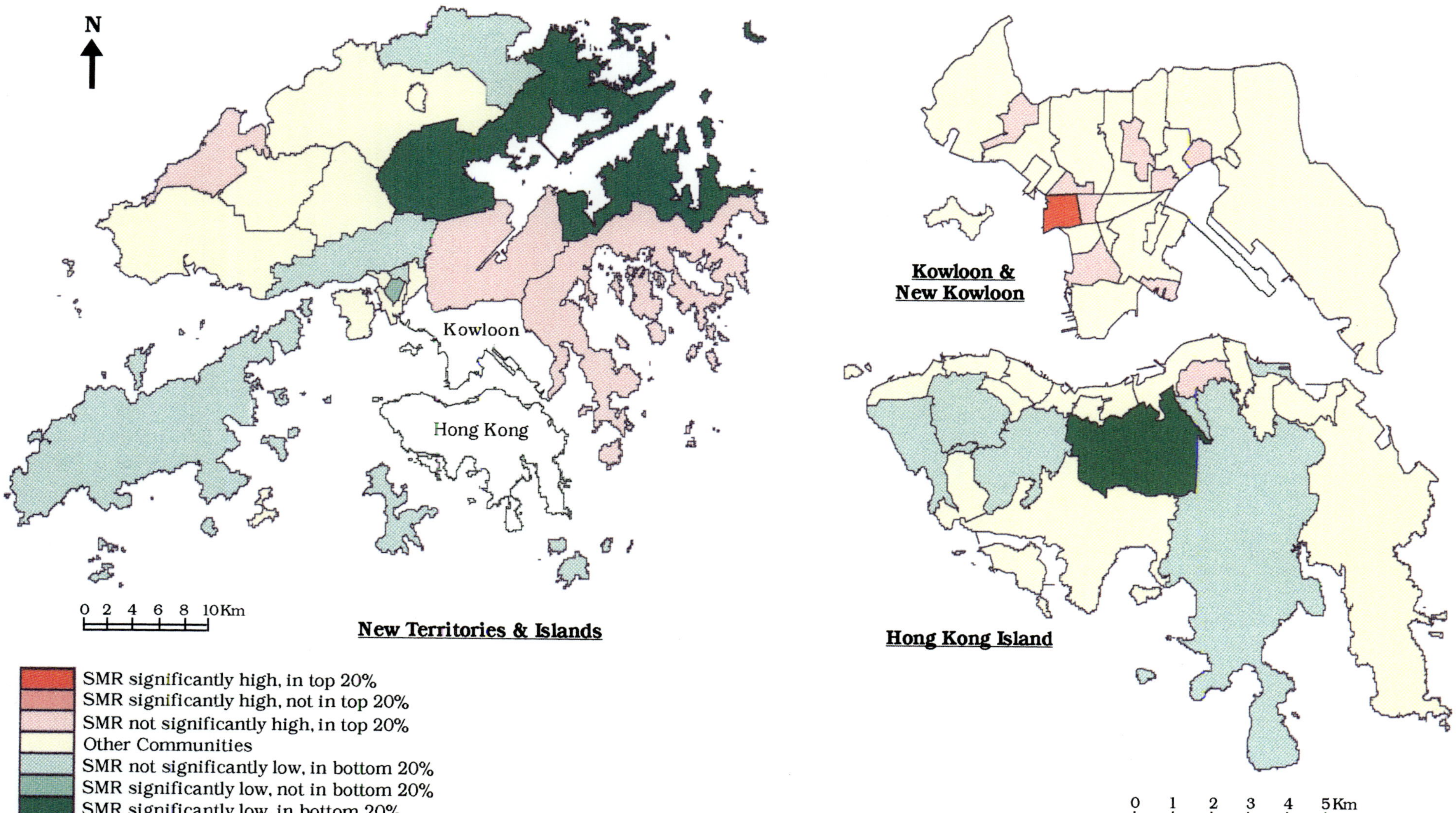

HBP (Female, 1979 - 1983)

Number of Deaths, Standardised Mortality Ratio (SMR) and 95% Confidence Interval of HBP by 65 Communities in 1979–1983

Community	Male			Female		
	Number of deaths	SMR	95% C.I.	Number of deaths	SMR	95% C.I.
HK1	22	67.4	42.1 - 102.1	29	102.6	65.3 - 139.9
HK2	53	98.6	72.1 - 125.2	32	76.5	50.0 - 103.0
HK3	19	89.1	53.7 - 139.2	15	95.9	53.6 - 158.2
HK4	30	93.9	60.3 - 127.5	20	75.2	45.9 - 116.3
HK5	24	76.2	48.8 - 113.3	21	82.0	50.6 - 125.3
HK6	20	77.9	47.5 - 120.4	16	54.4	31.1 - 88.3
HK7	7	136.6	54.9 - 281.7	2	33.8	4.1 - 122.0
HK8	9	87.9	40.3 - 166.7	13	107.0	56.9 - 182.9
HK9	3	67.0	13.8 - 195.9	3	57.5	11.9 - 168.2
HK10	66	93.7	71.1 - 116.3	73	101.5	78.2 - 124.8
HK11	6	99.6	36.5 - 216.9	2	41.1	5.0 - 148.5
HK12	5	101.2	32.8 - 236.5	9	136.2	62.5 - 258.5
HK13	5	62.3	20.1 - 145.5	8	101.4	43.7 - 199.6
HK14	13	65.5	34.9 - 112.0	13	69.5	37.0 - 118.8
HK15	10	128.7	61.9 - 236.6	7	90.0	36.2 - 185.7
HK16	35	93.8	62.7 - 124.9	31	99.5	64.5 - 134.6
HK17	28	67.6	42.6 - 92.7	34	98.2	65.2 - 131.2
HK18	2	34.6	4.2 - 125.1	4	67.2	18.3 - 171.8
HK19	16	85.5	48.9 - 138.8	13	74.0	39.3 - 126.4
HK20	52	120.3	87.6 - 153.1	34	93.9	62.3 - 125.4
HK21	6	120.1	44.0 - 261.6	2	49.4	6.0 - 178.2
KL1	39	142.1	97.5 - 186.7	23	101.9	64.5 - 153.0
KL2	56	100.7	74.3 - 127.1	65	133.8	101.3 - 166.4
KL3	21	127.3	78.6 - 194.6	23	144.5	91.4 - 216.9
KL4	46	101.2	71.9 - 130.4	44	115.8	81.6 - 150.1
KL5	47	121.1	86.5 - 155.8	38	122.2	83.3 - 161.0
KL6	6	59.9	22.0 - 130.6	9	73.5	33.7 - 139.4
KL7	7	98.1	39.4 - 202.3	8	97.4	42.0 - 191.6
KL8	26	110.3	67.9 - 152.7	24	105.8	67.8 - 157.4
KL9	98	112.2	90.0 - 134.4	88	105.4	83.3 - 127.4
KL10	9	103.8	47.6 - 196.9	12	136.5	70.4 - 238.2
KL11	17	69.3	40.3 - 110.8	19	78.0	47.0 - 121.8
KL12	5	65.2	21.1 - 152.4	8	127.1	54.8 - 250.2
KL13	91	99.4	79.0 - 119.8	84	107.0	84.2 - 129.9
KL14	58	101.4	75.3 - 127.5	41	95.2	66.1 - 124.3
KL15	5	119.0	38.5 - 278.1	2	51.7	6.3 - 186.6
KL16	26	119.6	73.7 - 165.6	30	151.4	97.2 - 205.6
KL17	5	80.4	26.0 - 187.9	10	119.0	57.2 - 218.7
KL18	2	52.0	6.3 - 187.7	7	172.6	69.3 - 356.0
KL19	81	102.7	80.3 - 125.1	80	106.8	83.4 - 130.2
KL20	25	87.9	53.4 - 122.3	24	95.3	61.1 - 141.8
KL21	43	91.9	64.4 - 119.4	43	104.6	73.3 - 135.8
KL22	8	103.6	44.7 - 204.0	9	149.4	68.5 - 283.5
KL23	16	66.7	38.1 - 108.2	29	144.4	91.8 - 197.0
KL24	20	143.4	87.4 - 221.6	11	89.5	44.7 - 160.1
KL25	254	118.0	103.5 - 132.5	199	103.9	89.4 - 118.3
NT1	10	90.7	43.6 - 166.7	5	47.1	15.3 - 110.1
NT2	10	64.2	30.9 - 118.1	14	106.2	58.0 - 178.2
NT3	26	82.1	50.5 - 113.6	28	119.7	75.4 - 164.0
NT4	15	93.0	52.0 - 153.5	10	62.3	29.9 - 114.4
NT5	57	93.9	69.5 - 118.3	39	73.1	50.2 - 96.1
NT6	17	58.6	34.1 - 93.8	26	95.1	58.5 - 131.6
NT7	8	80.7	34.8 - 158.8	6	70.1	25.7 - 152.8
NT8	34	101.2	67.2 - 135.2	22	79.5	49.7 - 120.5
NT9	21	191.9	118.4 - 293.4	11	126.4	63.2 - 226.2
NT10	45	99.5	70.4 - 128.6	41	115.0	79.8 - 150.2
NT11	11	116.6	58.3 - 208.6	6	84.7	31.0 - 184.6
NT12	41	94.8	65.7 - 123.8	35	98.6	65.9 - 131.2
NT13	12	148.4	76.5 - 259.0	8	113.5	48.9 - 223.4
NT14	8	104.7	45.2 - 206.2	4	54.2	14.8 - 138.6
NT15	36	119.9	80.7 - 159.1	17	62.4	36.3 - 99.9
NT16	46	131.8	93.7 - 169.9	46	139.0	98.8 - 179.2
NT17	26	144.6	89.0 - 200.2	23	147.3	93.2 - 221.2
NT18	5	55.5	17.9 - 129.6	10	121.5	58.4 - 223.4
NT19	7	46.0	18.5 - 94.8	7	49.3	19.8 - 101.7

HBP

Sex-Age specific mortality rate (1/100,000) of HBP in Hong Kong (1979–1983)

Age	Male No. of deaths	Male Mortality rate	Female No. of deaths	Female Mortality rate
0–4	0	0.00	0	0.00
5–9	0	0.00	0	0.00
10–14	0	0.00	0	0.00
15–19	0	0.00	0	0.00
20–24	1	0.07	0	0.00
25–29	1	0.08	2	0.17
30–34	8	0.73	2	0.22
35–39	8	1.11	4	0.72
40–44	18	2.56	14	2.53
45–49	71	9.84	46	7.60
50–54	113	16.45	70	11.48
55–59	179	31.47	106	19.82
60–64	274	59.96	148	32.44
65+	1204	176.60	1277	126.50
TOTAL	1877	14.24	1669	13.71

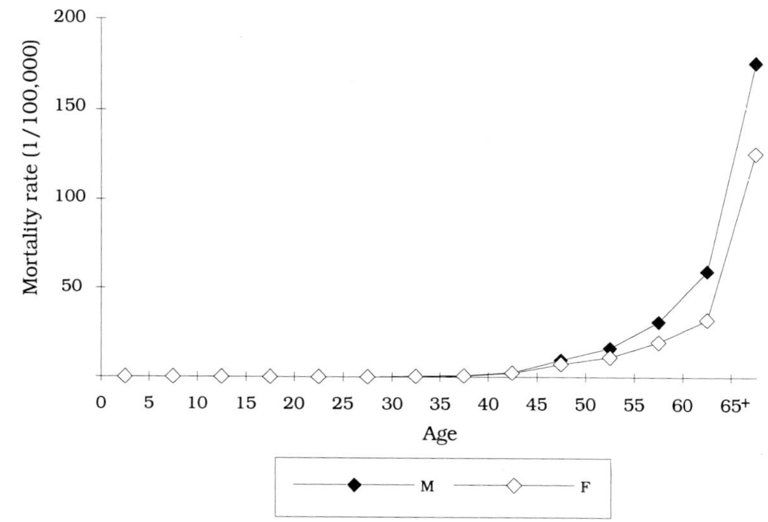

Number of communities on map by category based on standardized mortality ratio (SMR) during 1979–1983

Category	Number of communities Male	Number of communities Female
SMR significantly high, in top 20%	1	1
SMR significantly high , not in top 20%	1	0
SMR not significantly high, in top 20%	12	12
SMR not significantly low, in bottom 20%	10	10
SMR significantly low, not in bottom 20%	1	1
SMR significantly low, in bottom 20%	2	2
other communities	38	39

Values of the standardized mortality ratio (SMR) which divide the 65 communities into quintile

Percentile	Male	Female
20th	67.35	69.52
40th	91.92	93.88
60th	101.15	103.86
80th	119.64	121.53
Lowest SMR	34.64	33.80
Highest SMR	191.88	172.64
No. of communities with zero death	0	0

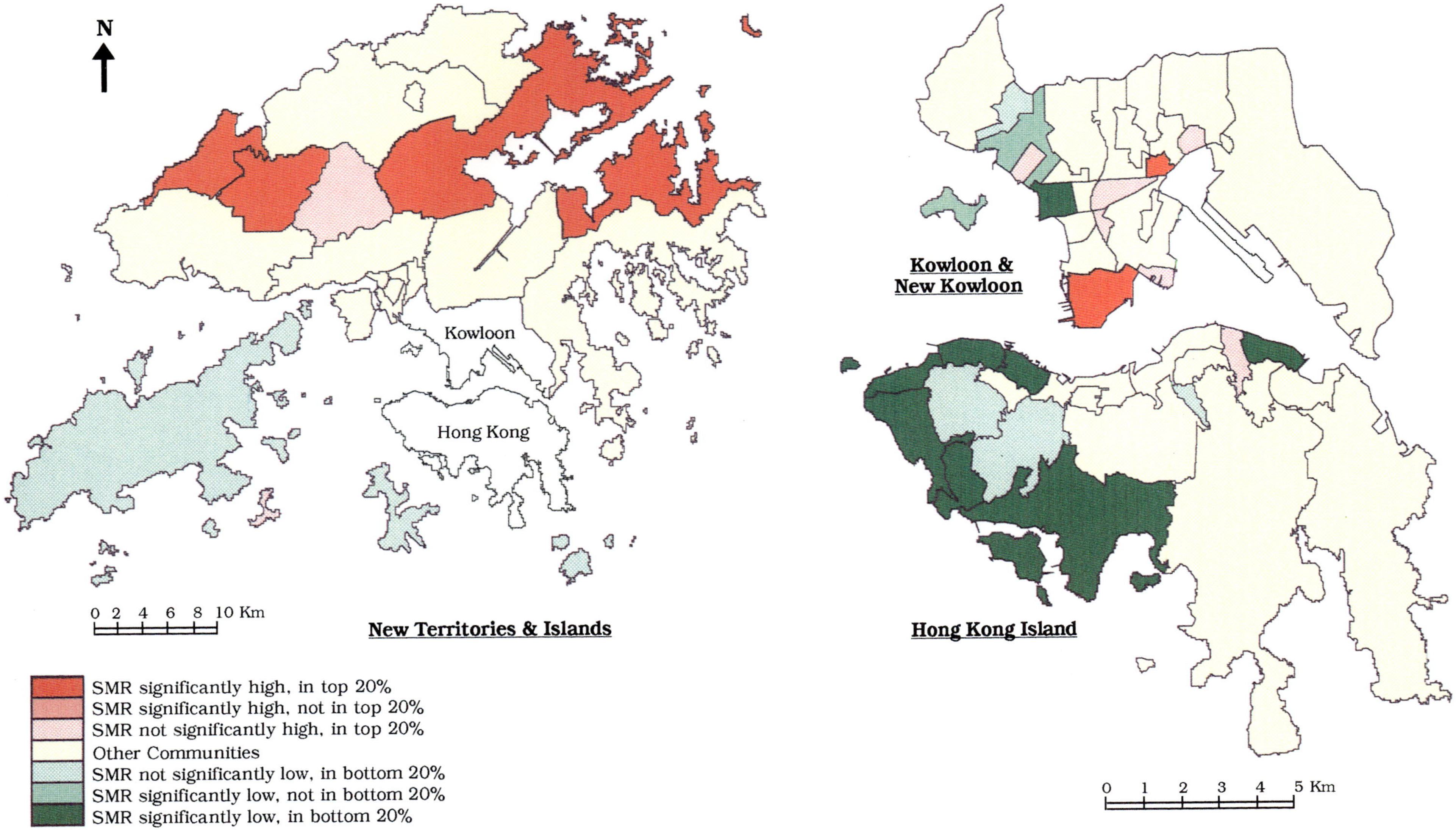

HBP (Male, 1984 -1988)

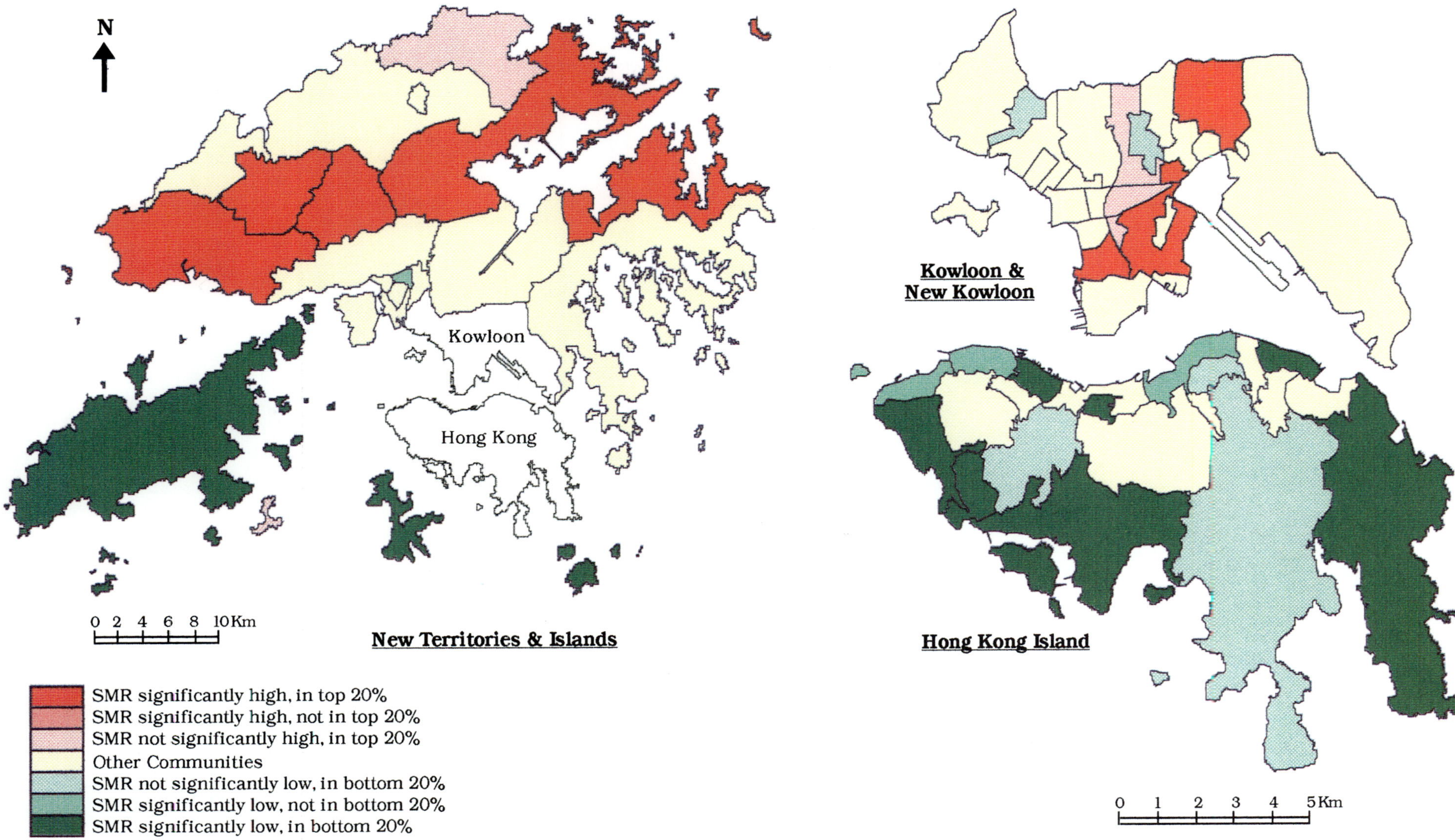

HBP (Female, 1984 – 1988)

Number of Deaths, Standardised Mortality Ratio (SMR) and 95% Confidence Interval of HBP by 65 Communities in 1984–1988

Community	Male			Female		
	Number of deaths	SMR	95% C.I.	Number of deaths	SMR	95% C.I.
HK1	19	48.4	26.7 - 70.2	24	68.5	41.1 - 95.9
HK2	33	59.0	38.9 - 79.2	37	73.9	50.1 - 97.7
HK3	12	57.2	29.5 - 99.7	7	41.8	16.8 - 86.2
HK4	33	99.2	65.4 - 133.1	22	73.1	42.5 - 103.6
HK5	36	122.0	82.2 - 161.9	14	49.3	23.5 - 75.1
HK6	25	82.5	50.2 - 114.9	26	75.0	46.2 - 103.8
HK7	4	64.8	17.7 - 165.7	7	102.3	41.1 - 211.0
HK8	9	79.4	36.4 - 150.7	10	80.7	38.8 - 148.3
HK9	3	63.9	13.2 - 186.9	2	33.4	4.0 - 120.7
HK10	68	82.4	62.8 - 101.9	70	77.4	59.3 - 95.5
HK11	4	53.9	14.7 - 137.8	4	70.4	19.2 - 180.1
HK12	6	89.6	32.8 - 195.2	4	55.6	15.2 - 142.3
HK13	15	149.1	83.3 - 246.1	9	105.8	48.5 - 200.7
HK14	19	62.2	34.2 - 90.1	18	55.7	30.0 - 81.5
HK15	9	96.2	44.1 - 182.5	8	75.3	32.5 - 148.2
HK16	35	83.1	55.6 - 110.7	33	85.5	56.3 - 114.7
HK17	49	85.6	61.6 - 109.5	35	67.4	45.1 - 89.8
HK18	0	0.0	...	1	14.5	0.4 - 80.4
HK19	16	62.0	31.6 - 92.4	14	55.9	26.6 - 85.1
HK20	40	68.2	47.0 - 89.3	30	56.4	36.2 - 76.6
HK21	7	105.6	42.4 - 217.7	2	29.2	3.5 - 105.6
KL1	46	154.5	109.8 - 199.1	28	108.6	68.4 - 148.9
KL2	36	64.7	43.5 - 85.8	45	87.5	61.9 - 113.0
KL3	13	73.8	39.2 - 126.1	13	72.3	38.4 - 123.5
KL4	46	86.6	61.6 - 111.6	42	95.9	66.9 - 124.9
KL5	53	133.6	97.7 - 169.6	48	141.4	101.4 - 181.4
KL6	17	147.5	85.8 - 236.0	20	151.2	92.2 - 233.6
KL7	11	137.5	68.7 - 246.0	10	129.1	62.1 - 237.3
KL8	33	124.1	81.8 - 166.5	24	97.4	62.4 - 144.9
KL9	107	101.4	82.2 - 120.6	130	129.7	107.4 - 152.0
KL10	14	137.9	75.3 - 231.3	10	95.9	46.1 - 176.3
KL11	32	102.3	66.9 - 137.8	26	86.2	53.0 - 119.3
KL12	3	34.7	7.2 - 101.6	5	66.9	21.7 - 156.4
KL13	69	72.3	55.2 - 89.3	85	98.5	77.5 - 119.4
KL14	76	102.2	79.2 - 125.1	70	112.6	86.2 - 138.9
KL15	17	147.2	85.6 - 235.6	8	68.0	29.3 - 133.9
KL16	19	79.4	47.8 - 124.1	22	106.3	66.4 - 161.1
KL17	15	128.2	71.6 - 211.5	25	142.6	92.0 - 210.3
KL18	5	116.7	37.8 - 272.7	2	48.9	5.9 - 176.5
KL19	110	110.7	90.0 - 131.3	122	132.6	109.1 - 156.2
KL20	24	97.9	62.8 - 145.7	27	112.6	74.1 - 163.9
KL21	53	121.8	89.0 - 154.6	44	120.9	85.2 - 156.6
KL22	14	166.8	91.1 - 279.8	7	93.2	37.4 - 192.2
KL23	40	189.3	135.2 - 258.0	38	204.4	144.4 - 280.8
KL24	20	98.7	60.2 - 152.5	19	120.4	72.6 - 188.2
KL25	320	104.6	93.1 - 116.0	285	102.9	91.0 - 114.9
NT1	12	71.4	36.8 - 124.6	20	122.9	74.9 - 189.9
NT2	17	79.9	46.4 - 127.8	15	80.8	45.2 - 133.4
NT3	49	129.9	93.5 - 166.2	24	83.9	50.4 - 117.5
NT4	22	72.1	42.0 - 102.2	20	67.8	38.1 - 97.5
NT5	56	82.3	60.8 - 103.9	54	92.3	67.7 - 116.9
NT6	39	97.0	66.5 - 127.4	33	95.8	63.1 - 128.5
NT7	19	98.9	59.6 - 154.5	13	83.7	44.5 - 143.0
NT8	69	101.9	77.8 - 125.9	85	127.3	100.3 - 154.4
NT9	23	180.8	114.4 - 271.4	15	120.7	67.4 - 199.1
NT10	87	139.9	110.5 - 169.3	86	163.0	128.5 - 197.4
NT11	15	138.4	77.3 - 228.4	19	174.8	105.3 - 273.2
NT12	60	110.9	82.8 - 138.9	57	110.2	81.6 - 138.8
NT13	15	105.9	59.2 - 174.8	8	73.6	31.7 - 144.9
NT14	10	110.2	53.0 - 202.6	12	139.2	71.8 - 243.0
NT15	66	134.3	101.9 - 166.7	74	145.2	112.1 - 178.3
NT16	111	108.1	88.0 - 128.2	122	106.6	87.6 - 125.5
NT17	25	113.3	73.1 - 167.1	17	86.5	50.3 - 138.4
NT18	16	144.3	82.5 - 234.3	14	130.2	71.2 - 218.5
NT19	9	53.6	24.6 - 101.7	5	32.1	10.4 - 75.0

HBP

Sex-Age specific mortality rate (1/100,000) of HBP in Hong Kong (1984–1988)

	Male		Female	
Age	No. of deaths	Mortality rate	No. of deaths	Mortality rate
0–4	0	0.00	0	0.00
5–9	0	0.00	0	0.00
10–14	0	0.00	0	0.00
15–19	0	0.00	1	0.09
20–24	0	0.00	0	0.00
25–29	1	0.06	0	0.00
30–34	4	0.30	2	0.16
35–39	21	1.89	6	0.62
40–44	17	2.32	7	1.17
45–49	52	7.39	21	3.60
50–54	114	15.55	67	10.61
55–59	202	30.41	113	18.60
60–64	348	64.43	206	38.48
65+	1664	184.30	1817	147.22
TOTAL	2423	16.99	2240	16.69

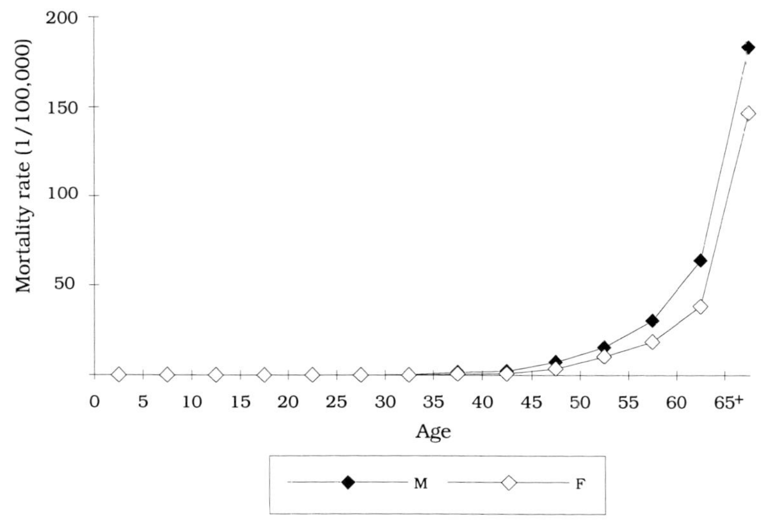

Number of communities on map by category based on standardized mortality ratio (SMR) during 1984–1988

Category	Number of communities Male	Female
SMR significantly high, in top 20%	5	8
SMR significantly high , not in top 20%	0	0
SMR not significantly high, in top 20%	8	5
SMR not significantly low, in bottom 20%	5	5
SMR significantly low, not in bottom 20%	1	4
SMR significantly low, in bottom 20%	8	8
other communities	38	35

Values of the standardized mortality ratio (SMR) which divide the 65 communities into quintile

Percentile	Male	Female
20th	68.17	67.43
40th	86.60	80.84
60th	105.57	98.46
80th	133.64	122.86
Lowest SMR	0.00	14.48
Highest SMR	189.34	204.42
No. of communities with zero death	1	0

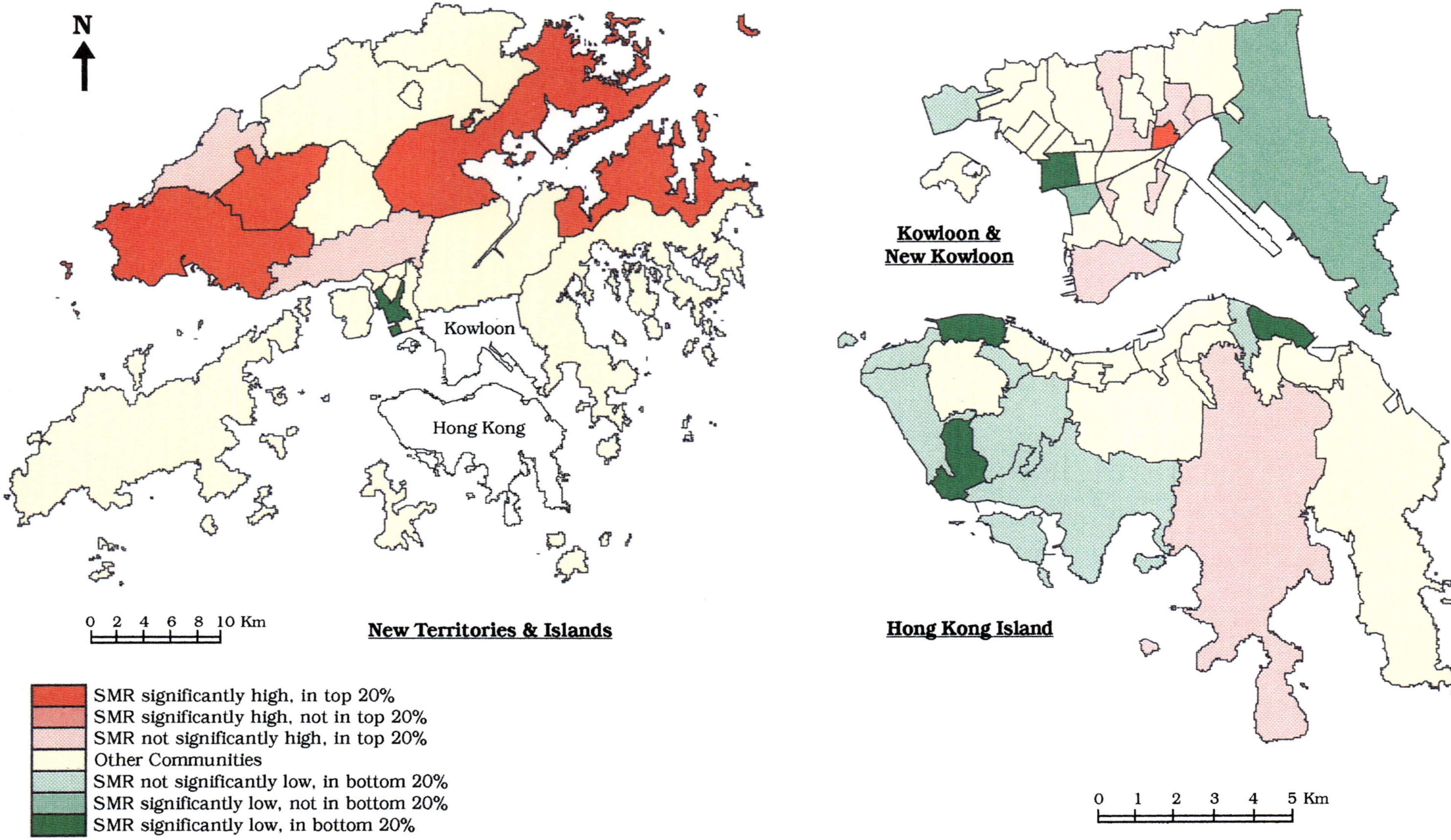

HBP (Male, 1989 -1993)

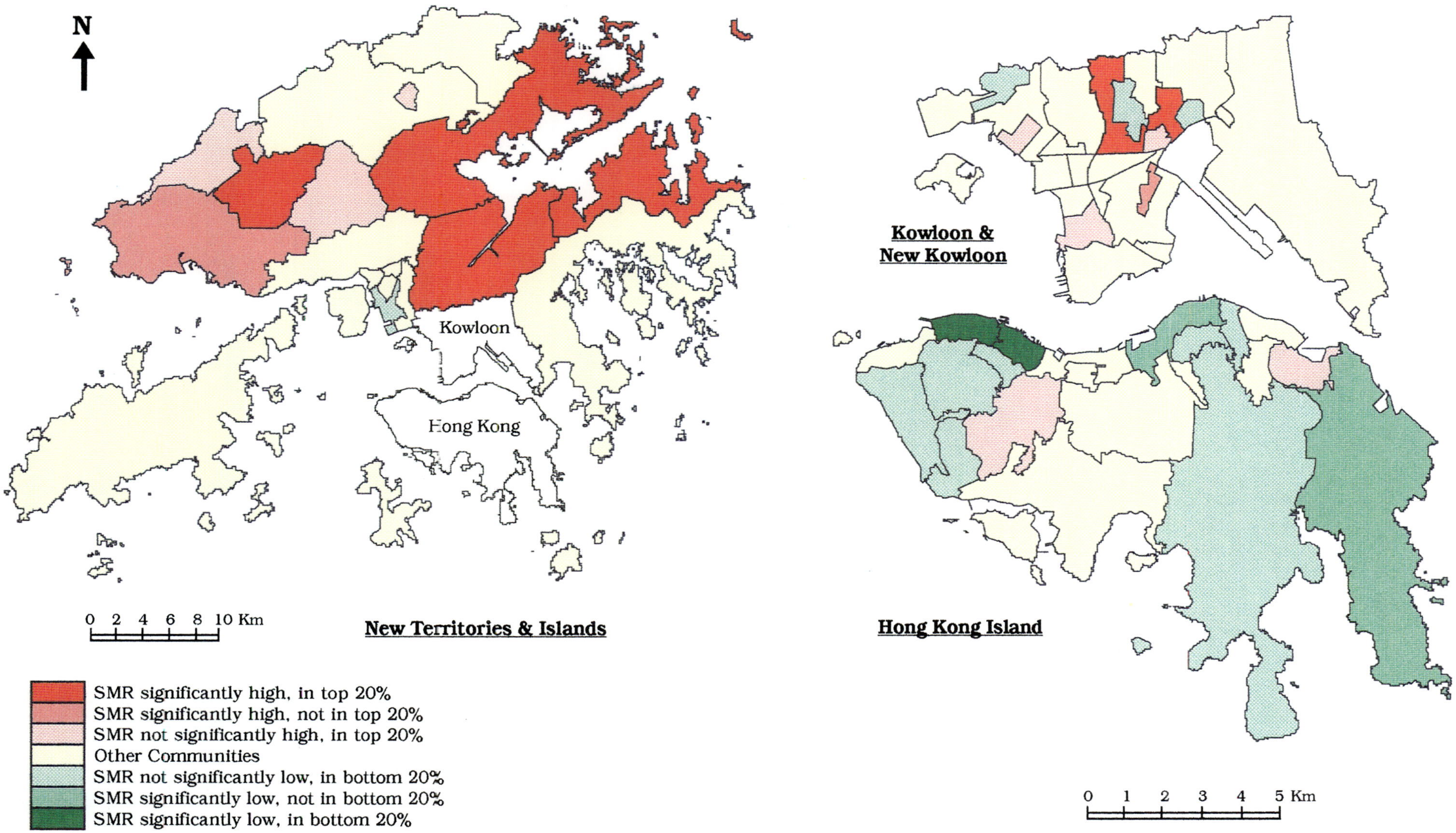

HBP (Female, 1989 -1993)

Number of Deaths, Standardised Mortality Ratio (SMR) and 95% Confidence Interval of HBP by 65 Communities in 1989–1993

Community	Male			Female		
	Number of deaths	SMR	95% C.I.	Number of deaths	SMR	95% C.I.
HK1	24	68.4	43.8 - 101.9	23	70.3	44.6 - 105.5
HK2	32	67.4	44.1 - 90.8	20	50.4	30.8 - 77.6
HK3	16	96.8	55.4 - 156.9	6	45.6	16.7 - 99.5
HK4	19	71.1	42.8 - 111.0	19	81.3	48.9 - 126.8
HK5	19	74.3	44.7 - 115.9	21	95.3	59.0 - 145.7
HK6	26	90.2	55.5 - 124.8	30	93.1	59.8 - 126.4
HK7	5	80.6	26.1 - 187.8	5	66.1	21.4 - 154.0
HK8	7	68.6	27.5 - 141.4	7	68.4	27.4 - 141.0
HK9	3	69.7	8.3 - 203.4	6	128.4	47.1 - 279.9
HK10	87	108.8	86.0 - 131.7	71	81.0	62.1 - 99.8
HK11	7	93.9	37.6 - 193.4	6	99.3	36.5 - 216.6
HK12	7	111.4	44.7 - 229.5	4	58.9	16.0 - 150.9
HK13	4	44.8	12.2 - 114.8	4	50.8	13.8 - 130.0
HK14	11	35.5	17.7 - 63.5	25	83.1	53.7 - 122.9
HK15	16	90.1	51.6 - 146.0	13	72.8	38.7 - 124.5
HK16	35	107.4	71.8 - 142.9	40	132.9	91.7 - 174.1
HK17	59	86.0	64.0 - 107.9	47	72.7	51.9 - 93.5
HK18	5	66.5	21.5 - 155.0	3	32.6	6.7 - 95.2
HK19	16	58.7	33.6 - 95.0	16	65.6	37.5 - 106.2
HK20	39	63.2	33.2 - 222.9	53	89.2	65.2 - 113.2
HK21	7	128.1	51.4 - 263.8	2	42.6	5.2 - 153.8
KL1	30	142.7	91.6 - 193.7	17	90.7	52.9 - 145.1
KL2	33	69.3	45.6 - 92.9	40	94.1	64.9 - 123.2
KL3	17	117.9	68.7 - 188.7	14	97.5	53.3 - 163.9
KL4	29	71.1	45.2 - 97.0	23	70.5	44.7 - 105.8
KL5	33	109.9	72.4 - 147.4	34	132.1	87.7 - 176.5
KL6	13	109.7	58.4 - 187.6	14	93.6	51.1 - 157.3
KL7	13	165.5	88.0 - 283.0	7	93.6	37.5 - 192.9
KL8	32	132.9	86.8 - 178.9	26	119.1	119.1 - 164.9
KL9	104	107.1	86.5 - 127.7	73	81.5	81.5 - 100.2
KL10	8	51.6	22.3 - 101.7	21	121.3	75.1 - 185.5
KL11	15	67.4	37.7 - 111.1	18	79.9	47.4 - 126.3
KL12	7	97.5	39.1 - 200.9	2	29.5	3.6 - 106.4

Community	Male			Female		
	Number of deaths	SMR	95% C.I.	Number of deaths	SMR	95% C.I.
KL13	97	107.0	85.7 - 128.3	68	86.9	66.2 - 107.5
KL14	53	85.1	62.2 - 108.0	59	102.6	76.4 - 128.8
KL15	11	99.5	49.6 - 178.0	16	147.4	84.3 - 238.8
KL16	19	94.8	57.1 - 147.9	16	91.5	52.3 - 148.3
KL17	12	127.1	65.7 - 222.4	40	301.6	208.1 - 395.1
KL18	4	99.2	27.0 - 253.9	2	42.8	5.2 - 154.4
KL19	88	91.4	72.3 - 110.4	101	103.4	83.3 - 123.6
KL20	22	102.0	64.0 - 154.0	22	112.0	70.2 - 169.1
KL21	47	132.8	94.8 - 170.7	36	159.4	117.1 - 201.7
KL22	9	130.3	59.7 - 247.5	3	47.1	9.7 - 137.6
KL23	24	167.1	107.1 - 249.0	21	159.4	98.6 - 243.8
KL24	17	86.0	50.2 - 137.6	12	78.3	40.5 - 136.9
KL25	244	86.6	75.7 - 97.5	242	89.9	78.5 - 101.2
NT1	26	124.6	76.7 - 172.5	18	82.6	49.0 - 130.5
NT2	11	47.4	23.7 - 84.9	16	70.2	40.1 - 113.7
NT3	44	107.0	75.4 - 138.7	26	79.0	48.6 - 109.4
NT4	30	107.1	68.8 - 145.4	22	79.3	49.7 - 119.8
NT5	67	108.8	82.8 - 134.9	55	99.5	73.2 - 125.8
NT6	44	110.3	77.7 - 142.9	33	88.0	58.0 - 118.0
NT7	30	83.8	53.8 - 113.7	37	113.9	77.2 - 150.6
NT8	109	125.9	102.2 - 149.5	106	124.8	101.1 - 148.6
NT9	19	149.2	89.8 - 232.7	18	137.5	81.5 - 217.2
NT10	111	183.4	149.3 - 217.5	83	150.0	117.7 - 182.3
NT11	13	111.1	59.1 - 189.9	19	161.2	97.0 - 251.5
NT12	69	124.5	95.1 - 153.8	62	108.8	81.0 - 136.7
NT13	11	97.2	48.5 - 174.0	16	132.7	75.9 - 215.0
NT14	5	74.7	24.2 - 174.1	9	125.2	57.4 - 237.9
NT15	92	150.5	119.7 - 181.2	111	171.5	139.6 - 203.4
NT16	170	116.4	98.9 - 133.9	220	133.2	115.6 - 150.8
NT17	35	94.3	63.1 - 125.6	31	79.2	51.3 - 107.0
NT18	10	90.0	43.2 - 165.6	11	101.5	50.6 - 181.6
NT19	12	90.2	46.6 - 157.9	10	72.3	34.7 - 133.0

HBP

Sex-Age specific mortality rate (1/100,000) of HBP in Hong Kong (1989–1993)

	Male		Female	
Age	No. of deaths	Mortality rate	No. of deaths	Mortality rate
0–4	0	0.00	0	0.00
5–9	0	0.00	0	0.00
10–14	0	0.00	0	0.00
15–19	0	0.00	0	0.00
20–24	1	0.09	2	0.18
25–29	1	0.07	0	0.00
30–34	4	0.26	2	0.13
35–39	8	0.60	7	0.56
40–44	20	1.82	13	1.34
45–49	32	4.38	20	3.35
50–54	86	12.40	43	7.55
55–59	166	23.76	88	14.45
60–64	293	47.46	198	34.26
65+	1722	155.46	1878	133.67
TOTAL	2333	15.95	2251	16.09

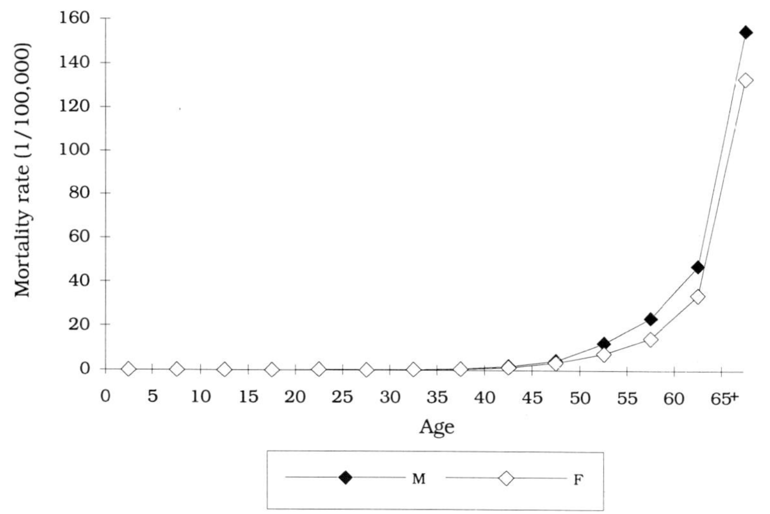

Number of communities on map by category based on standardized mortality ratio (SMR) during 1989–1993

Category	Number of communities Male	Female
SMR significantly high, in top 20%	4	5
SMR significantly high , not in top 20%	0	2
SMR not significantly high, in top 20%	9	8
SMR not significantly low, in bottom 20%	8	11
SMR significantly low, not in bottom 20%	2	2
SMR significantly low, in bottom 20%	5	2
other communities	37	35

Values of the standardized mortality ratio (SMR) which divide the 65 communities into quintile

Percentile	Male	Female
20th	69.66	70.16
40th	90.18	81.48
60th	107.03	95.25
80th	124.46	125.23
Lowest SMR	35.48	29.46
Highest SMR	183.38	301.62
No. of communities with zero cases	0	0

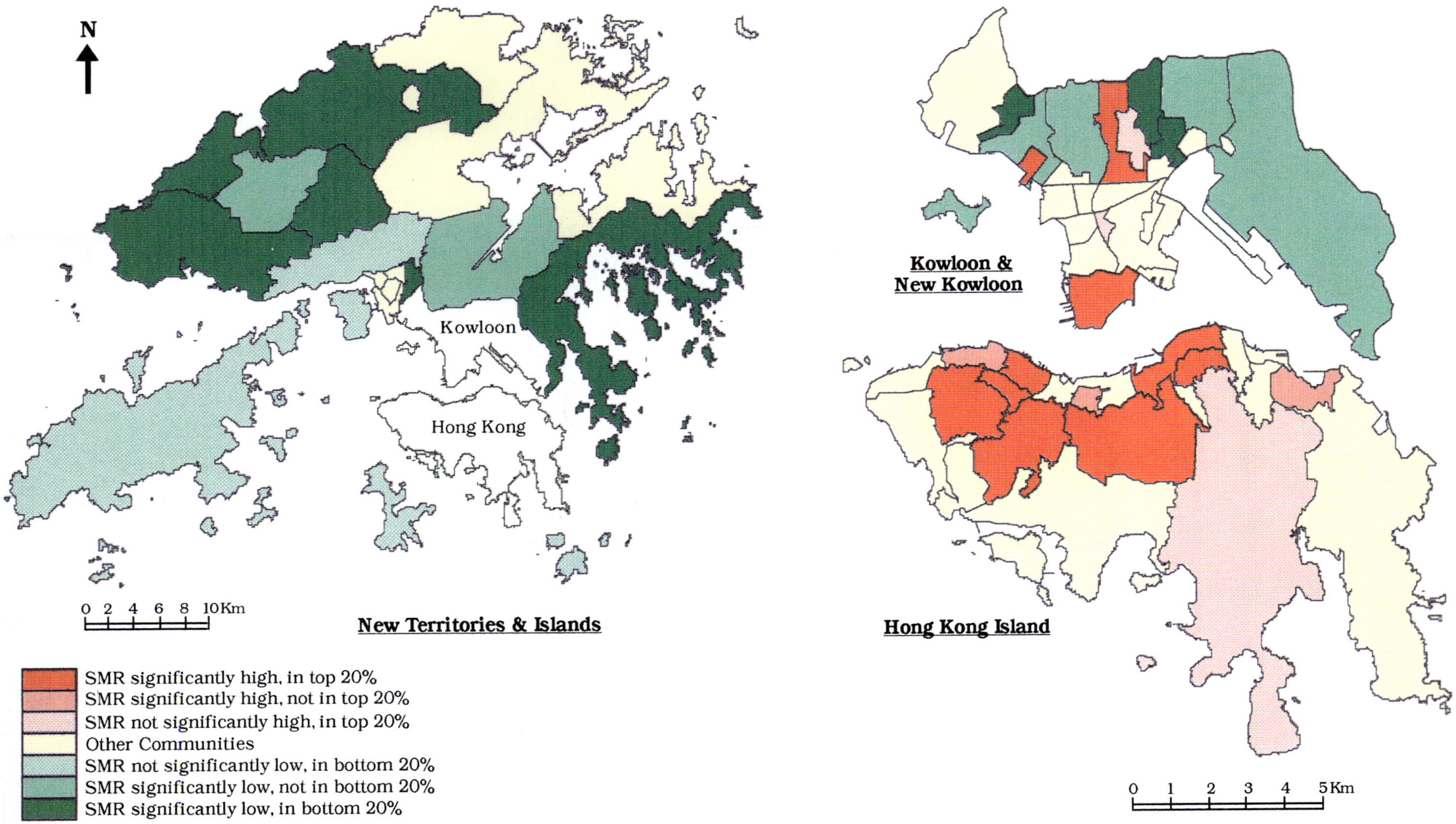

IHD (Male, 1979 – 1983)

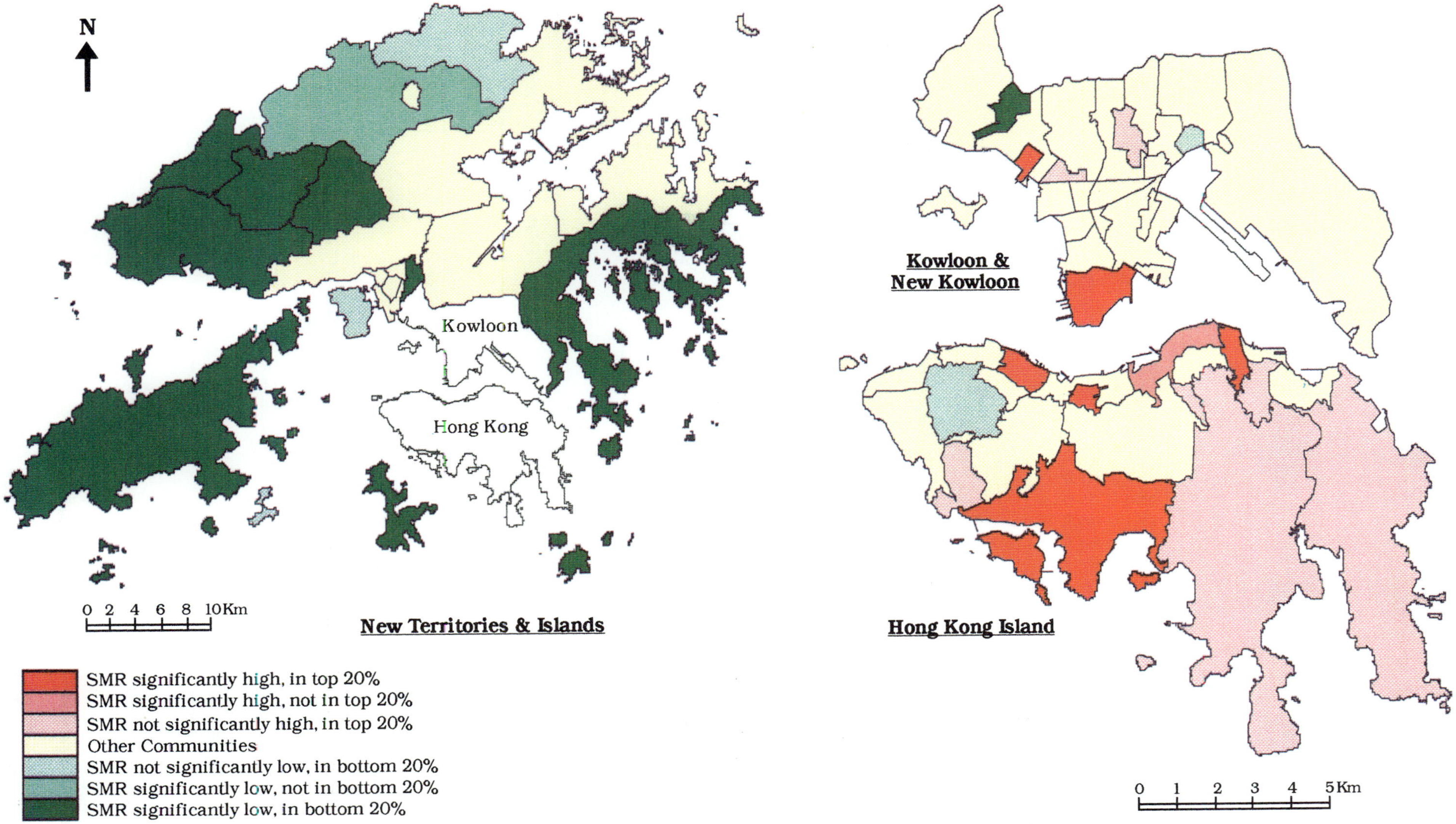

IHD (Female, 1979 – 1983)

Number of Deaths, Standardised Mortality Ratio (SMR) and 95% Confidence Interval of IHD by 65 Communities in 1979–1983

Community	Male			Female		
	Number of deaths	SMR	95% C.I.	Number of deaths	SMR	95% C.I.
HK1	114	115.5	94.3 - 136.7	89	107.9	85.5 - 130.3
HK2	205	126.0	108.8 - 143.3	144	116.5	97.5 - 135.6
HK3	84	130.2	102.4 - 158.1	65	139.5	105.6 - 173.4
HK4	105	108.8	88.0 - 129.6	86	110.0	86.8 - 133.3
HK5	121	127.1	104.5 - 149.8	105	138.3	111.9 - 164.8
HK6	105	135.3	109.5 - 161.2	92	106.6	84.8 - 128.4
HK7	29	187.2	119.0 - 255.3	13	75.3	40.0 - 128.7
HK8	57	184.1	136.3 - 231.9	34	95.0	63.1 - 127.0
HK9	23	170.8	108.1 - 256.4	14	93.5	51.1 - 156.9
HK10	315	148.0	131.7 - 164.3	246	117.1	102.4 - 131.7
HK11	18	99.2	58.7 - 156.8	17	123.8	72.0 - 198.1
HK12	36	242.1	163.0 - 321.2	16	83.1	47.5 - 135.0
HK13	25	103.6	63.0 - 144.2	35	153.2	102.4 - 203.9
HK14	61	101.7	76.2 - 127.3	58	106.5	79.1 - 134.0
HK15	26	111.0	68.4 - 153.7	29	129.8	82.6 - 177.1
HK16	140	124.2	103.6 - 144.8	98	108.2	86.8 - 129.7
HK17	136	108.4	90.2 - 126.6	122	120.8	99.3 - 142.2
HK18	15	86.1	48.1 - 142.0	14	79.8	43.6 - 133.9
HK19	59	104.8	78.1 - 131.6	60	118.3	88.3 - 148.2
HK20	150	114.8	96.4 - 133.1	131	124.2	102.9 - 145.4
HK21	22	146.6	91.6 - 222.1	14	122.3	66.8 - 205.1
KL1	163	196.8	166.6 - 227.1	85	129.0	101.5 - 156.4
KL2	148	88.4	74.1 - 102.6	139	96.5	80.5 - 112.6
KL3	58	116.5	86.5 - 146.5	49	103.6	74.6 - 132.6
KL4	150	109.4	91.9 - 126.9	122	108.5	89.3 - 127.8
KL5	137	117.0	97.4 - 136.5	91	98.7	78.4 - 119.0
KL6	39	128.8	88.3 - 169.2	38	104.5	71.3 - 137.8
KL7	28	129.9	81.8 - 178.1	21	86.6	53.4 - 132.4
KL8	70	98.9	75.7 - 122.0	77	116.0	90.1 - 141.9
KL9	293	111.4	98.6 - 124.1	249	102.6	89.9 - 115.3
KL10	31	118.6	76.9 - 160.4	27	105.7	65.8 - 145.5
KL11	81	109.2	85.4 - 133.0	66	92.0	69.8 - 114.2
KL12	12	51.9	26.7 - 90.5	10	52.7	25.4 - 97.0
KL13	231	83.7	72.9 - 94.5	220	95.5	82.9 - 108.1
KL14	140	80.6	67.3 - 94.0	114	90.7	74.1 - 107.4
KL15	24	189.8	121.7 - 282.4	20	173.9	106.0 - 268.8
KL16	83	126.7	99.4 - 153.9	73	124.0	95.5 - 152.4
KL17	33	176.2	116.1 - 236.3	26	105.2	64.7 - 145.6
KL18	17	147.3	85.7 - 235.8	15	126.8	70.8 - 209.2
KL19	190	79.9	68.5 - 91.2	237	108.6	94.8 - 122.4
KL20	62	72.0	54.1 - 89.9	66	89.9	68.2 - 111.5
KL21	105	74.1	59.9 - 88.2	113	93.8	76.5 - 111.1
KL22	28	120.2	75.7 - 164.7	13	73.4	39.0 - 125.4
KL23	64	88.3	66.6 - 109.9	60	102.1	76.2 - 127.9
KL24	44	105.3	74.2 - 136.4	40	116.1	80.1 - 152.1
KL25	523	80.7	73.8 - 87.6	523	94.2	86.1 - 102.3
NT1	26	78.0	48.0 - 108.0	28	88.9	55.9 - 121.8
NT2	39	83.1	57.0 - 109.2	36	94.5	63.6 - 125.4
NT3	105	110.2	89.1 - 131.3	71	105.7	81.1 - 130.3
NT4	43	89.1	62.5 - 115.8	37	79.4	53.8 - 105.0
NT5	159	87.0	73.5 - 100.5	167	108.1	91.7 - 124.5
NT6	56	64.4	47.5 - 81.2	62	78.3	58.8 - 97.8
NT7	21	70.3	43.4 - 107.5	15	60.6	33.9 - 100.1
NT8	76	74.8	58.0 - 91.6	58	71.2	52.9 - 89.5
NT9	19	57.4	34.5 - 89.6	7	27.4	11.0 - 56.5
NT10	109	79.6	64.7 - 94.6	71	67.9	52.1 - 83.6
NT11	15	52.5	29.3 - 86.6	7	33.6	13.5 - 69.4
NT12	83	63.3	49.7 - 76.9	85	81.0	63.8 - 98.2
NT13	25	102.1	62.1 - 142.1	20	95.8	58.4 - 148.1
NT14	24	103.7	66.5 - 154.3	16	72.7	41.5 - 118.0
NT15	85	93.4	73.6 - 113.3	66	81.7	62.0 - 101.4
NT16	83	78.7	61.8 - 95.7	86	88.6	69.9 - 107.3
NT17	41	75.2	52.2 - 98.2	34	73.3	48.7 - 98.0
NT18	21	76.6	47.3 - 117.2	18	73.5	43.5 - 116.1
NT19	36	78.0	52.5 - 103.5	23	53.8	34.1 - 80.8

IHD

Sex-Age specific mortality rate (1/100,000) of IHD in Hong Kong (1979–1983)

	Male		Female	
Age	No. of deaths	Mortality rate	No. of deaths	Mortality rate
0–4	0	0.00	1	0.10
5–9	0	0.00	1	0.10
10–14	2	0.17	0	0.00
15–19	1	0.07	1	0.08
20–24	7	0.46	0	0.00
25–29	5	0.38	4	0.34
30–34	19	1.72	8	0.87
35–39	30	4.16	8	1.44
40–44	64	9.09	13	2.35
45–49	145	20.10	56	9.25
50–54	315	45.85	108	17.71
55–59	553	97.22	211	39.45
60–64	827	180.99	411	90.10
65+	3698	542.41	4061	402.30
TOTAL	5666	42.97	4883	40.11

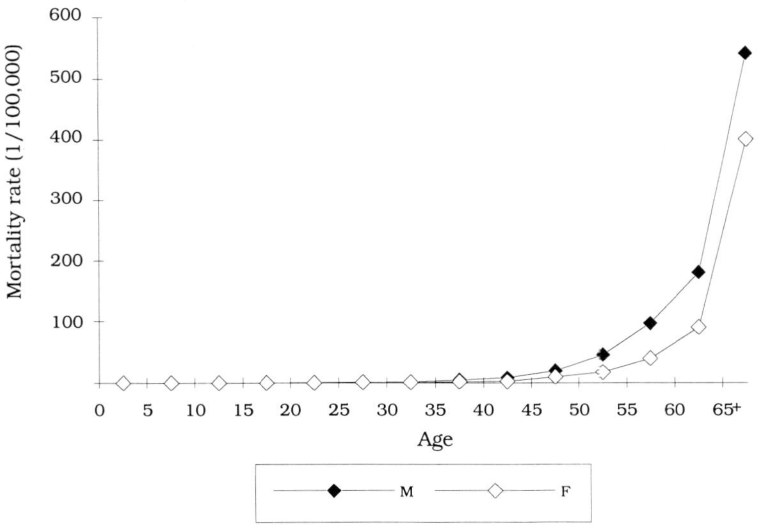

Number of communities on map by category based on standardized mortality ratio (SMR) during 1979–1983

Category	Number of communities Male	Female
SMR significantly high, in top 20%	10	6
SMR significantly high , not in top 20%	3	1
SMR not significantly high, in top 20%	3	7
SMR not significantly low, in bottom 20%	4	5
SMR significantly low, not in bottom 20%	6	1
SMR significantly low, in bottom 20%	9	8
other communities	30	37

Values of the standardized mortality ratio (SMR) which divide the 65 communities into quintile

Percentile	Male	Female
20th	78.04	78.34
40th	93.43	93.83
60th	110.20	105.65
80th	128.76	117.05
Lowest SMR	51.88	27.38
Highest SMR	242.10	173.90
No. of communities with zero death	0	0

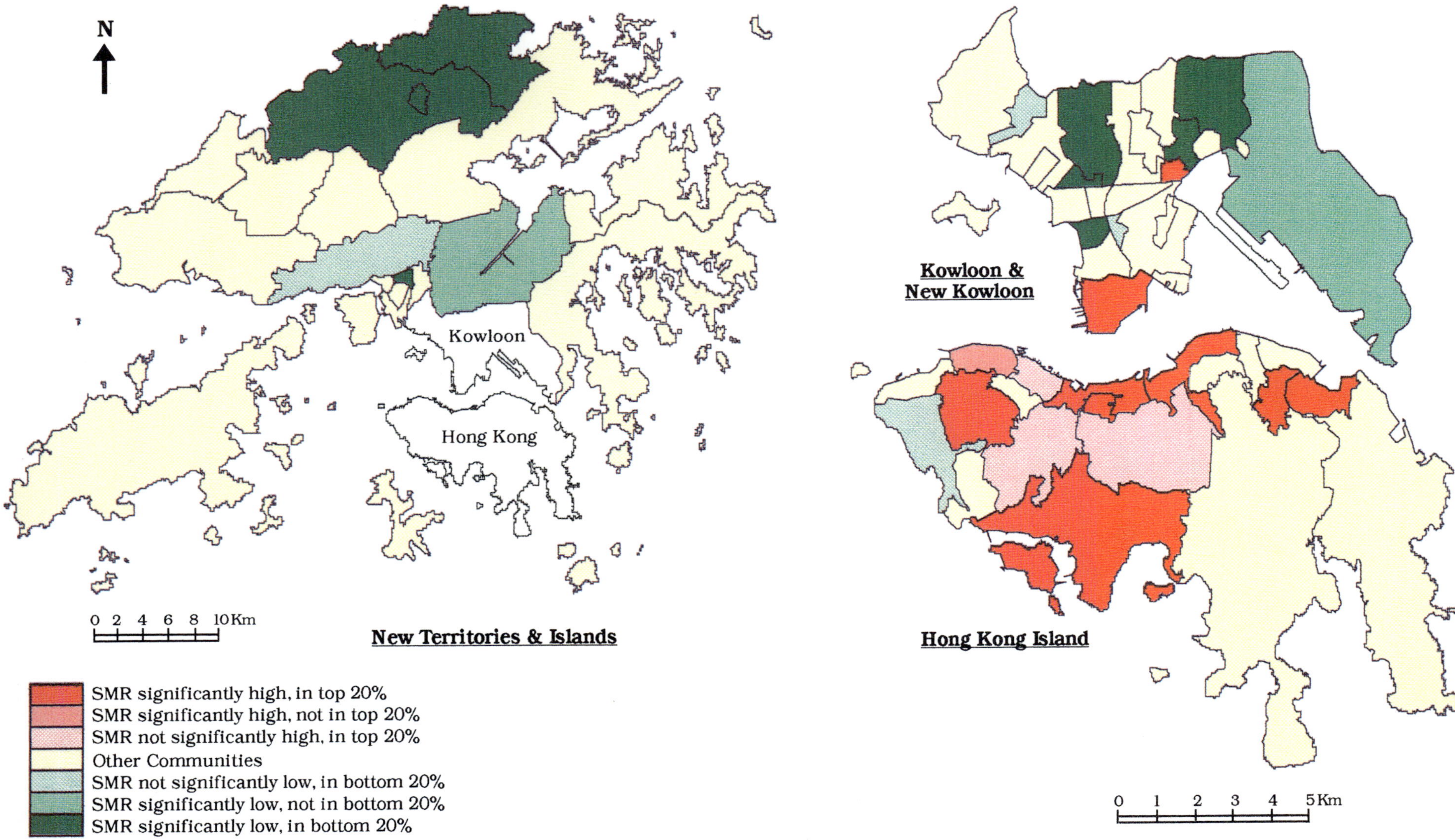

IHD (Male, 1984 – 1988)

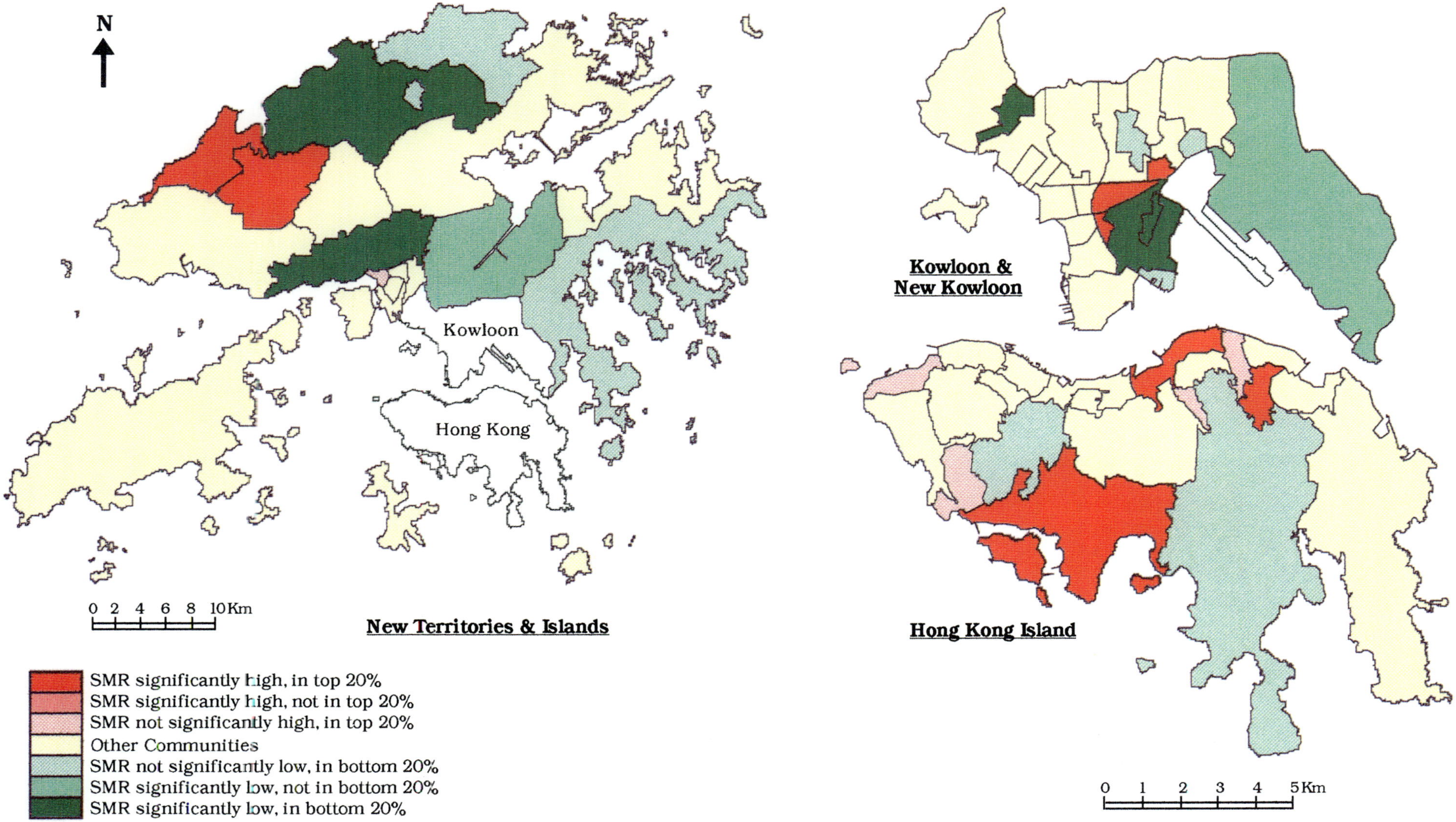

IHD (Female, 1984 – 1988)

Number of Deaths, Standardised Mortality Ratio (SMR) and 95% Confidence Interval of IHD by 65 Communities in 1984–1988

Community	Male			Female		
	Number of deaths	SMR	95% C.I.	Number of deaths	SMR	95% C.I.
HK1	131	116.9	96.9 - 136.9	111	122.0	99.3 - 144.7
HK2	187	116.8	100.1 - 133.5	126	95.9	79.2 - 112.7
HK3	76	126.5	98.1 - 155.0	46	105.0	74.7 - 135.4
HK4	118	123.9	101.5 - 146.2	80	101.5	79.2 - 123.7
HK5	119	141.5	116.0 - 166.9	85	114.3	90.0 - 138.6
HK6	107	123.3	99.9 - 146.7	108	119.0	96.5 - 141.4
HK7	36	202.8	141.6 - 280.9	20	112.4	68.5 - 173.8
HK8	36	110.8	74.6 - 146.9	36	112.1	75.5 - 148.7
HK9	19	141.4	85.2 - 220.9	12	78.0	40.2 - 136.1
HK10	355	150.0	134.4 - 165.6	292	124.1	109.9 - 138.3
HK11	36	169.9	118.7 - 235.3	17	120.9	70.3 - 193.4
HK12	21	109.9	67.8 - 168.1	22	118.5	74.1 - 179.6
HK13	34	118.1	78.4 - 157.8	30	137.0	92.6 - 195.7
HK14	78	89.0	69.3 - 108.8	73	86.9	67.0 - 106.9
HK15	41	153.3	106.4 - 200.2	49	177.9	128.1 - 227.7
HK16	153	127.1	107.0 - 147.2	108	107.7	87.4 - 128.0
HK17	184	112.5	96.2 - 128.7	157	116.3	98.1 - 134.5
HK18	13	74.0	39.3 - 126.4	17	93.2	54.2 - 149.2
HK19	79	107.1	83.4 - 130.7	80	123.9	96.8 - 151.1
HK20	222	132.1	114.7 - 149.5	196	141.5	121.7 - 161.3
HK21	17	89.9	52.3 - 143.9	14	78.8	43.0 - 132.2
KL1	154	180.4	151.9 - 208.9	73	109.1	84.1 - 134.2
KL2	166	104.5	88.6 - 120.4	119	88.5	72.6 - 104.4
KL3	42	82.9	57.9 - 108.0	47	99.2	70.8 - 127.5
KL4	124	81.7	67.3 - 96.1	114	99.3	81.1 - 117.5
KL5	121	106.7	87.7 - 125.8	76	85.7	66.4 - 104.9
KL6	34	102.9	68.3 - 137.5	57	164.2	121.6 - 206.9
KL7	15	65.4	36.5 - 107.9	30	149.9	101.3 - 214.2
KL8	69	90.9	69.5 - 112.4	47	73.6	52.5 - 94.6
KL9	300	99.3	88.1 - 110.6	213	82.4	71.3 - 93.4
KL10	28	96.4	60.7 - 132.1	22	81.8	47.6 - 115.9
KL11	94	105.0	83.7 - 126.2	72	91.7	70.5 - 112.8
KL12	18	73.0	43.2 - 115.4	5	25.3	8.2 - 59.1
KL13	246	90.3	79.0 - 101.5	205	91.1	78.7 - 103.6
KL14	153	71.8	60.4 - 83.1	156	96.1	81.0 - 111.1
KL15	30	91.4	58.7 - 124.2	29	94.8	60.3 - 129.3
KL16	53	77.4	56.6 - 98.3	48	88.9	63.7 - 114.0
KL17	37	109.3	74.1 - 144.6	47	100.0	71.4 - 128.6
KL18	10	81.8	39.3 - 150.4	7	66.5	26.7 - 137.1
KL19	232	81.8	71.2 - 92.3	254	106.8	93.7 - 120.0
KL20	68	97.4	74.3 - 120.6	54	86.9	63.7 - 110.1
KL21	86	69.2	54.6 - 83.8	87	92.5	73.1 - 112.0
KL22	20	83.4	50.8 - 128.8	16	81.5	46.6 - 132.3
KL23	92	152.2	121.1 - 183.4	66	137.0	103.9 - 170.0
KL24	60	104.5	78.1 - 130.9	46	115.9	82.4 - 149.4
KL25	736	84.2	78.1 - 90.3	597	83.8	77.1 - 90.6
NT1	38	78.7	53.7 - 103.8	31	73.3	47.5 - 99.1
NT2	57	93.3	69.1 - 117.5	47	98.3	70.2 - 126.5
NT3	122	113.1	93.0 - 133.1	89	122.5	97.0 - 147.9
NT4	64	73.5	55.5 - 91.5	72	95.0	73.1 - 117.0
NT5	204	105.2	90.7 - 119.6	160	106.9	90.4 - 123.5
NT6	103	89.6	72.3 - 106.9	92	104.4	83.0 - 125.7
NT7	49	89.2	64.2 - 114.2	38	96.0	65.4 - 126.5
NT8	189	97.3	83.4 - 111.2	161	92.3	78.0 - 106.6
NT9	42	115.9	80.9 - 151.0	52	160.0	116.5 - 203.5
NT10	186	104.4	89.4 - 119.4	193	140.4	120.6 - 160.2
NT11	26	83.9	51.7 - 116.2	34	119.9	79.6 - 160.2
NT12	115	74.2	60.7 - 87.8	104	76.6	61.9 - 91.4
NT13	28	68.9	43.4 - 94.4	22	78.2	45.5 - 110.9
NT14	17	65.6	34.4 - 96.8	15	66.1	36.9 - 109.1
NT15	135	95.8	79.7 - 112.0	122	91.3	75.1 - 107.5
NT16	248	84.3	73.8 - 94.8	261	87.5	76.9 - 98.1
NT17	68	107.2	81.7 - 132.7	43	83.3	58.4 - 108.2
NT18	34	106.9	71.0 - 142.9	30	105.9	68.0 - 143.8
NT19	41	85.1	59.0 - 111.1	45	109.2	77.3 - 141.1

IHD

Sex-Age specific mortality rate (1/100,000) of IHD in Hong Kong (1984–1988)

	Male		Female	
Age	No. of deaths	Mortality rate	No. of deaths	Mortality rate
0–4	1	0.09	0	0.00
5–9	0	0.00	0	0.00
10–14	0	0.00	1	0.10
15–19	6	0.50	1	0.09
20–24	4	0.28	1	0.07
25–29	11	0.70	4	0.27
30–34	15	1.11	11	0.89
35–39	39	3.52	14	1.44
40–44	76	10.37	6	1.00
45–49	144	20.45	31	5.31
50–54	328	44.75	89	14.09
55–59	565	85.06	183	30.12
60–64	874	161.82	446	83.32
65+	4872	539.59	5035	407.96
TOTAL	6935	48.63	5822	43.38

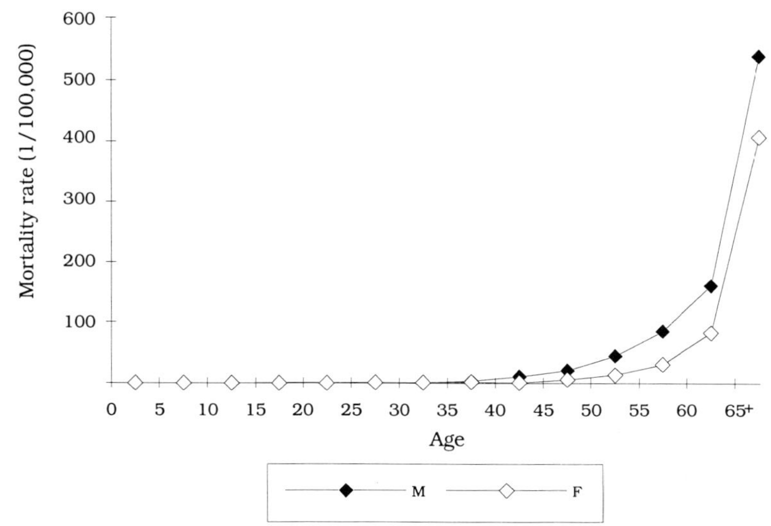

Number of communities on map by category based on standardized mortality ratio (SMR) during 1984–1988

Category	Number of communities Male	Female
SMR significantly high, in top 20%	10	8
SMR significantly high , not in top 20%	1	0
SMR not significantly high, in top 20%	3	5
SMR not significantly low, in bottom 20%	4	8
SMR significantly low, not in bottom 20%	2	2
SMR significantly low, in bottom 20%	9	5
other communities	36	37

Values of the standardized mortality ratio (SMR) which divide the 65 communities into quintile

Percentile	Male	Female
20th	81.76	83.29
40th	90.91	93.25
60th	105.15	105.87
80th	118.10	119.91
Lowest SMR	65.42	25.29
Highest SMR	202.82	177.85
No. of communities with zero death	0	0

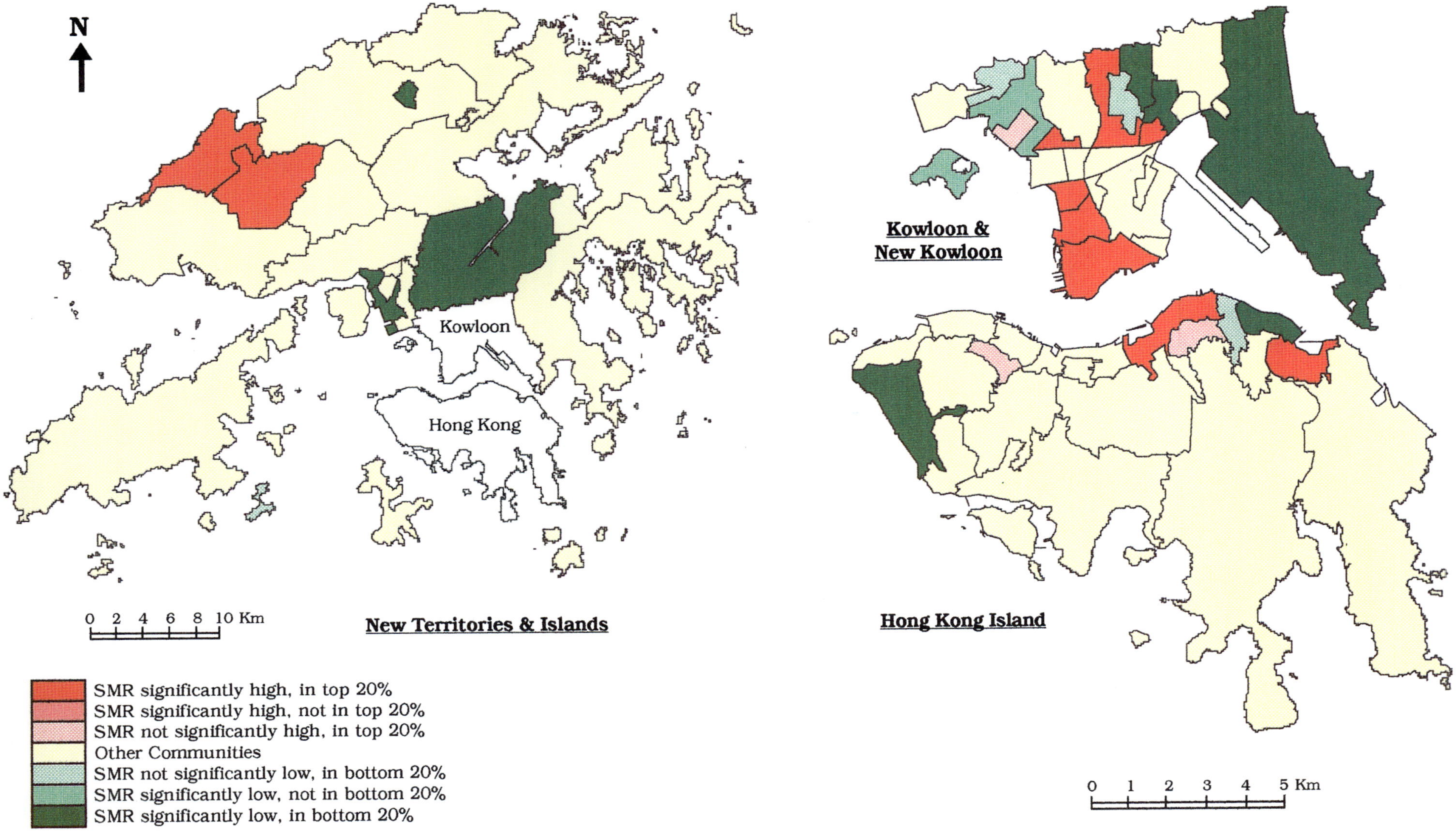

IHD (Male, 1989 -1993)

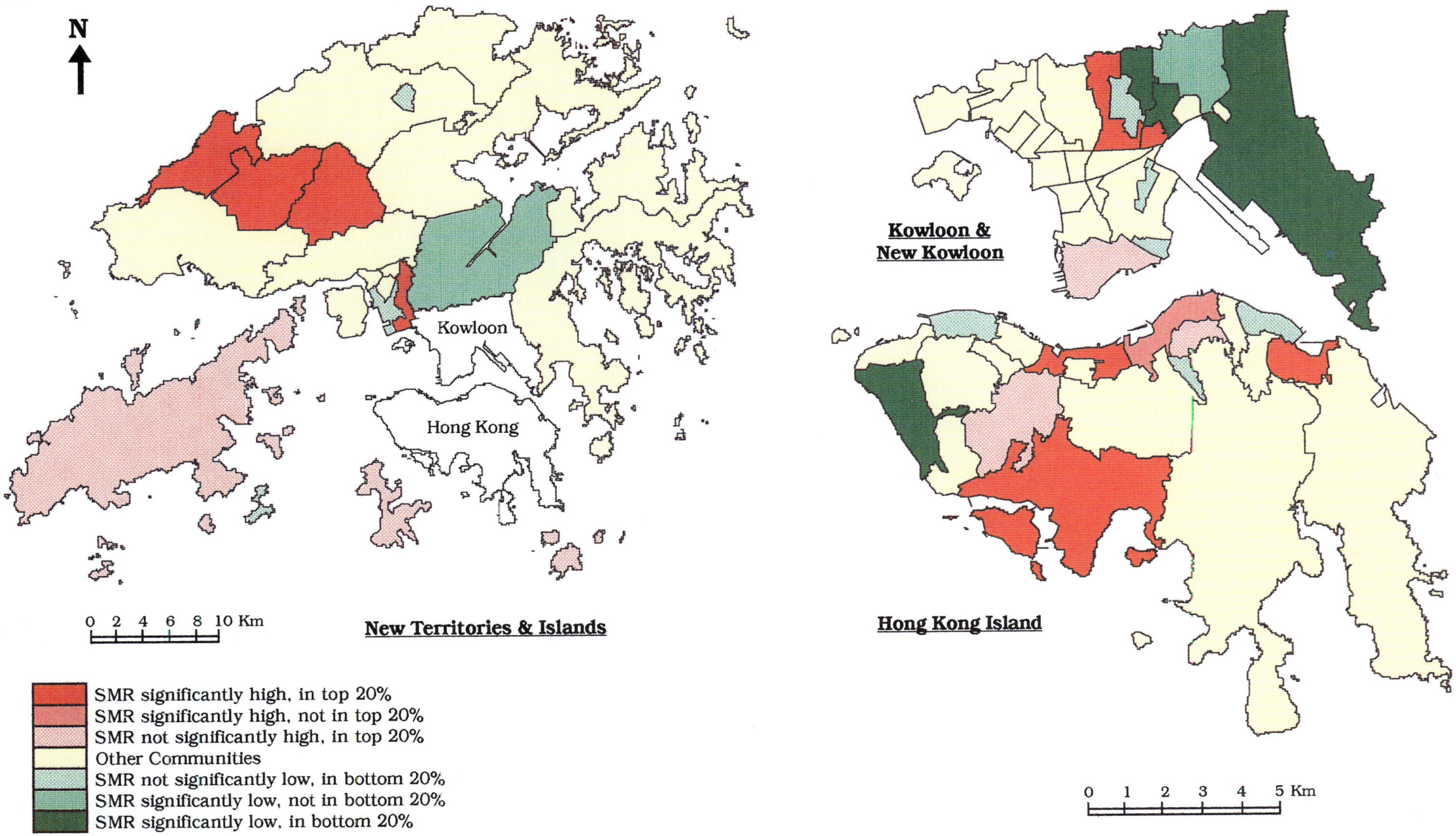

IHD (Female, 1989 -1993)

Number of Deaths, Standardised Mortality Ratio (SMR) and 95% Confidence Interval of IHD by 65 Communities in 1989–1993

Community	Male			Female		
	Number of deaths	SMR	95% C.I.	Number of deaths	SMR	95% C.I.
HK1	133	109.7	91.1 - 128.3	96	95.1	76.1 - 114.2
HK2	175	106.7	90.9 - 122.5	105	85.7	69.3 - 102.0
HK3	51	89.4	64.9 - 114.0	36	87.5	58.9 - 116.1
HK4	106	115.0	93.1 - 136.8	94	128.7	102.7 - 154.8
HK5	94	106.4	84.9 - 127.9	82	119.0	93.2 - 144.7
HK6	118	117.4	96.2 - 138.6	113	111.9	91.3 - 132.6
HK7	25	115.2	74.6 - 170.5	21	88.8	55.0 - 135.8
HK8	44	123.5	87.0 - 160.0	30	95.4	61.2 - 129.5
HK9	16	106.2	60.7 - 172.0	18	129.2	76.6 - 204.1
HK10	360	129.7	116.3 - 143.1	314	115.6	102.8 - 128.3
HK11	29	113.3	72.1 - 154.6	14	78.2	42.7 - 131.3
HK12	32	146.1	95.5 - 196.7	25	120.1	77.7 - 177.7
HK13	21	68.3	42.3 - 104.6	28	115.0	72.4 - 157.6
HK14	79	73.4	57.2 - 89.5	75	82.1	63.5 - 100.7
HK15	65	105.6	79.9 - 131.3	59	110.7	82.5 - 139.0
HK16	141	125.4	104.7 - 146.1	134	144.4	120.0 - 168.9
HK17	234	98.7	86.0 - 111.3	183	91.8	78.5 - 105.1
HK18	9	34.1	15.6 - 64.8	14	47.0	25.7 - 78.9
HK19	111	118.4	96.3 - 140.4	73	98.8	76.1 - 121.5
HK20	234	109.6	95.5 - 123.6	239	128.5	112.2 - 144.8
HK21	22	114.5	71.8 - 172.9	14	99.8	54.5 - 167.7
KL1	137	188.3	156.8 - 219.8	73	125.5	96.7 - 154.3
KL2	174	106.1	90.3 - 121.9	150	112.8	94.7 - 130.8
KL3	48	96.3	69.1 - 123.5	49	108.4	78.0 - 138.7
KL4	167	118.8	100.8 - 136.8	99	97.4	78.2 - 116.6
KL5	129	124.6	103.1 - 146.1	80	98.8	77.1 - 120.4
KL6	40	96.8	66.8 - 126.8	49	101.1	72.8 - 129.4
KL7	25	91.3	59.1 - 135.2	27	90.7	56.5 - 124.9
KL8	83	100.4	78.8 - 122.0	57	84.8	62.8 - 106.8
KL9	319	95.4	84.9 - 105.8	267	97.1	85.5 - 108.8
KL10	56	103.8	76.6 - 131.0	43	81.9	57.4 - 106.3
KL11	86	111.3	87.7 - 134.8	61	87.5	65.6 - 109.5
KL12	18	72.5	43.0 - 114.6	22	99.6	62.4 - 150.4
KL13	276	88.5	78.1 - 99.0	223	91.3	79.3 - 103.3
KL14	196	91.0	78.3 - 103.7	182	100.9	86.2 - 115.6
KL15	52	136.4	99.3 - 173.5	38	112.2	76.5 - 147.9
KL16	92	132.7	105.6 - 159.8	56	102.5	75.7 - 129.3
KL17	62	186.7	140.2 - 233.2	84	193.8	152.3 - 235.2
KL18	8	57.0	24.6 - 112.3	12	80.7	41.7 - 141.3
KL19	302	91.1	80.8 - 101.3	265	86.4	76.0 - 96.8
KL20	47	63.5	45.3 - 81.7	39	65.0	44.6 - 85.5
KL21	90	73.9	58.6 - 89.2	79	74.0	57.7 - 90.4
KL22	22	92.1	57.7 - 139.0	21	105.4	65.2 - 161.2
KL23	79	158.5	123.6 - 193.5	70	169.2	129.6 - 208.8
KL24	74	110.1	85.0 - 135.2	51	111.5	80.9 - 142.1
KL25	832	85.8	80.0 - 91.6	665	79.9	73.8 - 86.0
NT1	84	115.4	90.7 - 140.1	63	94.1	70.9 - 117.4
NT2	50	62.3	45.0 - 79.6	57	80.0	59.2 - 100.8
NT3	103	72.5	58.5 - 86.6	99	99.7	80.1 - 119.4
NT4	101	104.8	84.4 - 125.3	77	90.1	70.0 - 110.2
NT5	212	100.1	86.6 - 113.6	149	87.6	73.5 - 101.6
NT6	142	103.4	86.4 - 120.4	150	129.6	108.8 - 150.3
NT7	130	104.0	86.1 - 121.9	100	101.9	81.9 - 121.8
NT8	303	99.8	88.6 - 111.0	262	99.7	87.6 - 111.7
NT9	64	144.8	109.4 - 180.3	62	146.2	109.8 - 182.6
NT10	266	126.5	111.3 - 141.7	328	188.2	167.8 - 208.5
NT11	37	90.9	61.6 - 120.2	62	162.4	122.0 - 202.8
NT12	181	94.1	80.4 - 107.8	170	100.0	85.0 - 115.1
NT13	27	68.9	42.9 - 95.0	28	73.7	46.4 - 101.0
NT14	25	108.1	69.9 - 160.0	26	112.8	69.4 - 156.1
NT15	219	102.7	89.1 - 116.4	196	96.2	82.7 - 109.6
NT16	431	84.9	76.8 - 92.9	445	86.4	78.4 - 94.4
NT17	112	86.7	70.6 - 102.7	112	91.8	74.8 - 108.8
NT18	29	75.2	47.8 - 102.6	24	69.7	44.6 - 103.8
NT19	41	88.5	61.4 - 115.6	55	123.2	90.6 - 155.7

IHD

Sex-Age specific mortality rate (1/100,000) of IHD in Hong Kong (1989–1993)

	Male		Female	
Age	No. of deaths	Mortality rate	No. of deaths	Mortality rate
0–4	1	0.10	0	0.00
5–9	0	0.00	0	0.00
10–14	0	0.00	0	0.00
15–19	2	0.18	1	0.10
20–24	1	0.09	2	0.18
25–29	9	0.62	7	0.47
30–34	25	1.60	6	0.39
35–39	43	3.21	8	0.64
40–44	94	8.54	14	1.44
45–49	134	18.34	26	4.35
50–54	294	42.38	74	13.00
55–59	551	78.85	159	26.10
60–64	959	155.35	433	74.93
65+	5957	537.78	6265	445.94
TOTAL	8070	55.18	6995	49.99

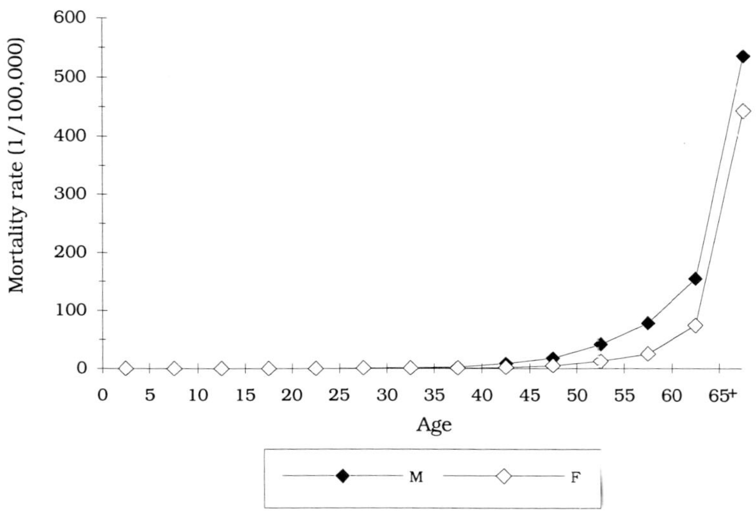

Number of communities on map by category based on standardized mortality ratio (SMR) during 1989–1993

Category	Number of communities Male	Female
SMR significantly high, in top 20%	10	9
SMR significantly high , not in top 20%	0	1
SMR not significantly high, in top 20%	3	4
SMR not significantly low, in bottom 20%	4	9
SMR significantly low, not in bottom 20%	1	2
SMR significantly low, in bottom 20%	9	4
other communities	38	36

Values of the standardized mortality ratio (SMR) which divide the 65 communities into quintile

Percentile	Male	Female
20th	85.79	85.66
40th	96.79	95.15
60th	106.41	101.12
80th	118.35	118.97
Lowest SMR	34.11	46.99
Highest SMR	188.29	193.78
No. of communities with zero cases	0	0

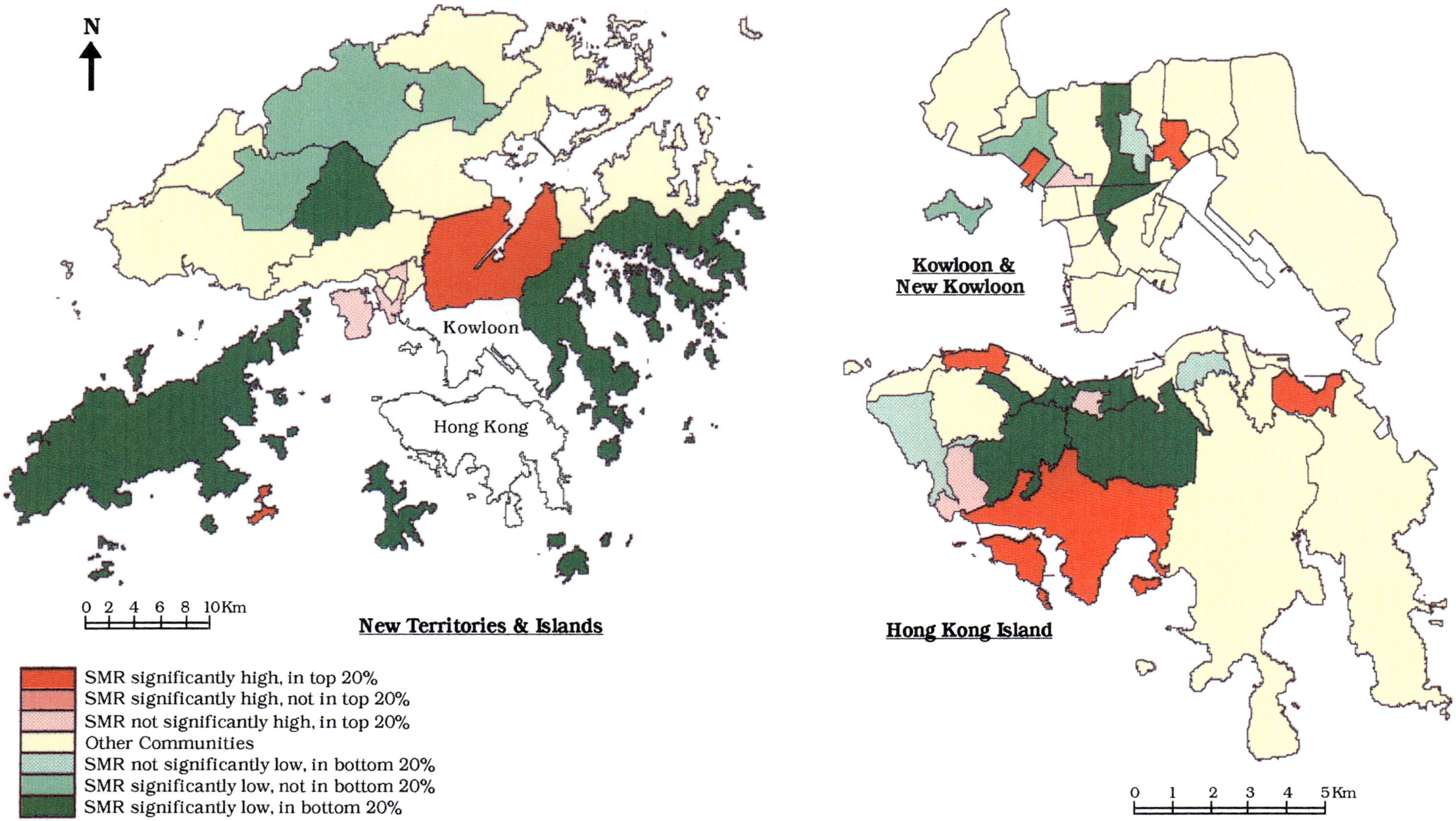

CVA (Male, 1979 - 1983)

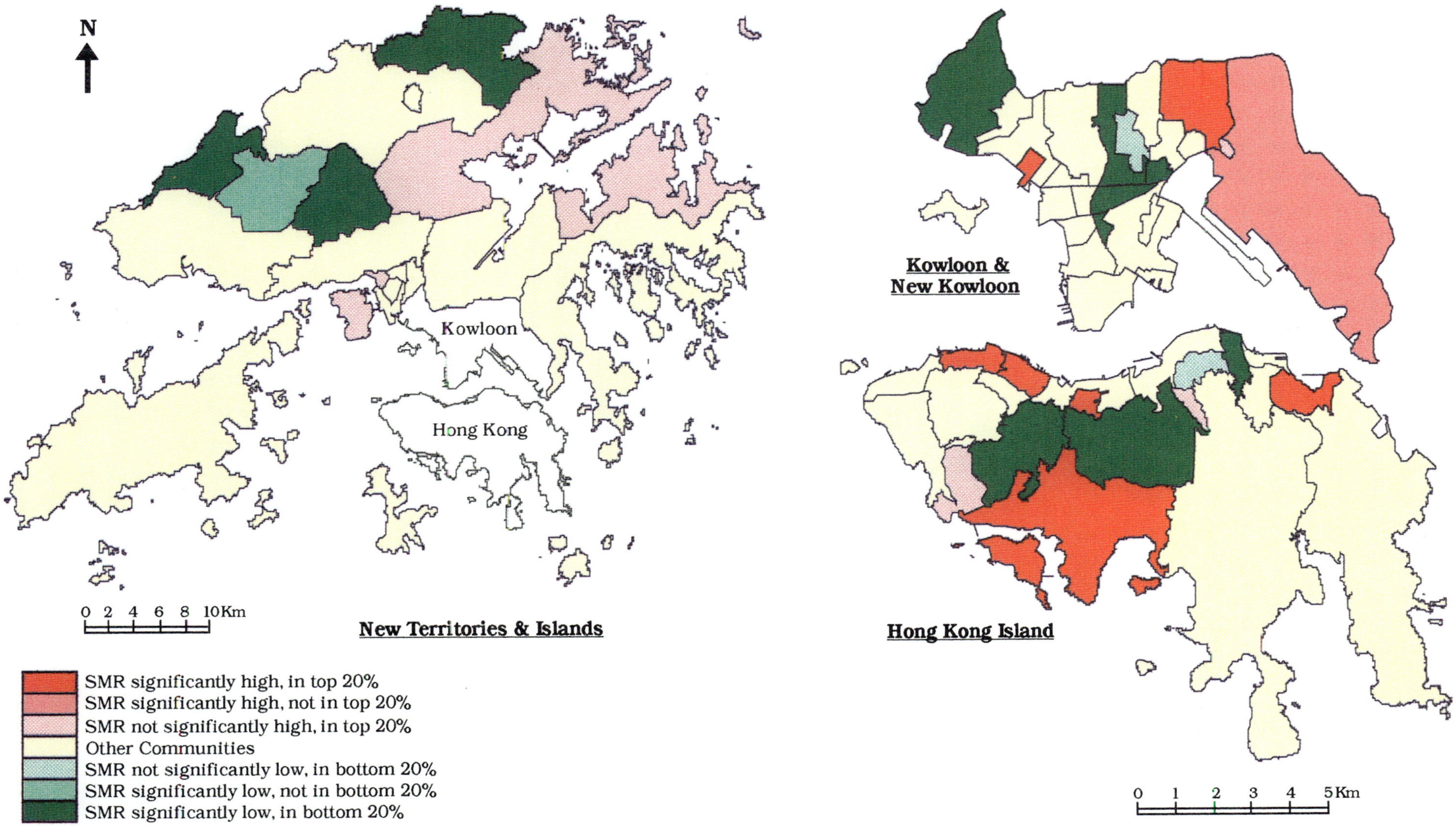

CVA (Female, 1979 - 1983)

Number of Deaths, Standardised Mortality Ratio (SMR) and 95% Confidence Interval of CVA by 65 Communities in 1979–1983

	Male			Female		
Community	Number of deaths	SMR	95% C.I.	Number of deaths	SMR	95% C.I.
HK1	148	111.1	93.2 - 129.0	138	96.7	80.6 - 112.8
HK2	275	126.3	111.4 - 141.2	252	119.3	104.6 - 134.0
HK3	83	96.3	75.6 - 117.0	109	138.1	112.2 - 164.0
HK4	84	64.6	50.8 - 78.4	116	86.4	70.7 - 102.2
HK5	150	117.4	98.6 - 136.2	178	137.7	117.5 - 158.0
HK6	66	63.3	48.0 - 78.6	105	70.8	57.2 - 84.3
HK7	19	91.2	55.0 - 142.6	28	93.7	59.0 - 128.4
HK8	24	57.8	37.1 - 86.1	49	79.9	57.6 - 102.3
HK9	9	49.2	22.6 - 93.3	9	34.3	15.7 - 65.1
HK10	287	100.2	88.6 - 111.8	344	94.8	84.8 - 104.9
HK11	19	76.5	46.1 - 119.6	29	118.6	75.5 - 161.8
HK12	12	59.1	30.5 - 103.2	24	71.8	46.1 - 106.9
HK13	27	82.1	51.1 - 113.0	29	73.0	46.4 - 99.6
HK14	77	95.2	74.0 - 116.5	82	86.6	67.9 - 105.4
HK15	34	106.7	70.8 - 142.5	29	73.6	46.8 - 100.4
HK16	204	133.8	115.5 - 152.2	190	121.0	103.8 - 138.2
HK17	178	105.6	90.1 - 121.1	187	107.0	91.7 - 122.3
HK18	17	72.4	42.1 - 115.8	22	73.2	45.7 - 110.9
HK19	95	123.6	98.7 - 148.4	104	116.9	94.5 - 139.4
HK20	224	127.1	110.4 - 143.7	248	135.5	118.7 - 152.4
HK21	16	77.1	44.1 - 125.2	23	112.3	71.1 - 168.7
KL1	122	109.2	89.8 - 128.6	112	98.3	80.1 - 116.6
KL2	248	109.2	95.6 - 122.8	231	94.2	82.0 - 106.3
KL3	74	110.2	85.1 - 135.4	70	87.1	66.7 - 107.5
KL4	183	98.6	84.3 - 112.9	208	108.5	93.7 - 123.2
KL5	170	107.8	91.6 - 124.0	155	98.6	83.1 - 114.2
KL6	29	71.7	45.6 - 97.9	33	53.4	35.2 - 71.7
KL7	13	44.9	23.9 - 76.7	26	62.6	38.6 - 86.7
KL8	90	93.0	73.8 - 112.3	104	90.9	73.4 - 108.4
KL9	349	97.4	87.1 - 107.6	445	105.6	95.8 - 115.4
KL10	26	73.2	45.1 - 101.3	47	105.6	75.4 - 135.8
KL11	84	84.2	66.2 - 102.2	83	67.3	52.8 - 81.8
KL12	28	89.9	56.6 - 123.2	33	103.9	68.4 - 139.3

	Male			Female		
Community	Number of deaths	SMR	95% C.I.	Number of deaths	SMR	95% C.I.
KL13	311	83.1	73.9 - 92.3	367	92.9	83.4 - 102.4
KL14	234	101.0	88.1 - 114.0	208	95.7	82.7 - 108.7
KL15	29	168.1	106.9 - 229.3	35	179.0	119.7 - 238.4
KL16	107	120.8	97.9 - 143.7	108	108.0	87.7 - 128.4
KL17	15	59.2	33.1 - 97.7	30	70.8	45.5 - 96.1
KL18	9	56.9	26.1 - 107.9	13	63.2	33.6 - 108.1
KL19	307	94.9	84.3 - 105.5	432	114.4	103.7 - 125.2
KL20	119	102.5	84.1 - 120.9	111	87.5	71.2 - 103.8
KL21	220	115.7	100.4 - 131.0	206	99.4	85.9 - 113.0
KL22	30	95.2	61.1 - 129.3	27	88.7	55.2 - 122.1
KL23	93	94.8	75.6 - 114.1	73	71.9	55.4 - 88.4
KL24	61	105.4	78.9 - 131.8	76	123.9	96.1 - 151.8
KL25	928	104.9	98.1 - 111.6	1062	109.8	103.2 - 116.4
NT1	40	88.4	61.0 - 115.8	51	94.9	68.8 - 120.9
NT2	81	126.1	98.7 - 153.6	59	88.3	65.8 - 110.9
NT3	150	115.0	96.6 - 133.4	134	113.4	94.2 - 132.7
NT4	79	117.7	91.7 - 143.6	83	102.0	80.1 - 123.9
NT5	239	95.7	83.6 - 107.8	266	98.8	86.9 - 110.7
NT6	102	85.1	68.6 - 101.6	122	88.3	72.6 - 103.9
NT7	55	134.0	98.6 - 169.5	54	124.2	91.1 - 157.4
NT8	132	95.9	79.5 - 112.2	130	92.5	76.6 - 108.4
NT9	49	110.0	79.2 - 140.8	31	70.6	45.7 - 95.4
NT10	159	86.4	73.0 - 99.9	150	83.3	70.0 - 96.6
NT11	18	46.9	27.7 - 74.0	13	36.3	19.3 - 62.1
NT12	137	77.9	64.8 - 90.9	167	93.2	79.1 - 107.4
NT13	28	85.1	53.6 - 116.7	40	112.4	77.6 - 147.3
NT14	27	87.3	54.4 - 120.3	21	56.3	34.8 - 86.1
NT15	139	114.1	95.1 - 133.1	156	113.4	95.6 - 131.1
NT16	169	118.1	100.3 - 135.9	183	109.3	93.5 - 125.1
NT17	52	71.5	52.1 - 90.9	70	88.6	67.9 - 109.4
NT18	51	140.3	101.8 - 178.9	46	110.7	78.7 - 142.7
NT19	34	55.3	36.7 - 73.9	59	82.5	61.4 - 103.5

CVA

Sex-Age specific mortality rate (1/100,000) of CVA in Hong Kong (1979–1983)

	Male		Female	
Age	No. of deaths	Mortality rate	No. of deaths	Mortality rate
0–4	5	0.47	7	0.71
5–9	3	0.28	7	0.71
10–14	6	0.52	11	1.03
15–19	18	1.26	20	1.50
20–24	24	1.57	15	1.08
25–29	17	1.29	19	1.63
30–34	29	2.63	21	2.29
35–39	52	7.20	26	4.68
40–44	111	15.77	80	14.46
45–49	269	37.29	169	27.92
50–54	523	76.13	301	49.36
55–59	815	143.28	529	98.92
60–64	1115	244.01	789	172.96
65+	4681	686.60	6431	637.08
TOTAL	7668	58.16	8425	69.20

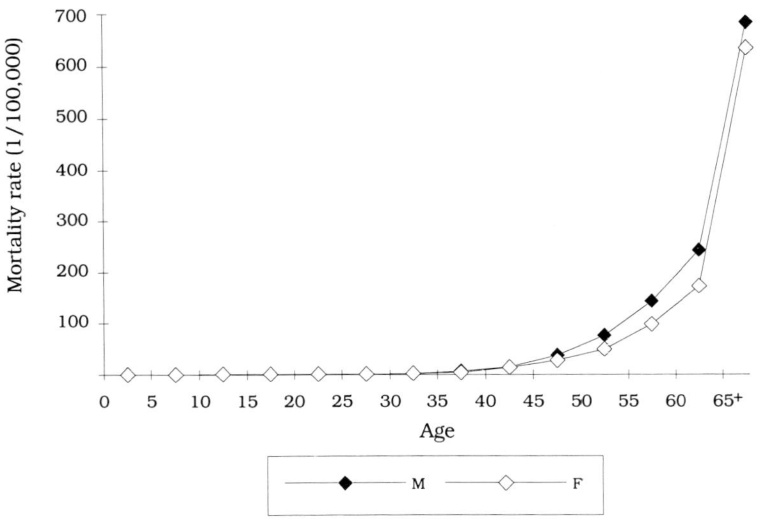

Number of communities on map by category based on standardized mortality ratio (SMR) during 1979–1983

Category	Number of communities Male	Number of communities Female
SMR significantly high, in top 20%	7	7
SMR significantly high , not in top 20%	0	1
SMR not significantly high, in top 20%	6	6
SMR not significantly low, in bottom 20%	3	2
SMR significantly low, not in bottom 20%	3	1
SMR significantly low, in bottom 20%	10	11
other communities	36	37

Values of the standardized mortality ratio (SMR) which divide the 65 communities into quintile

Percentile	Male	Female
20th	72.38	73.01
40th	89.90	88.66
60th	101.05	98.78
80th	114.99	112.43
Lowest SMR	44.88	34.31
Highest SMR	168.12	179.05
No. of communities with zero death	0	0

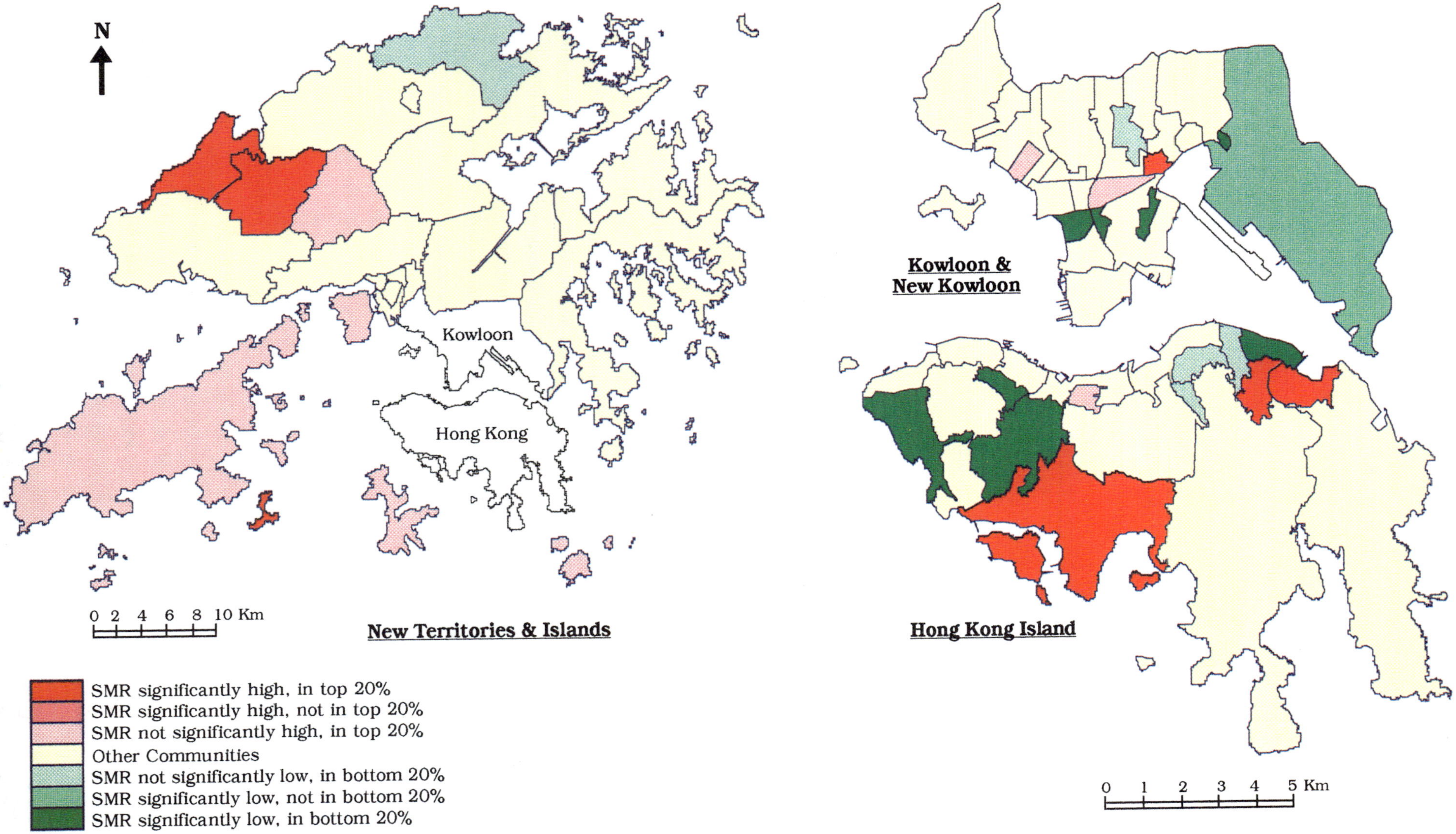

CVA (Male, 1984 -1988)

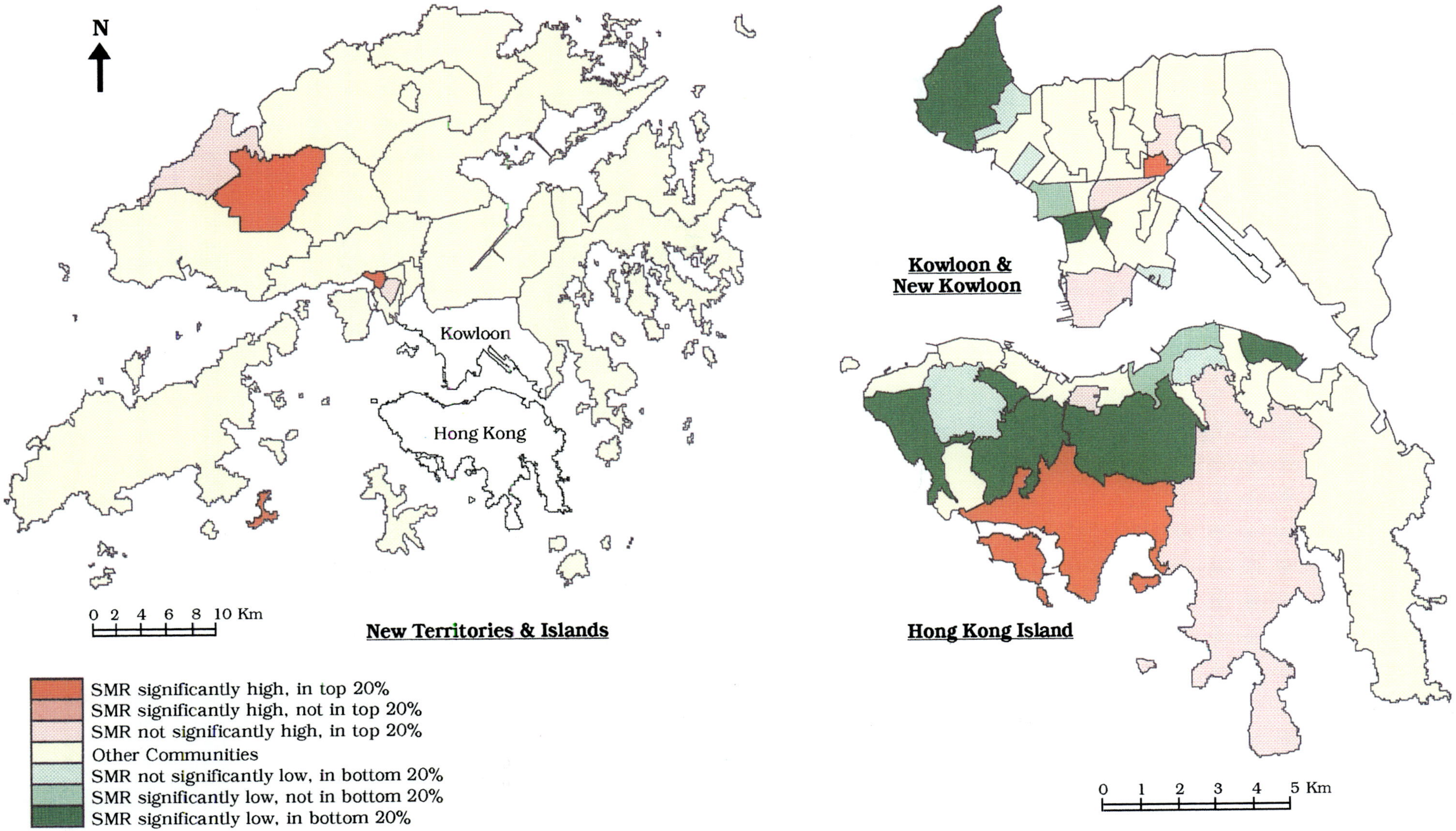

CVA (Female, 1984 -1988)

Number of Deaths, Standardised Mortality Ratio (SMR) and 95% Confidence Interval of CVA by 65 Communities in 1984–1988

Community	Male			Female			Community	Male			Female		
	Number of deaths	SMR	95% C.I.	Number of deaths	SMR	95% C.I.		Number of deaths	SMR	95% C.I.	Number of deaths	SMR	95% C.I.
HK1	125	107.5	88.6 - 126.3	122	95.5	78.6 - 112.5	KL13	266	93.6	82.4 - 104.9	311	98.8	87.8 - 109.8
HK2	175	105.6	90.0 - 121.3	175	95.7	81.5 - 109.8	KL14	235	107.9	94.1 - 121.7	229	101.7	88.5 - 114.9
HK3	65	104.6	79.2 - 130.0	64	105.1	79.3 - 130.8	KL15	38	110.7	75.5 - 145.9	34	79.0	52.5 - 105.6
HK4	99	100.4	80.6 - 120.2	104	94.7	76.5 - 112.9	KL16	58	81.4	60.4 - 102.3	70	92.7	71.0 - 114.4
HK5	103	117.7	95.0 - 140.5	118	114.2	93.6 - 134.8	KL17	35	102.2	68.3 - 136.0	69	107.4	82.1 - 132.8
HK6	82	91.5	71.7 - 111.3	104	82.1	66.3 - 97.8	KL18	7	54.4	21.8 - 112.1	13	86.6	46.1 - 148.0
HK7	15	82.0	45.8 - 135.4	18	72.0	42.6 - 113.8	KL19	296	100.4	89.0 - 111.9	353	105.5	94.5 - 116.5
HK8	23	68.6	40.5 - 96.6	29	64.2	40.8 - 87.5	KL20	76	104.9	81.3 - 128.4	75	86.1	66.6 - 105.6
HK9	5	35.6	11.5 - 83.2	7	31.8	12.8 - 65.7	KL21	122	95.4	78.5 - 112.3	151	114.6	96.3 - 132.9
HK10	256	104.2	91.5 - 117.0	289	87.6	77.5 - 97.8	KL22	26	103.2	63.6 - 142.9	24	87.3	52.4 - 122.2
HK11	13	58.9	31.3 - 100.6	21	102.8	63.5 - 157.2	KL23	105	166.4	134.6 - 198.3	98	144.3	115.7 - 172.8
HK12	15	75.3	42.1 - 124.3	19	72.5	39.9 - 105.1	KL24	38	63.4	43.3 - 83.6	68	119.0	90.7 - 147.3
HK13	22	73.6	42.8 - 104.3	30	96.7	62.1 - 131.4	KL25	851	93.0	86.7 - 99.2	982	97.1	91.0 - 103.2
HK14	66	72.6	55.1 - 90.2	81	68.8	53.8 - 83.7	NT1	48	94.6	67.8 - 121.3	57	95.0	70.4 - 119.7
HK15	44	157.1	110.7 - 203.5	42	108.0	75.3 - 140.6	NT2	67	104.9	79.8 - 130.0	68	100.1	76.3 - 123.8
HK16	150	119.7	100.6 - 138.9	153	108.5	91.3 - 125.7	NT3	121	106.7	87.7 - 125.7	130	124.0	102.7 - 145.3
HK17	164	96.9	82.1 - 111.8	207	109.5	94.6 - 124.4	NT4	81	87.2	68.2 - 106.2	109	99.9	81.1 - 118.6
HK18	8	43.9	18.9 - 86.4	16	62.7	32.0 - 93.5	NT5	212	103.9	89.9 - 117.9	242	113.1	98.9 - 127.4
HK19	77	99.5	77.3 - 121.7	97	105.4	84.4 - 126.4	NT6	101	83.7	67.4 - 100.0	119	94.4	77.4 - 111.3
HK20	226	129.7	112.8 - 146.6	322	165.2	147.2 - 183.3	NT7	64	109.9	82.9 - 136.8	61	106.2	79.6 - 132.9
HK21	20	100.0	61.0 - 154.5	28	111.1	70.0 - 152.3	NT8	203	98.9	85.3 - 112.6	235	95.2	83.1 - 107.4
KL1	91	102.8	81.7 - 123.9	108	115.1	93.4 - 136.8	NT9	58	153.1	113.7 - 192.5	59	129.8	96.7 - 162.9
KL2	172	103.5	88.0 - 119.0	157	83.7	70.6 - 96.7	NT10	254	137.8	120.9 - 154.8	257	133.4	117.1 - 149.7
KL3	54	103.2	75.7 - 130.7	62	94.1	70.7 - 117.6	NT11	41	127.0	88.1 - 165.9	43	108.3	76.0 - 140.7
KL4	126	79.8	65.9 - 93.8	127	79.5	65.6 - 93.3	NT12	162	100.9	85.4 - 116.5	171	90.5	76.9 - 104.0
KL5	113	96.2	78.4 - 113.9	114	92.3	75.3 - 109.2	NT13	43	102.3	71.7 - 132.9	37	93.3	63.2 - 123.3
KL6	38	112.0	76.4 - 147.6	63	130.4	98.2 - 162.6	NT14	20	74.8	42.0 - 107.6	26	82.7	50.9 - 114.5
KL7	11	46.3	23.2 - 82.9	17	60.1	31.6 - 88.7	NT15	155	105.7	89.1 - 122.4	199	106.6	91.8 - 121.4
KL8	57	71.7	53.1 - 90.3	90	99.7	79.1 - 120.3	NT16	312	100.6	89.5 - 111.8	393	93.3	84.1 - 102.5
KL9	290	92.1	81.5 - 102.7	330	90.4	80.6 - 100.1	NT17	64	98.3	74.2 - 122.4	77	107.2	83.2 - 131.1
KL10	32	105.1	68.7 - 141.5	28	73.5	46.2 - 100.7	NT18	46	141.3	100.5 - 182.1	55	140.1	103.0 - 177.1
KL11	80	86.1	67.2 - 105.0	89	80.7	63.9 - 97.4	NT19	56	113.3	83.6 - 142.9	63	110.8	83.5 - 138.2
KL12	21	81.8	46.8 - 116.8	20	73.4	41.3 - 105.6							

CVA

Sex-Age specific mortality rate (1/100,000) of CVA in Hong Kong (1984–1988)

	Male		Female	
Age	No. of deaths	Mortality rate	No. of deaths	Mortality rate
0–4	0	0.00	4	0.40
5–9	6	0.55	7	0.69
10–14	7	0.61	7	0.67
15–19	13	1.09	16	1.45
20–24	16	1.11	14	1.01
25–29	17	1.08	22	1.49
30–34	51	3.77	18	1.45
35–39	52	4.69	32	3.30
40–44	78	10.64	48	8.01
45–49	196	27.84	107	18.34
50–54	392	53.49	252	39.90
55–59	676	101.78	349	57.45
60–64	959	177.56	620	115.82
65+	4783	529.74	6682	541.40
TOTAL	7246	50.82	8178	60.93

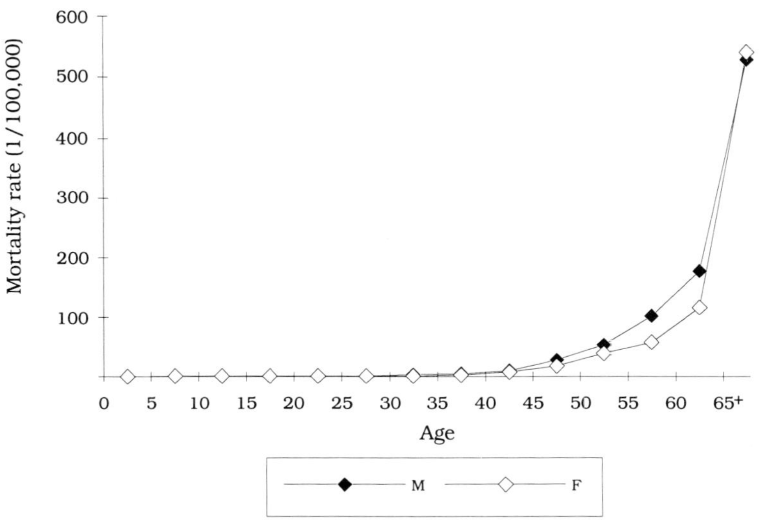

Number of communities on map by category based on standardized mortality ratio (SMR) during 1984–1988

Category	Number of communities Male	Female
SMR significantly high, in top 20%	7	5
SMR significantly high , not in top 20%	0	0
SMR not significantly high, in top 20%	6	8
SMR not significantly low, in bottom 20%	5	5
SMR significantly low, not in bottom 20%	1	2
SMR significantly low, in bottom 20%	8	8
other communities	38	37

Values of the standardized mortality ratio (SMR) which divide the 65 communities into quintile

Percentile	Male	Female
20th	79.83	82.05
40th	96.15	94.12
60th	103.21	101.68
80th	107.90	110.85
Lowest SMR	35.62	31.85
Highest SMR	166.42	165.22
No. of communities with zero death	0	0

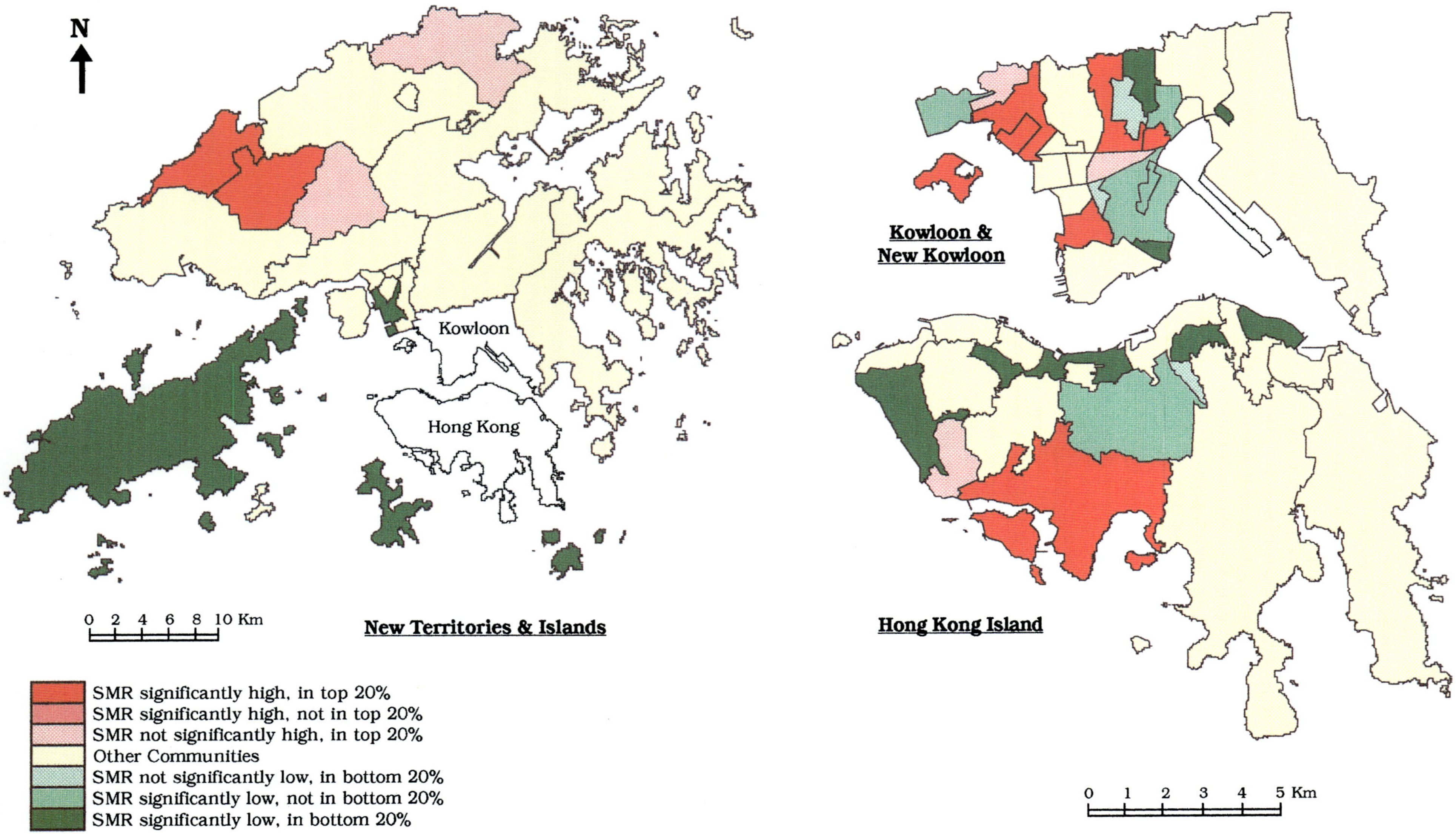

CVA (Male, 1989 -1993)

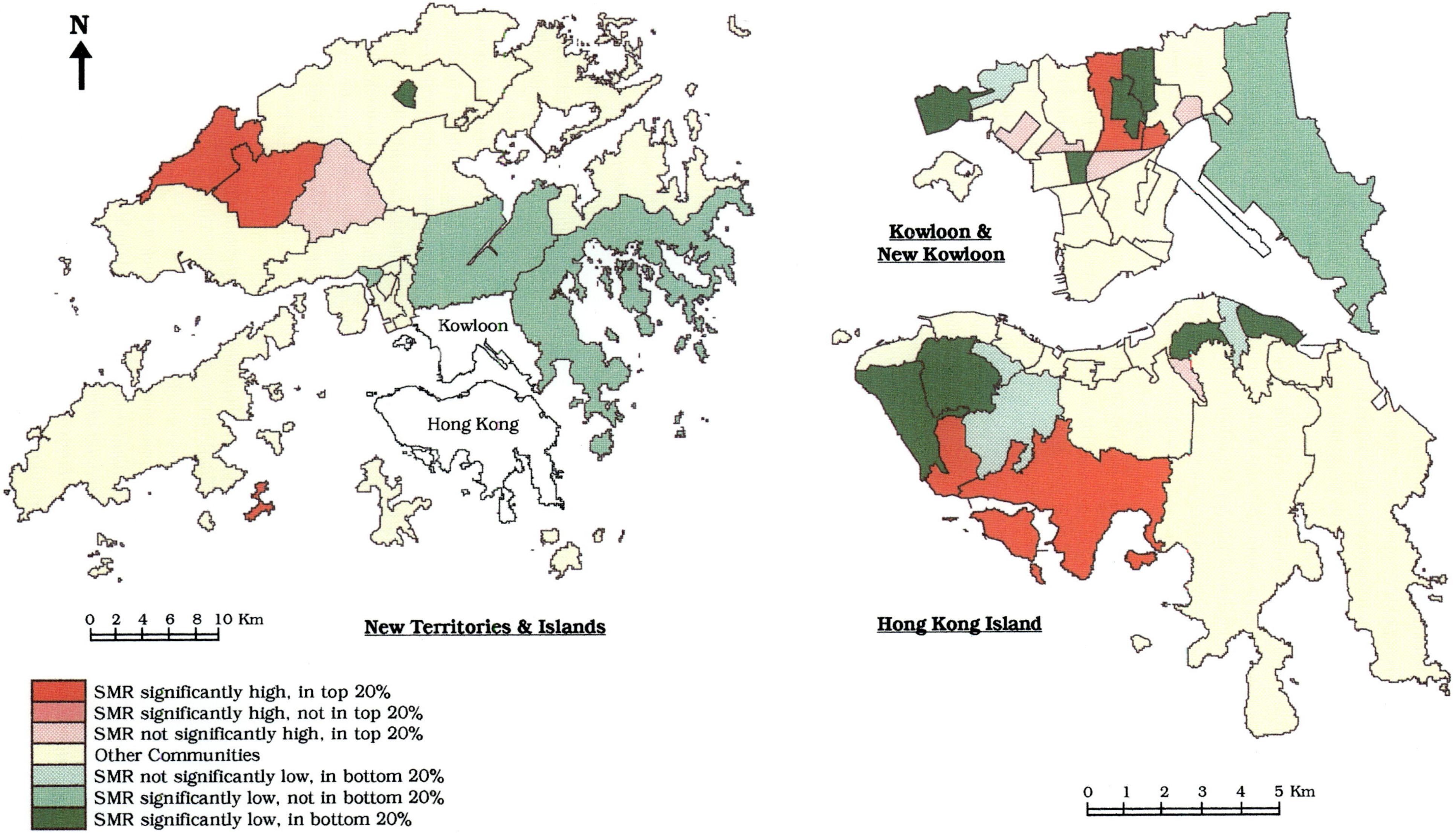

CVA (Female, 1989 -1993)

Number of Deaths, Standardised Mortality Ratio (SMR) and 95% Confidence Interval of CVA by 65 Communities in 1989–1993

Community	Male			Female		
	Number of deaths	SMR	95% C.I.	Number of deaths	SMR	95% C.I.
HK1	107	99.8	80.9 - 118.7	100	86.8	69.8 - 103.9
HK2	131	90.4	74.9 - 105.8	157	112.4	94.8 - 129.9
HK3	52	103.5	75.4 - 131.6	51	109.4	79.4 - 139.5
HK4	61	74.9	56.1 - 93.7	74	89.2	68.9 - 109.6
HK5	78	100.1	77.9 - 122.3	77	98.6	76.5 - 120.6
HK6	69	77.7	59.4 - 96.0	104	90.4	73.0 - 107.7
HK7	18	93.4	54.4 - 147.5	16	59.1	33.8 - 95.8
HK8	12	38.1	19.7 - 66.6	28	77.4	48.7 - 106.1
HK9	12	88.8	45.9 - 155.4	12	72.8	37.6 - 127.3
HK10	231	93.8	81.7 - 105.9	286	92.2	81.5 - 102.9
HK11	15	66.3	37.1 - 109.4	30	144.0	92.5 - 195.5
HK12	8	41.0	17.7 - 80.8	13	54.1	28.8 - 92.5
HK13	24	88.7	56.9 - 132.2	19	68.3	41.1 - 106.6
HK14	65	67.8	51.3 - 84.3	80	75.8	59.2 - 92.5
HK15	48	87.1	62.5 - 111.7	69	111.2	85.0 - 137.5
HK16	106	106.7	86.4 - 127.0	123	115.9	95.5 - 136.4
HK17	202	96.2	82.9 - 109.5	210	92.4	79.9 - 104.8
HK18	11	47.2	23.5 - 84.5	21	62.5	38.7 - 95.6
HK19	92	110.4	87.9 - 133.0	139	162.5	135.5 - 189.5
HK20	265	140.2	123.3 - 157.1	267	126.1	111.0 - 141.2
HK21	16	91.7	52.4 - 148.5	14	84.5	46.1 - 142.0
KL1	55	85.4	62.8 - 108.0	74	111.2	85.9 - 136.6
KL2	142	97.5	81.5 - 113.5	160	105.8	89.4 - 122.2
KL3	36	81.8	55.1 - 108.5	38	74.2	50.6 - 97.8
KL4	115	92.5	75.6 - 109.4	109	94.3	76.6 - 112.0
KL5	116	127.0	103.9 - 150.1	86	93.8	74.0 - 113.6
KL6	42	116.1	81.0 - 151.2	69	127.0	97.0 - 157.0
KL7	17	70.2	40.9 - 112.3	36	106.4	71.6 - 141.1
KL8	57	77.6	57.5 - 97.8	67	86.8	66.0 - 107.6
KL9	248	83.6	73.2 - 94.0	283	89.7	79.2 - 100.1
KL10	30	61.9	39.7 - 84.0	50	82.3	59.5 - 105.1
KL11	53	77.3	56.5 - 98.1	56	70.1	51.8 - 88.5
KL12	26	118.3	72.8 - 163.8	17	68.6	40.0 - 109.8
KL13	312	113.3	100.7 - 125.8	295	106.4	94.2 - 118.5
KL14	191	101.3	87.0 - 115.7	186	91.8	78.6 - 105.0
KL15	58	172.0	127.7 - 216.2	49	127.5	91.8 - 163.2
KL16	58	94.4	70.1 - 118.7	73	117.5	90.5 - 144.4
KL17	64	219.9	166.0 - 273.8	98	201.9	162.0 - 241.9
KL18	6	48.0	17.6 - 104.7	5	29.5	9.6 - 68.7
KL19	285	97.7	86.3 - 109.0	321	92.7	82.5 - 102.8
KL20	47	71.9	51.3 - 92.5	45	65.5	46.4 - 84.7
KL21	84	78.6	61.8 - 95.4	120	99.5	81.7 - 117.3
KL22	19	89.7	54.0 - 139.9	27	119.1	74.2 - 164.0
KL23	89	201.9	160.0 - 243.9	93	198.5	158.1 - 238.8
KL24	43	73.1	51.3 - 95.0	52	98.7	71.9 - 125.6
KL25	833	96.8	90.2 - 103.4	860	90.3	84.3 - 96.3
NT1	59	89.7	66.8 - 112.6	70	90.2	69.1 - 111.3
NT2	51	71.5	51.9 - 91.1	66	81.1	61.5 - 100.6
NT3	124	97.7	80.5 - 114.9	92	79.5	63.3 - 95.8
NT4	91	105.4	83.7 - 127.0	97	97.9	78.4 - 117.4
NT5	194	103.2	88.7 - 117.7	175	97.9	78.4 - 117.4
NT6	107	87.3	70.8 - 103.9	127	95.2	78.7 - 111.8
NT7	107	94.2	76.4 - 112.1	108	93.8	76.1 - 111.5
NT8	266	96.9	85.3 - 108.6	322	105.9	94.4 - 117.5
NT9	56	144.2	106.4 - 181.9	72	151.5	116.5 - 186.5
NT10	359	192.7	172.7 - 212.6	410	207.0	186.9 - 227.0
NT11	45	125.7	89.0 - 162.5	52	121.4	88.4 - 154.5
NT12	175	102.5	87.3 - 117.7	176	91.3	77.8 - 104.8
NT13	33	94.8	62.4 - 127.1	30	69.5	44.6 - 94.4
NT14	27	133.0	82.8 - 183.1	25	96.8	62.7 - 143.3
NT15	204	107.3	92.6 - 122.1	262	112.9	99.2 - 126.6
NT16	450	98.8	89.7 - 107.9	525	89.0	81.4 - 96.6
NT17	101	87.3	70.3 - 104.3	115	82.3	67.2 - 97.3
NT18	35	103.5	69.2 - 137.7	57	147.1	108.9 - 185.2
NT19	29	70.9	45.1 - 96.7	50	99.9	72.2 - 127.5

CVA

Sex-Age specific mortality rate (1/100,000) of CVA in Hong Kong (1989–1993)

	Male		Female	
Age	No. of deaths	Mortality rate	No. of deaths	Mortality rate
0–4	6	0.63	3	0.34
5–9	4	0.38	1	0.10
10–14	3	0.27	6	0.60
15–19	8	0.73	9	0.90
20–24	13	1.14	5	0.44
25–29	22	1.53	9	0.61
30–34	32	2.05	18	1.18
35–39	58	4.33	36	2.86
40–44	101	9.17	53	5.45
45–49	157	21.49	84	14.07
50–54	304	43.82	165	28.98
55–59	513	73.41	272	44.66
60–64	814	131.86	489	84.62
65+	5129	463.03	6840	486.87
TOTAL	7164	48.98	7990	57.10

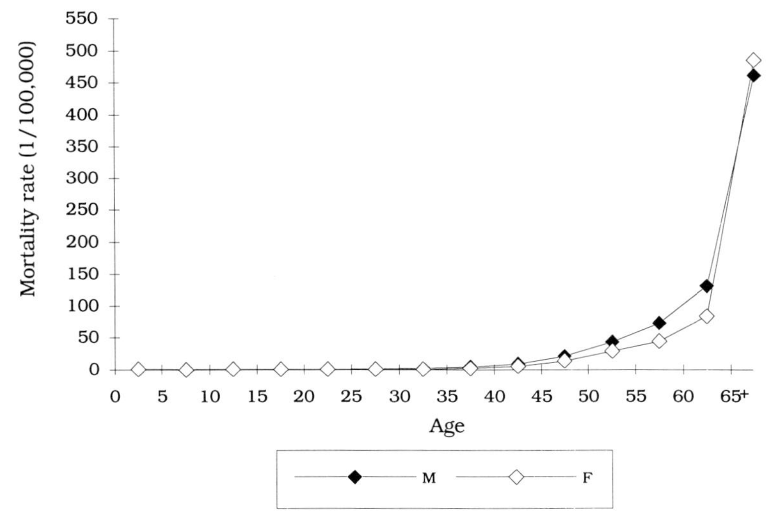

Number of communities on map by category based on standardized mortality ratio (SMR) during 1989–1993

Category	Number of communities Male	Female
SMR significantly high, in top 20%	8	7
SMR significantly high , not in top 20%	0	0
SMR not significantly high, in top 20%	5	6
SMR not significantly low, in bottom 20%	3	4
SMR significantly low, not in bottom 20%	5	4
SMR significantly low, in bottom 20%	10	9
other communities	34	35

Values of the standardized mortality ratio (SMR) which divide the 65 communities into quintile

Percentile	Male	Female
20th	74.91	77.22
40th	89.65	85.23
60th	97.50	99.38
80th	107.32	119.05
Lowest SMR	38.08	49.76
Highest SMR	219.90	201.79
No. of communities with zero cases	0	0

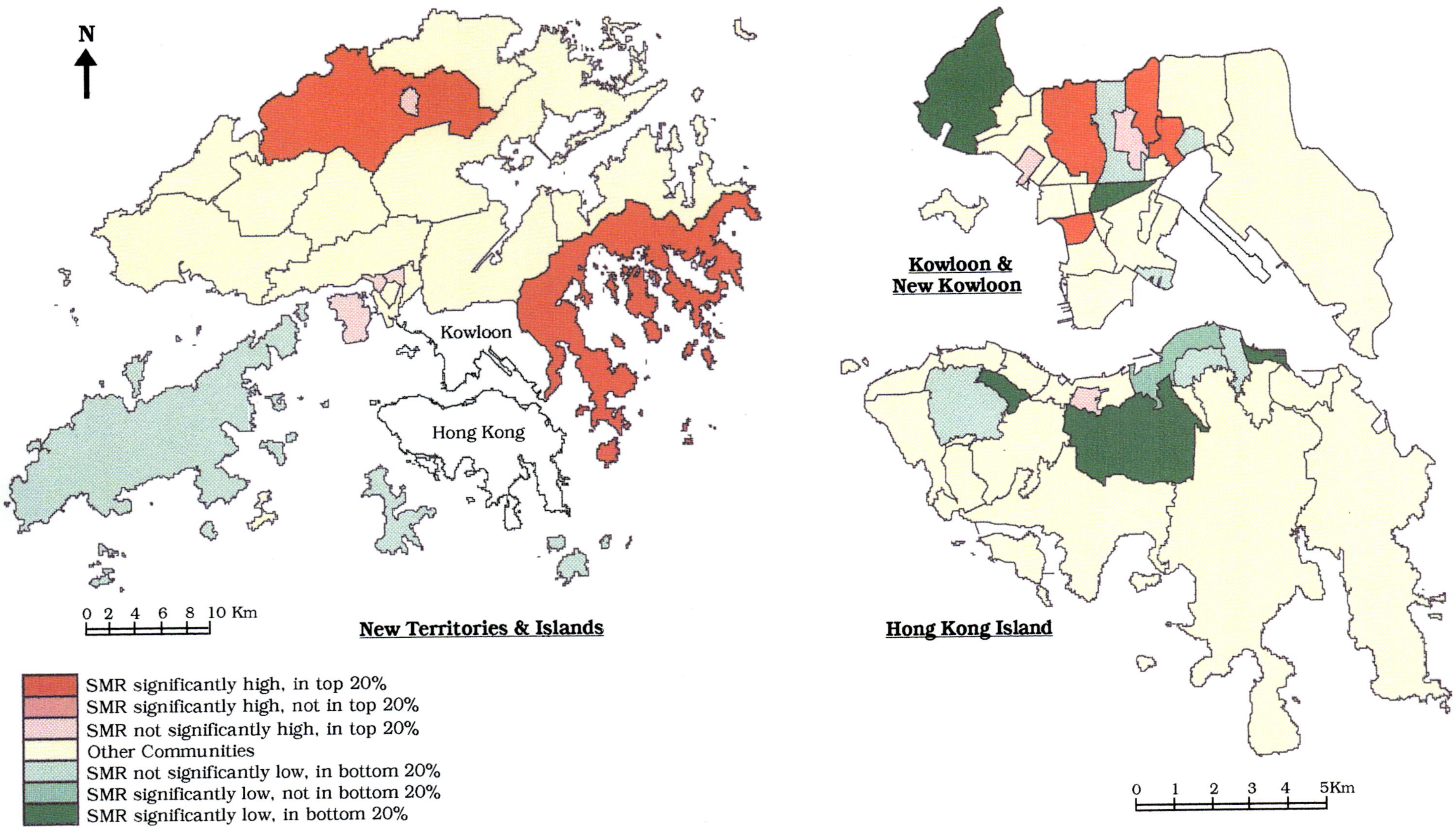

TB (Male, 1979 -1983)

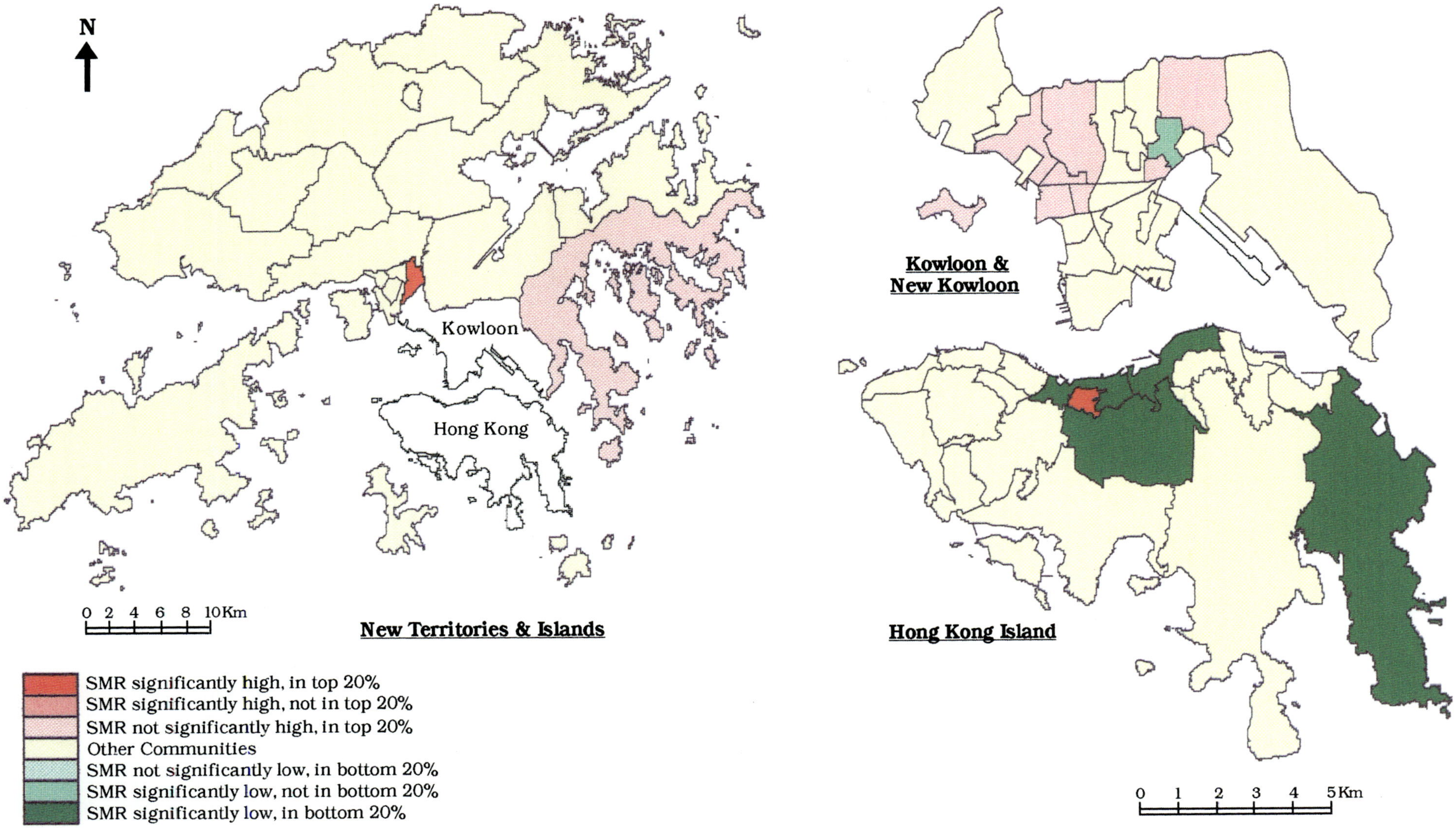

TB (Female, 1979 - 1983)

Number of Deaths, Standardised Mortality Ratio (SMR) and 95% Confidence Interval of TB by 65 Communities in 1979–1983

	Male			Female		
Community	Number of deaths	SMR	95% C.I.	Number of deaths	SMR	95% C.I.
HK1	18	63.5	37.6 - 100.4	10	122.8	59.0 - 225.6
HK2	35	77.5	51.9 - 103.2	15	127.8	71.4 - 211.2
HK3	13	73.3	39.0 - 125.3	5	116.7	37.8 - 272.7
HK4	27	97.7	60.8 - 134.5	2	26.5	3.2 - 95.6
HK5	37	138.8	94.0 - 183.5	14	197.3	107.8 - 331.0
HK6	10	45.4	21.8 - 83.4	2	24.1	2.9 - 87.0
HK7	1	22.6	0.6 - 125.4	1	58.5	1.5 - 324.8
HK8	1	11.5	0.3 - 64.0	0	0.0	...
HK9	0	0.0	...	0	0.0	...
HK10	36	59.2	39.8 - 78.5	6	29.4	10.8 - 64.1
HK11	4	73.2	20.0 - 187.3	1	69.3	1.8 - 385.0
HK12	2	43.8	5.3 - 158.3	0	0.0	...
HK13	4	55.7	15.2 - 142.5	0	0.0	...
HK14	4	22.9	6.2 - 58.6	2	36.0	4.4 - 129.9
HK15	6	84.0	30.8 - 182.9	0	0.0	...
HK16	36	110.7	74.5 - 146.8	6	67.0	24.5 - 146.0
HK17	33	93.6	61.7 - 125.5	3	30.5	6.3 - 89.3
HK18	4	79.3	21.6 - 202.8	2	115.3	14.0 - 416.1
HK19	12	70.8	36.5 - 123.5	5	95.0	30.7 - 221.8
HK20	28	75.1	47.3 - 102.9	11	105.0	52.5 - 187.9
HK21	3	62.6	12.9 - 183.0	1	78.1	2.0 - 434.1
KL1	23	96.4	61.0 - 144.8	7	108.0	43.4 - 222.7
KL2	56	113.8	84.0 - 143.7	18	132.2	78.2 - 208.8
KL3	13	91.1	48.4 - 155.7	7	158.2	63.6 - 326.3
KL4	59	147.9	110.1 - 185.6	14	131.6	71.9 - 220.8
KL5	30	89.9	57.7 - 122.0	10	115.1	55.3 - 211.6
KL6	1	12.1	0.3 - 67.1	1	29.9	0.8 - 166.4
KL7	6	97.6	35.8 - 212.7	1	43.0	1.1 - 239.2
KL8	18	84.6	50.0 - 133.6	4	61.9	16.9 - 158.3
KL9	75	95.4	73.8 - 116.9	31	128.1	83.0 - 173.2
KL10	4	50.9	13.9 - 130.2	3	114.1	23.5 - 333.5
KL11	9	42.2	19.4 - 80.0	6	84.7	31.0 - 184.6
KL12	4	60.7	16.5 - 155.3	3	177.5	36.6 - 518.9
KL13	77	96.0	74.5 - 117.4	29	132.7	84.4 - 181.0
KL14	66	139.6	105.9 - 173.3	19	157.4	94.8 - 245.9
KL15	7	183.3	73.6 - 377.8	4	367.7	100.2 - 940.3
KL16	16	84.2	48.1 - 136.7	8	145.1	62.5 - 285.6
KL17	1	18.3	0.5 - 101.8	0	0.0	...
KL18	5	139.2	45.0 - 325.2	0	0.0	...
KL19	70	100.4	76.9 - 123.9	30	141.7	91.0 - 192.3
KL20	38	156.6	106.8 - 206.4	8	114.3	49.3 - 225.1
KL21	61	155.2	116.3 - 194.2	4	35.3	9.6 - 90.4
KL22	4	58.7	16.0 - 150.0	2	115.6	14.0 - 417.2
KL23	24	114.2	73.2 - 169.9	8	138.6	59.7 - 272.8
KL24	10	77.9	37.4 - 143.1	2	56.8	6.9 - 205.0
KL25	222	114.5	99.4 - 129.5	64	114.9	86.8 - 143.1
NT1	9	90.4	41.5 - 171.5	2	64.4	7.8 - 232.6
NT2	11	76.3	38.2 - 136.6	4	99.2	27.0 - 253.8
NT3	37	127.5	86.4 - 168.5	6	85.8	31.4 - 186.9
NT4	20	128.0	78.0 - 197.8	6	123.7	45.3 - 269.5
NT5	62	112.9	84.8 - 140.9	19	121.7	73.3 - 190.2
NT6	28	103.8	65.3 - 142.2	9	390.8	179.3 - 741.5
NT7	14	150.5	82.3 - 252.6	2	74.4	9.0 - 268.7
NT8	38	126.1	86.0 - 166.1	8	95.1	41.0 - 187.3
NT9	11	118.7	59.4 - 212.4	2	81.7	9.9 - 294.8
NT10	33	85.8	56.5 - 115.1	8	78.8	34.0 - 155.1
NT11	5	62.4	20.2 - 145.8	3	148.8	30.7 - 435.0
NT12	56	153.5	113.3 - 193.7	10	101.7	48.9 - 187.0
NT13	10	146.7	70.5 - 269.7	2	102.3	12.4 - 369.3
NT14	5	79.2	25.6 - 185.1	2	99.8	12.1 - 360.2
NT15	25	99.0	60.2 - 137.8	7	92.2	37.0 - 190.0
NT16	30	96.4	61.9 - 130.9	9	92.7	42.5 - 176.0
NT17	24	160.9	103.2 - 239.5	7	159.8	64.2 - 329.4
NT18	6	82.6	30.3 - 180.0	2	88.8	10.8 - 320.8
NT19	7	55.8	22.4 - 114.9	0	0.0	...

TB

Sex-Age specific mortality rate (1/100,000) of TB in Hong Kong (1979–1983)

Age	Male No. of deaths	Male Mortality rate	Female No. of deaths	Female Mortality rate
0–4	3	0.28	6	0.61
5–9	3	0.28	2	0.20
10–14	3	0.26	1	0.09
15–19	5	0.35	2	0.15
20–24	13	0.85	7	0.50
25–29	13	0.98	8	0.69
30–34	22	1.99	12	1.31
35–39	35	4.85	6	1.08
40–44	55	7.82	15	2.71
45–49	97	13.45	11	1.82
50–54	146	21.25	19	3.12
55–59	198	34.81	40	7.48
60–64	268	58.65	47	10.30
65+	783	114.85	301	29.82
TOTAL	1644	12.47	477	3.92

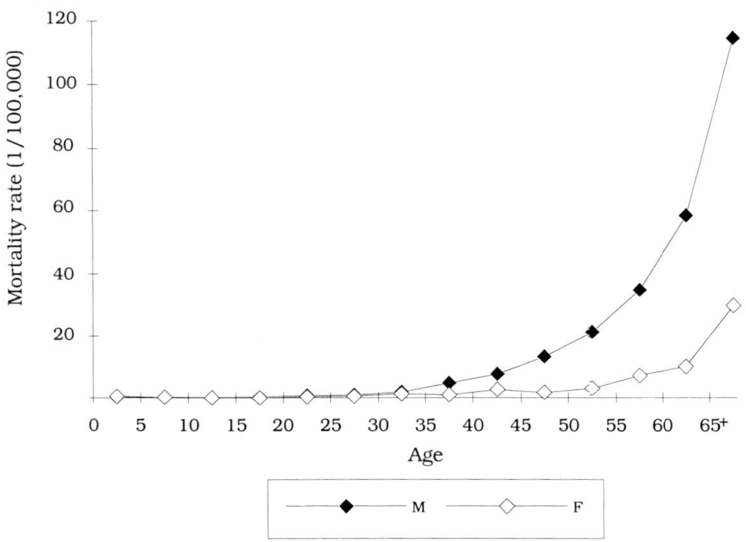

Number of communities on map by category based on standardized mortality ratio (SMR) during 1979–1983

Category	Number of communities Male	Number of communities Female
SMR significantly high, in top 20%	6	2
SMR significantly high , not in top 20%	0	0
SMR not significantly high, in top 20%	7	8
SMR not significantly low, in bottom 20%	7	0
SMR significantly low, not in bottom 20%	1	1
SMR significantly low, in bottom 20%	5	4
other communities	39	50

Values of the standardized mortality ratio (SMR) which divide the 65 communities into quintile

Percentile	Male	Female
20th	58.65	30.54
40th	79.23	81.65
60th	96.38	108.02
80th	126.05	131.50
Lowest SMR	0.00	0.00
Highest SMR	183.25	390.79
No. of communities with zero death	1	8

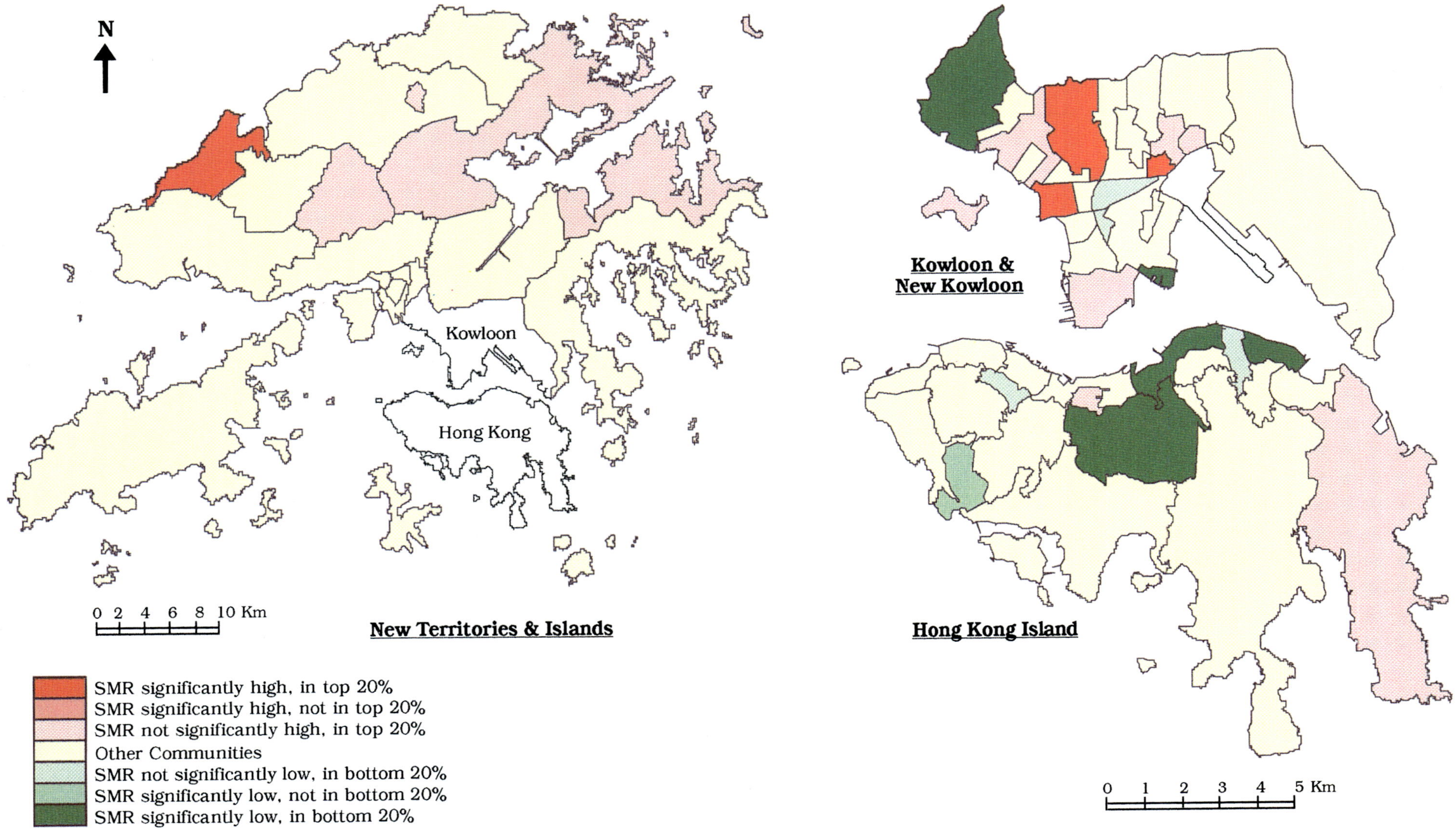

TB (Male, 1984 -1988)

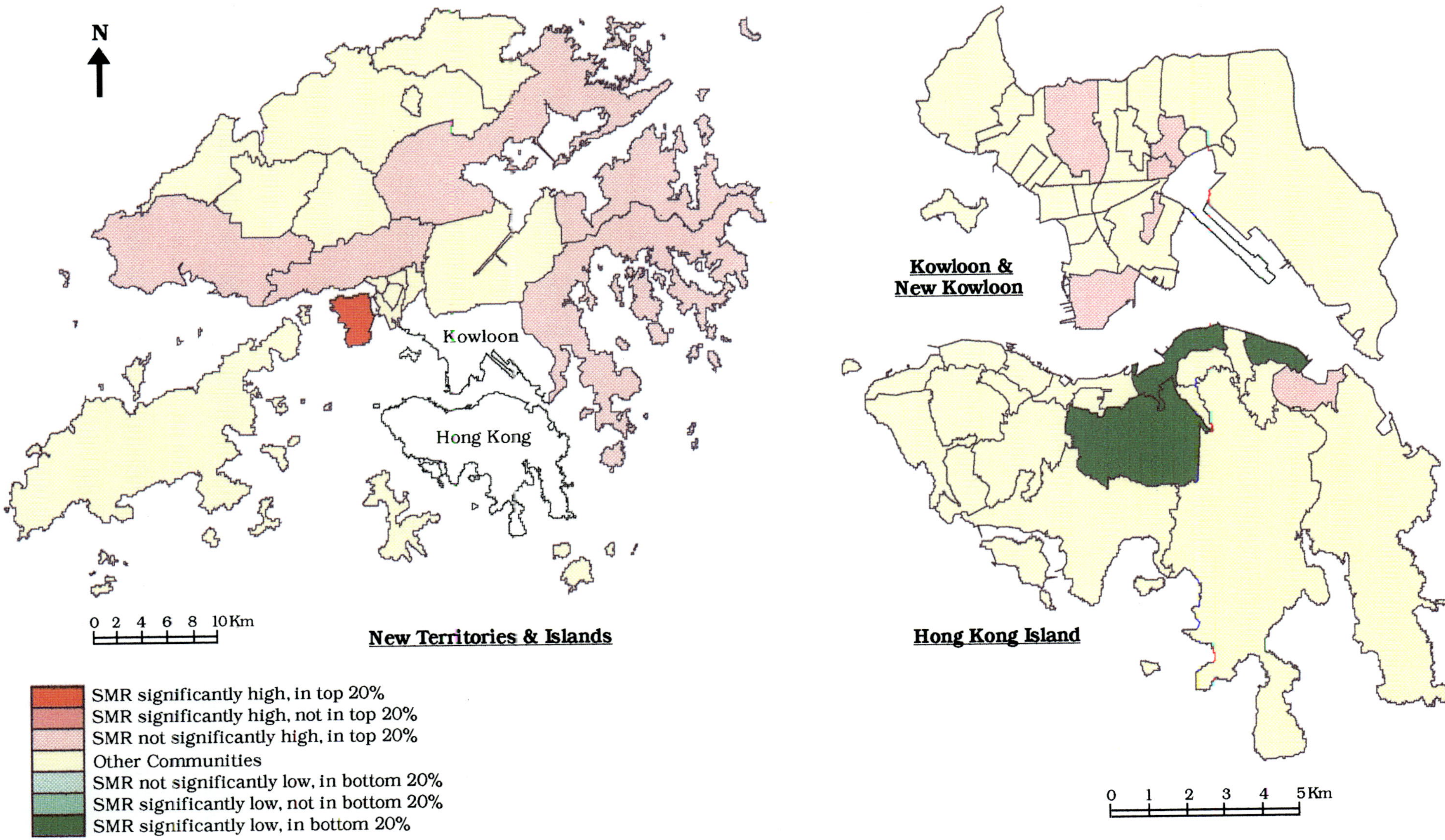

TB (Female, 1984 –1988)

Number of Deaths, Standardised Mortality Ratio (SMR) and 95% Confidence Interval of TB by 65 Communities in 1984–1988

Community	Male			Female		
	Number of deaths	SMR	95% C.I.	Number of deaths	SMR	95% C.I.
HK1	19	85.0	51.2 - 132.9	4	63.5	17.3 - 162.5
HK2	30	94.5	60.7 - 128.4	7	78.8	31.6 - 162.4
HK3	12	100.8	52.0 - 176.0	3	102.4	21.1 - 299.5
HK4	18	94.7	56.1 - 149.7	5	94.0	30.4 - 219.7
HK5	24	141.8	90.9 - 211.0	5	100.8	32.6 - 235.4
HK6	5	29.0	9.4 - 67.8	0	0.0	...
HK7	1	28.7	0.7 - 159.3	1	80.8	2.0 - 448.7
HK8	2	31.0	3.8 - 111.9	0	0.0	...
HK9	2	71.1	8.6 - 256.6	0	0.0	...
HK10	16	33.5	17.1 - 49.9	7	43.2	17.4 - 89.1
HK11	3	70.2	14.5 - 205.1	1	94.8	2.4 - 526.4
HK12	0	0.0	...	0	0.0	...
HK13	2	34.9	4.2 - 126.0	1	64.4	1.6 - 357.9
HK14	2	11.4	1.4 - 41.2	1	17.1	0.4 - 95.0
HK15	2	36.0	4.4 - 130.1	1	51.2	1.3 - 284.6
HK16	21	86.6	53.5 - 132.5	12	172.2	88.8 - 300.5
HK17	42	130.9	91.3 - 170.5	10	107.7	51.8 - 197.9
HK18	0	0.0	...	0	0.0	...
HK19	6	39.2	14.4 - 85.4	3	63.9	13.2 - 186.7
HK20	25	75.1	45.6 - 104.5	10	103.0	49.5 - 189.4
HK21	2	49.7	6.0 - 179.5	0	0.0	...
KL1	22	128.4	80.2 - 194.5	7	151.8	61.0 - 313.0
KL2	47	143.8	102.7 - 184.9	11	120.2	60.1 - 215.0
KL3	7	69.8	28.0 - 143.9	1	31.6	0.8 - 175.4
KL4	34	111.1	73.7 - 148.4	9	116.5	53.4 - 221.0
KL5	27	119.3	78.5 - 173.6	8	133.9	57.7 - 263.6
KL6	2	31.1	3.8 - 112.4	3	129.4	26.7 - 378.2
KL7	1	21.9	0.6 - 121.4	1	70.2	1.8 - 389.9
KL8	16	101.9	58.2 - 165.4	7	155.8	62.6 - 321.3
KL9	48	78.0	56.0 - 100.1	12	66.0	34.0 - 115.1
KL10	0	0.0	...	2	103.4	12.5 - 373.4
KL11	6	33.3	12.2 - 72.5	6	109.4	40.1 - 238.5
KL12	5	100.5	32.5 - 234.8	1	77.2	2.0 - 428.9
KL13	68	123.1	93.8 - 152.3	18	117.6	69.6 - 185.7
KL14	65	162.0	122.6 - 201.3	18	166.8	98.7 - 263.5
KL15	6	89.9	32.9 - 195.8	3	141.8	29.2 - 414.7
KL16	15	108.2	60.4 - 178.5	3	81.3	16.8 - 237.7
KL17	6	95.4	34.9 - 207.9	1	33.6	0.8 - 186.4
KL18	0	0.0	...	0	0.0	...
KL19	68	120.4	91.8 - 149.0	18	109.4	64.7 - 172.8
KL20	11	79.7	39.9 - 142.6	5	117.5	38.0 - 274.4
KL21	30	125.6	84.8 - 179.4	11	171.9	86.0 - 307.6
KL22	7	140.7	56.5 - 290.1	0	0.0	...
KL23	21	170.6	105.3 - 260.9	5	147.6	47.8 - 344.8
KL24	11	95.7	47.8 - 171.1	2	69.4	8.4 - 250.6
KL25	188	104.7	89.7 - 119.7	57	111.4	82.5 - 140.3
NT1	8	79.4	34.2 - 156.3	5	161.4	52.2 - 377.1
NT2	12	95.6	49.3 - 166.9	3	86.8	17.9 - 253.8
NT3	27	119.7	78.8 - 174.3	5	91.3	29.5 - 213.2
NT4	18	94.3	55.8 - 149.0	4	70.4	19.2 - 180.1
NT5	48	118.9	85.2 - 152.5	12	109.8	56.6 - 191.7
NT6	25	104.9	67.7 - 154.8	6	93.3	34.2 - 203.3
NT7	12	101.5	52.3 - 177.1	8	258.1	111.2 - 508.1
NT8	46	112.3	79.8 - 144.7	19	147.0	88.6 - 229.7
NT9	14	189.9	103.8 - 318.7	3	134.3	27.7 - 392.6
NT10	41	116.9	81.1 - 152.7	5	52.6	17.0 - 122.9
NT11	9	145.1	66.6 - 275.4	3	154.4	31.8 - 451.5
NT12	35	114.2	76.4 - 152.1	5	54.1	17.5 - 126.5
NT13	10	125.6	60.4 - 230.8	1	49.7	1.3 - 276.2
NT14	4	78.7	21.4 - 201.3	2	133.5	16.2 - 481.9
NT15	40	141.8	97.9 - 185.7	13	140.0	74.5 - 239.4
NT16	57	92.3	68.3 - 116.2	21	97.8	60.4 - 149.5
NT17	12	98.1	50.6 - 171.2	7	199.3	80.0 - 410.8
NT18	6	99.5	36.4 - 216.7	0	0.0	...
NT19	9	97.5	44.7 - 185.0	2	74.4	9.0 - 268.4

TB

Sex-Age specific mortality rate (1/100,000) of TB in Hong Kong (1984–1988)

	Male		Female	
Age	No. of deaths	Mortality rate	No. of deaths	Mortality rate
0–4	1	0.09	1	0.10
5–9	1	0.09	1	0.10
10–14	1	0.09	2	0.19
15–19	0	0.00	3	0.27
20–24	5	0.35	4	0.29
25–29	6	0.38	8	0.54
30–34	12	0.89	5	0.40
35–39	24	2.16	5	0.52
40–44	25	3.41	6	1.00
45–49	64	9.09	13	2.23
50–54	127	17.33	14	2.22
55–59	147	22.13	28	4.61
60–64	195	36.10	28	5.23
65+	801	88.71	287	23.25
TOTAL	1409	9.88	405	3.02

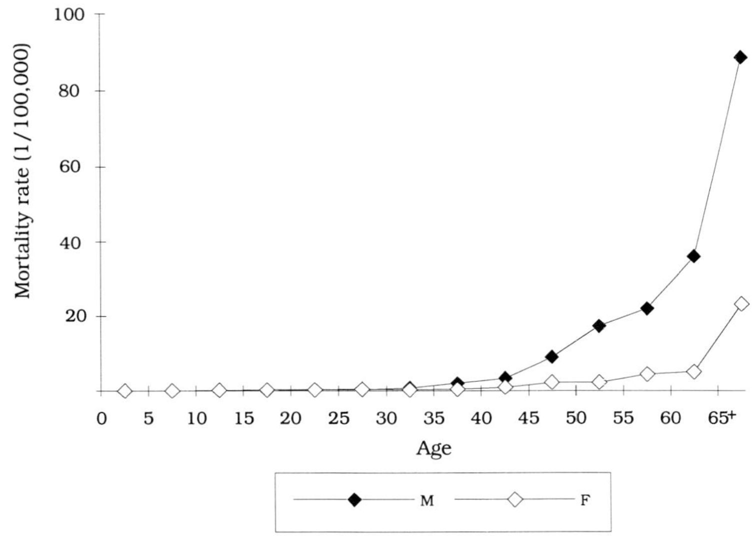

Number of communities on map by category based on standardized mortality ratio (SMR) during 1984–1988

Category	Number of communities Male	Female
SMR significantly high, in top 20%	4	1
SMR significantly high , not in top 20%	0	0
SMR not significantly high, in top 20%	9	10
SMR not significantly low, in bottom 20%	4	0
SMR significantly low, not in bottom 20%	1	0
SMR significantly low, in bottom 20%	5	3
other communities	42	51

Values of the standardized mortality ratio (SMR) which divide the 65 communities into quintile

Percentile	Male	Female
20th	34.89	43.23
40th	86.64	77.20
60th	100.85	103.44
80th	120.36	134.27
Lowest SMR	0.00	0.00
Highest SMR	189.94	258.09
No. of communities with zero death	4	9

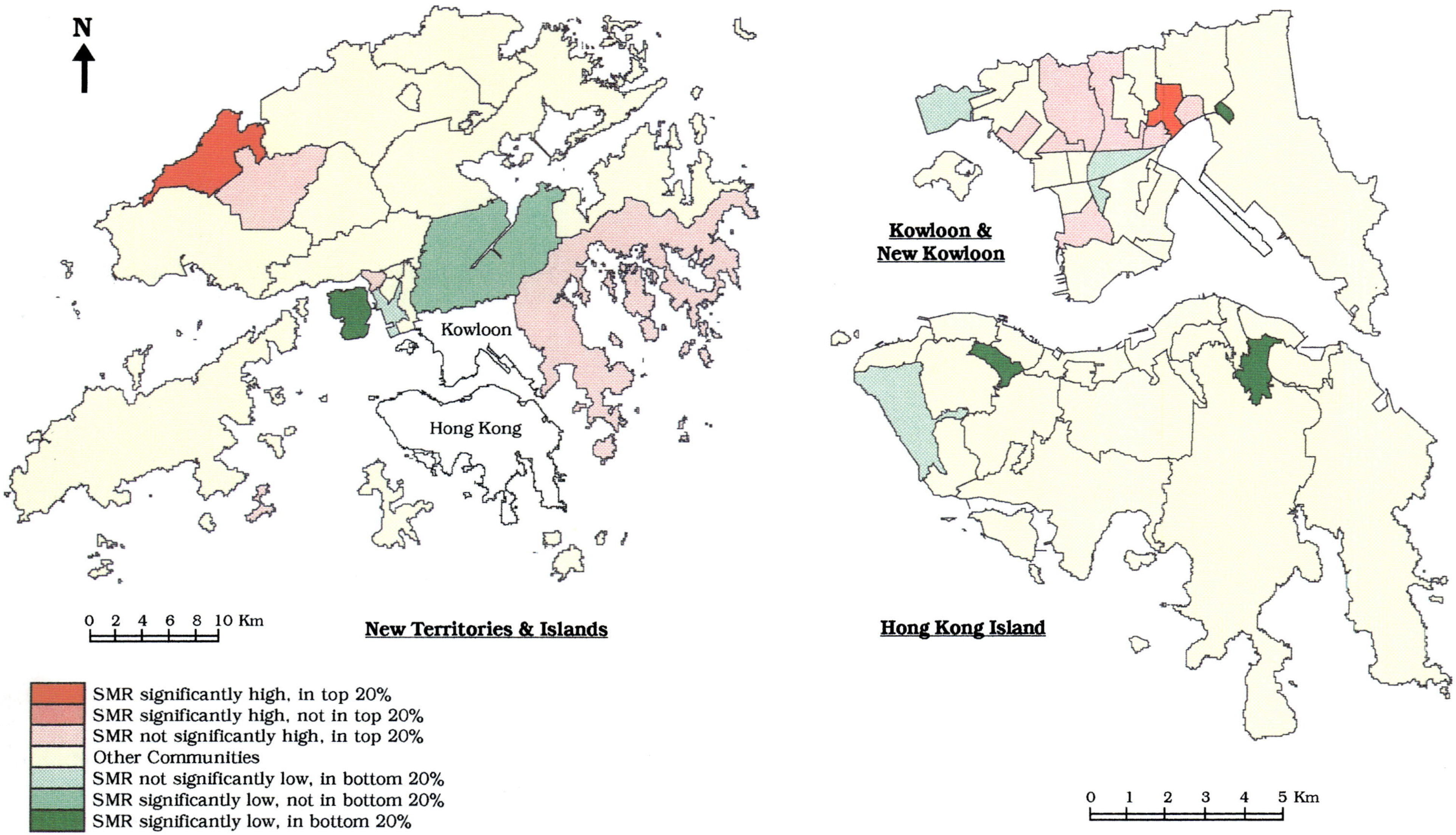

TB (Male, 1989 -1993)

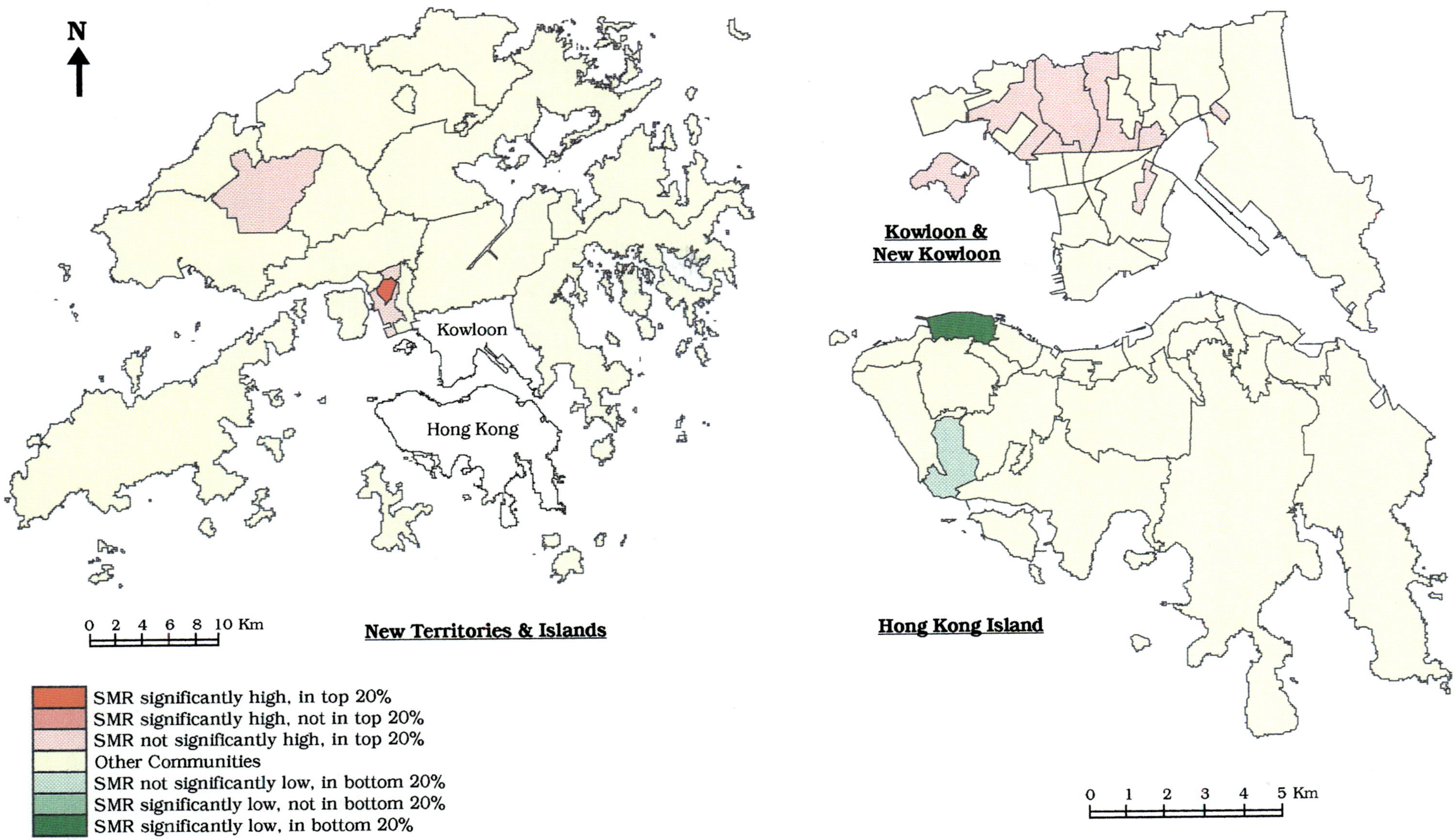

TB (Female, 1989 -1993)

Number of Deaths, Standardised Mortality Ratio (SMR) and 95% Confidence Interval of TB by 65 Communities in 1989–1993

Community	Male			Female		
	Number of deaths	SMR	95% C.I.	Number of deaths	SMR	95% C.I.
HK1	22	110.9	69.5 - 167.5	7	113.6	45.5 - 234.0
HK2	24	89.4	57.3 - 133.3	1	13.4	0.3 - 74.4
HK3	12	129.9	67.2 - 227.3	1	40.8	1.0 - 227.1
HK4	14	92.8	50.7 - 156.0	1	23.1	0.6 - 128.4
HK5	18	125.1	74.2 - 197.7	2	49.0	5.9 - 176.9
HK6	10	61.2	29.4 - 112.6	4	64.4	17.5 - 164.9
HK7	0	0.0	...	1	66.9	1.7 - 372.8
HK8	0	0.0	...	2	99.8	12.1 - 360.4
HK9	0	0.0	...	0	0.0	...
HK10	35	76.0	50.9 - 101.2	13	79.0	42.0 - 135.1
HK11	5	118.8	38.5 - 276.8	0	0.0	...
HK12	1	27.0	0.7 - 150.3	1	73.8	1.9 - 411.2
HK13	3	60.8	12.5 - 177.5	0	0.0	...
HK14	13	71.9	38.2 - 122.9	4	67.9	18.5 - 173.7
HK15	4	37.8	10.3 - 96.8	2	55.9	6.8 - 201.8
HK16	11	59.4	29.7 - 106.4	3	53.1	10.9 - 155.0
HK17	39	100.3	68.8 - 131.8	14	114.2	62.4 - 191.9
HK18	1	23.3	0.6 - 129.5	0	0.0	...
HK19	14	89.3	48.8 - 150.1	1	21.3	0.5 - 118.9
HK20	32	91.2	59.6 - 122.8	8	70.5	30.4 - 138.8
HK21	2	57.6	7.0 - 208.0	1	98.0	2.5 - 546.1
KL1	11	91.6	45.7 - 164.0	1	28.2	0.7 - 157.0
KL2	32	116.0	75.8 - 156.1	9	113.2	51.8 - 215.0
KL3	5	61.3	19.9 - 142.9	2	74.9	9.1 - 270.2
KL4	23	99.3	63.0 - 148.9	8	131.4	56.6 - 258.8
KL5	24	141.7	90.8 - 211.2	4	83.8	22.8 - 214.6
KL6	2	31.0	3.8 - 112.0	2	72.0	8.7 - 260.0
KL7	1	22.3	0.6 - 124.0	2	111.2	13.5 - 401.5
KL8	13	93.4	49.7 - 159.7	6	145.3	53.3 - 316.7
KL9	58	104.2	77.4 - 131.1	16	95.6	54.7 - 154.8
KL10	8	84.7	36.5 - 166.8	0	0.0	...
KL11	6	46.8	17.2 - 102.0	2	46.3	5.6 - 167.3
KL12	4	97.1	26.4 - 248.6	1	78.1	2.0 - 435.3
KL13	58	113.5	84.3 - 142.7	20	138.3	84.5 - 213.0
KL14	45	134.5	95.2 - 173.9	17	164.0	95.6 - 262.4
KL15	10	159.3	76.5 - 293.1	3	149.3	30.8 - 436.0
KL16	17	147.3	85.9 - 235.7	5	152.8	49.5 - 355.9
KL17	9	173.1	79.3 - 328.9	5	200.1	64.8 - 466.3
KL18	0	0.0	...	1	108.0	2.7 - 601.5
KL19	50	94.1	68.0 - 120.1	13	72.7	38.7 - 124.4
KL20	11	91.3	45.6 - 163.5	3	81.7	16.8 - 238.6
KL21	30	156.0	100.2 - 211.8	5	81.4	26.4 - 189.6
KL22	6	150.7	55.3 - 328.6	1	84.0	2.1 - 467.6
KL23	14	171.8	93.8 - 288.6	6	244.0	89.6 - 531.9
KL24	4	37.6	10.2 - 96.2	5	184.7	59.8 - 430.3
KL25	148	91.7	76.9 - 106.4	51	100.6	73.0 - 128.2
NT1	9	69.4	31.8 - 131.8	4	87.8	23.9 - 224.8
NT2	7	52.0	20.9 - 107.1	7	162.1	65.0 - 335.0
NT3	21	156.0	96.6 - 238.7	6	92.4	33.9 - 201.5
NT4	15	89.3	50.0 - 147.3	9	168.0	76.9 - 319.1
NT5	45	127.3	90.1 - 164.5	19	182.9	110.1 - 285.4
NT6	29	123.7	78.7 - 168.7	8	111.7	48.2 - 220.1
NT7	15	27.8	15.6 - 45.9	6	87.2	32.0 - 190.1
NT8	65	120.5	91.2 - 149.8	24	134.1	85.9 - 199.8
NT9	14	199.4	108.9 - 335.1	2	83.3	10.1 - 300.7
NT10	48	138.9	99.6 - 178.3	15	140.9	78.9 - 232.5
NT11	8	123.9	53.4 - 244.0	0	0.0	...
NT12	39	123.0	84.4 - 161.6	10	96.4	46.3 - 177.3
NT13	18	68.4	40.6 - 108.1	3	128.7	26.5 - 375.7
NT14	2	54.6	6.6 - 197.3	0	0.0	...
NT15	43	119.6	83.9 - 155.4	11	85.7	42.8 - 153.5
NT16	71	80.9	62.0 - 99.7	40	122.0	84.2 - 159.8
NT17	30	135.8	87.2 - 184.3	7	89.1	35.7 - 183.6
NT18	8	132.2	57.0 - 260.4	4	198.9	54.1 - 509.1
NT19	7	94.1	37.7 - 193.8	1	39.0	1.0 - 217.3

TB

Sex-Age specific mortality rate (1/100,000) of TB in Hong Kong (1989–1993)

	Male		Female	
Age	No. of deaths	Mortality rate	No. of deaths	Mortality rate
0–4	1	0.10	0	0.00
5–9	5	0.47	0	0.00
10–14	1	0.09	2	0.20
15–19	4	0.37	0	0.00
20–24	5	0.44	8	0.71
25–29	9	0.62	5	0.34
30–34	12	0.77	15	0.99
35–39	22	1.64	10	0.79
40–44	29	2.63	10	1.03
45–49	54	7.39	5	0.84
50–54	78	11.24	14	2.46
55–59	118	16.89	15	2.46
60–64	179	29.00	20	3.46
65+	826	74.57	326	23.20
TOTAL	1343	9.18	430	3.07

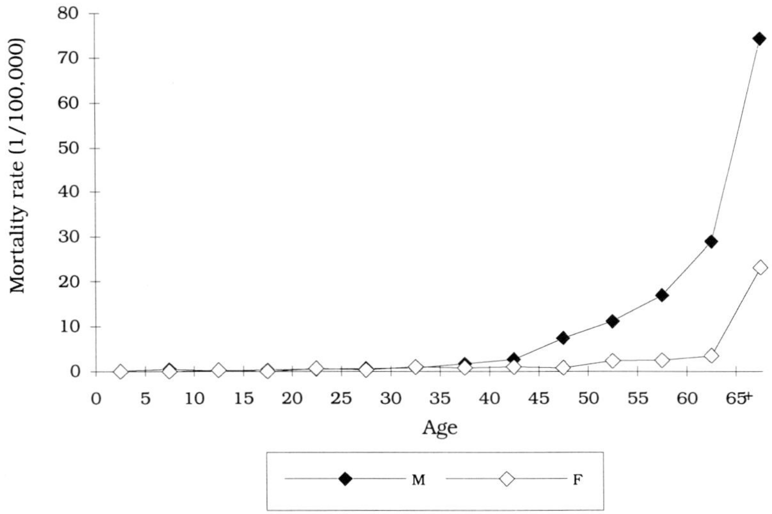

Number of communities on map by category based on standardized mortality ratio (SMR) during 1989–1993

Category	Number of communities Male	Female
SMR significantly high, in top 20%	2	1
SMR significantly high , not in top 20%	0	0
SMR not significantly high, in top 20%	11	10
SMR not significantly low, in bottom 20%	5	1
SMR significantly low, not in bottom 20%	1	0
SMR significantly low, in bottom 20%	4	1
other communities	42	52

Values of the standardized mortality ratio (SMR) which divide the 65 communities into quintile

Percentile	Male	Female
20th	52.01	40.78
40th	89.25	78.15
60th	100.30	96.39
80th	129.90	134.06
Lowest SMR	0.00	0.00
Highest SMR	199.44	244.01
No. of communities with zero cases	4	7

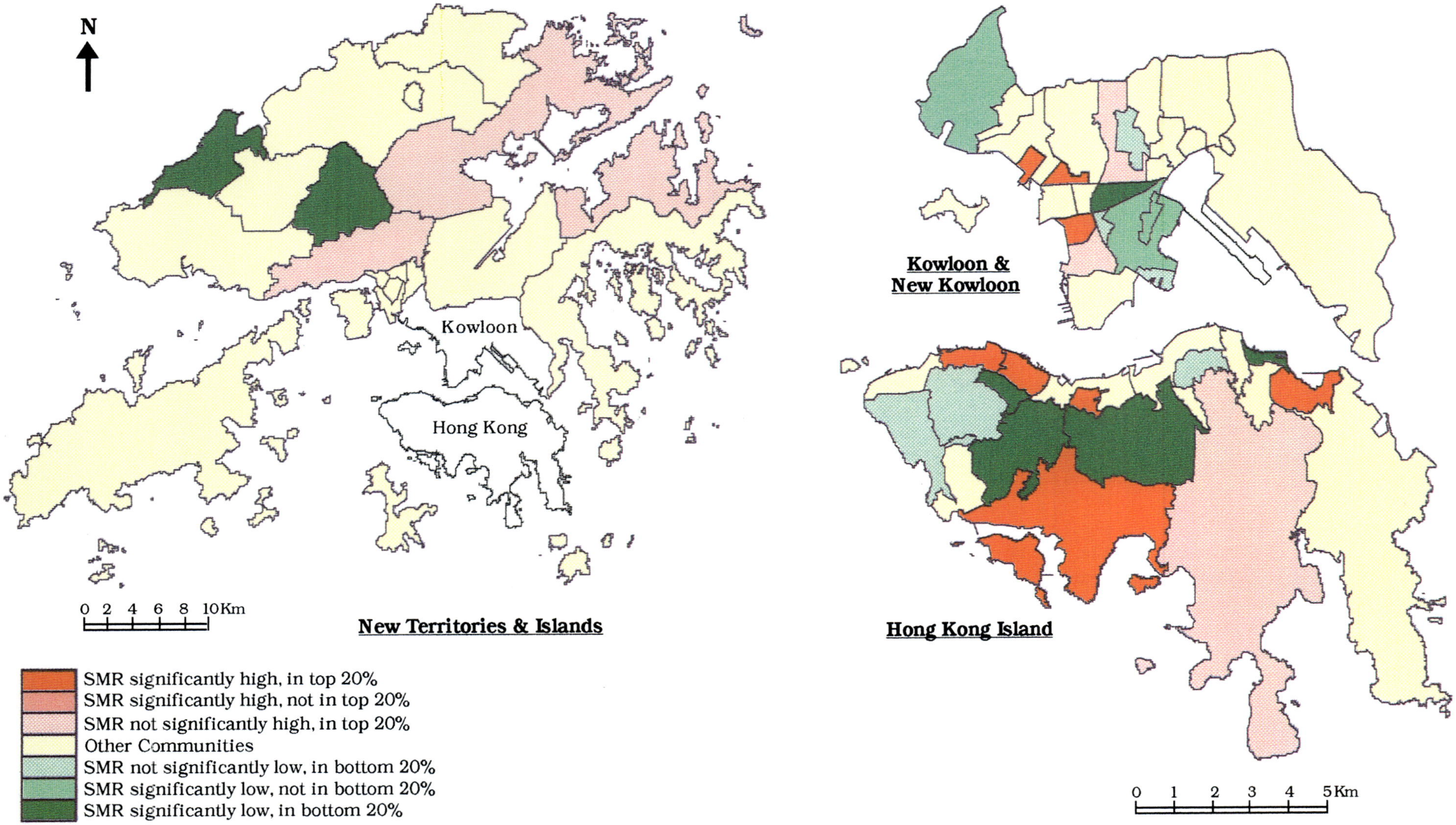

Pneumonia (Male, 1979 - 1983)

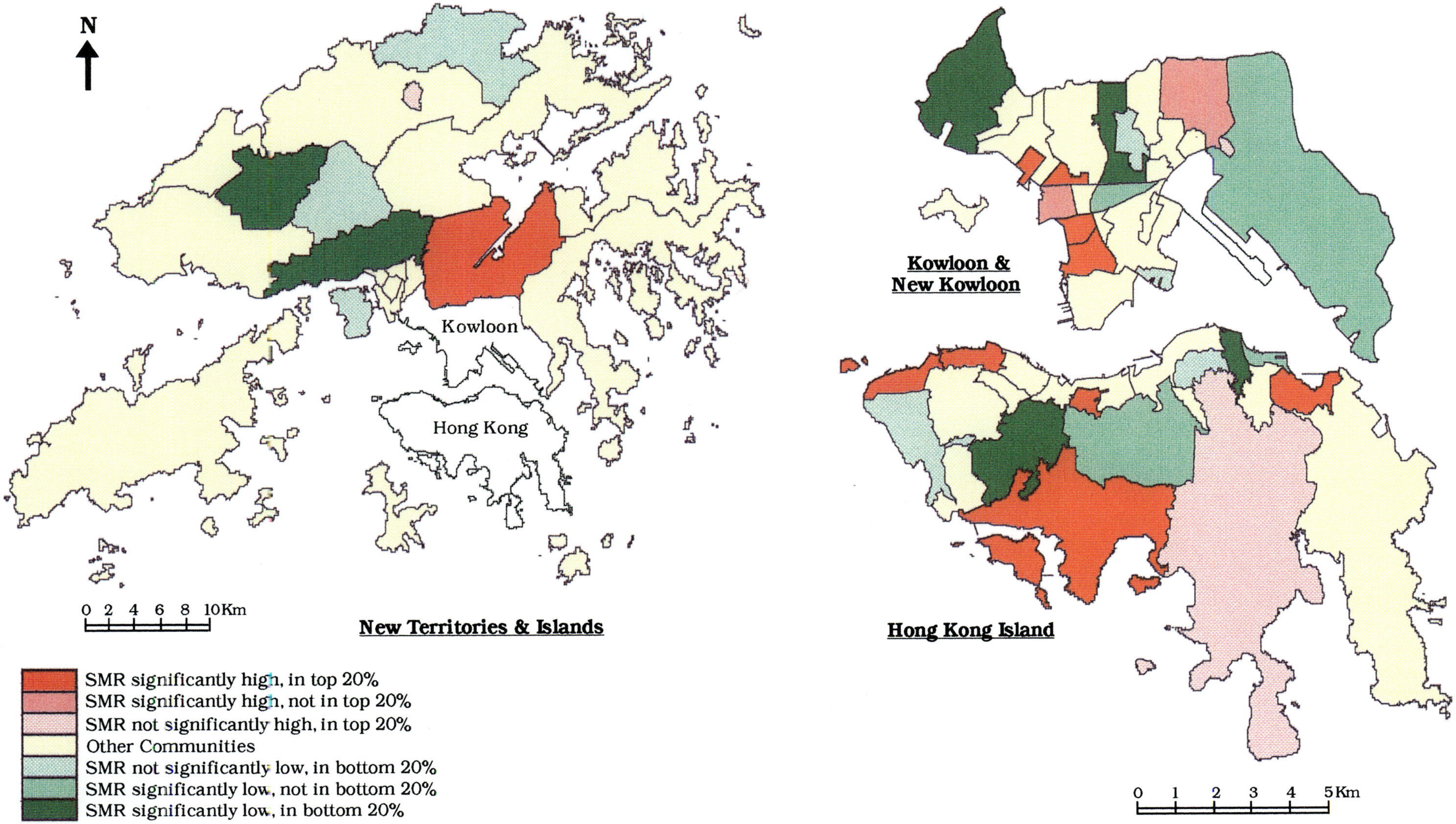

Pneumonia (Female, 1979 – 1983)

Number of Deaths, Standardised Mortality Ratio (SMR) and 95% Confidence Interval of Pneumonia by 65 Communities in 1979–1983

Community	Male			Female		
	Number of deaths	SMR	95% C.I.	Number of deaths	SMR	95% C.I.
HK1	96	107.2	85.7 - 128.6	111	126.6	103.0 - 150.2
HK2	175	120.8	102.9 - 138.7	171	130.5	111.0 - 150.1
HK3	74	130.3	100.6 - 160.0	53	107.8	78.8 - 136.8
HK4	79	91.3	71.2 - 111.4	83	100.7	79.0 - 122.3
HK5	108	127.8	103.7 - 151.9	100	125.0	100.5 - 149.5
HK6	48	69.1	49.6 - 88.7	67	74.6	56.7 - 92.4
HK7	10	70.6	33.9 - 129.8	17	94.1	54.7 - 150.5
HK8	16	57.4	32.8 - 93.2	31	83.2	53.9 - 112.5
HK9	5	41.2	13.3 - 96.2	7	45.3	18.2 - 93.5
HK10	216	112.4	97.4 - 127.4	193	88.0	75.6 - 100.4
HK11	17	105.7	61.4 - 169.0	11	76.3	38.2 - 136.6
HK12	10	71.5	34.4 - 131.5	12	59.1	30.5 - 103.1
HK13	17	78.6	45.7 - 125.8	13	53.8	28.6 - 92.0
HK14	35	62.8	42.0 - 83.7	40	69.1	47.7 - 90.5
HK15	22	98.5	61.6 - 149.2	18	75.5	44.7 - 119.3
HK16	132	129.1	107.1 - 151.2	119	123.0	100.9 - 145.2
HK17	129	114.3	94.5 - 134.0	123	114.8	94.5 - 135.1
HK18	10	61.4	29.5 - 112.9	12	63.5	32.7 - 110.8
HK19	47	89.1	63.7 - 114.6	59	107.7	80.2 - 135.1
HK20	159	132.2	111.7 - 152.8	176	154.4	131.6 - 177.2
HK21	18	127.1	75.2 - 200.8	20	160.8	12.2 - 248.6
KL1	68	91.6	69.9 - 113.4	72	103.6	79.7 - 127.6
KL2	159	104.7	88.4 - 121.0	182	118.1	100.9 - 135.2
KL3	42	93.4	65.2 - 121.7	52	103.6	75.4 - 131.7
KL4	152	123.3	103.7 - 142.9	165	137.9	116.8 - 158.9
KL5	126	120.7	99.6 - 141.7	123	126.1	103.8 - 148.4
KL6	13	48.6	25.8 - 83.1	27	71.6	44.6 - 98.6
KL7	13	66.3	35.3 - 113.4	21	82.4	50.9 - 126.1
KL8	48	74.5	53.4 - 95.5	72	101.6	78.1 - 125.0
KL9	210	87.0	75.3 - 98.8	235	90.7	79.1 - 102.3
KL10	18	72.1	42.7 - 113.9	18	65.5	38.7 - 103.4
KL11	51	74.2	53.9 - 94.6	49	63.9	46.0 - 81.7
KL12	15	73.3	41.0 - 121.0	16	79.0	45.2 - 128.3

Community	Male			Female		
	Number of deaths	SMR	95% C.I.	Number of deaths	SMR	95% C.I.
KL13	243	98.9	86.4 - 111.3	219	89.6	77.8 - 101.5
KL14	152	99.4	83.6 - 115.2	153	116.5	98.0 - 134.9
KL15	20	172.7	105.3 - 267.0	22	176.6	110.4 - 267.6
KL16	97	163.3	130.8 - 195.8	82	130.1	101.9 - 158.2
KL17	22	130.1	81.3 - 197.1	12	46.5	24.0 - 81.2
KL18	8	70.8	30.5 - 139.4	7	54.1	21.7 - 111.6
KL19	229	106.4	92.6 - 120.1	268	115.1	101.3 - 128.8
KL20	78	102.6	79.8 - 125.4	90	116.6	92.5 - 140.7
KL21	116	93.4	76.4 - 110.4	124	98.6	81.2 - 116.0
KL22	21	99.3	61.3 - 151.8	18	94.5	55.9 - 149.2
KL23	57	85.7	63.4 - 107.9	71	113.2	86.9 - 139.5
KL24	29	80.5	51.2 - 109.8	43	119.5	83.8 - 155.3
KL25	555	92.5	84.8 - 100.2	538	89.5	82.0 - 97.1
NT1	37	115.2	78.1 - 152.3	21	60.1	37.1 - 91.9
NT2	35	77.0	51.5 - 102.5	50	117.4	84.9 - 149.9
NT3	77	87.8	68.2 - 107.4	81	111.6	87.3 - 136.0
NT4	38	79.9	54.5 - 105.3	47	89.6	63.9 - 115.2
NT5	177	103.5	88.3 - 118.8	151	89.4	75.1 - 103.6
NT6	72	87.6	67.4 - 107.8	76	87.9	68.1 - 107.7
NT7	26	85.5	52.6 - 118.4	19	66.3	40.0 - 103.7
NT8	109	107.7	87.5 - 127.9	85	90.7	71.4 - 110.0
NT9	16	52.5	30.0 - 85.3	20	71.8	43.8 - 110.9
NT10	135	107.2	89.1 - 125.3	67	58.7	44.7 - 72.8
NT11	15	56.6	31.6 - 93.4	15	65.5	36.6 - 108.1
NT12	131	110.0	91.2 - 128.9	108	94.8	76.9 - 112.7
NT13	24	107.6	69.0 - 160.2	33	146.5	96.5 - 196.5
NT14	22	104.8	65.5 - 158.8	15	63.5	35.5 - 104.7
NT15	99	117.8	94.6 - 141.0	73	83.2	64.1 - 102.3
NT16	89	88.5	70.1 - 106.8	136	126.9	105.6 - 148.3
NT17	47	94.3	67.4 - 121.3	54	107.8	79.1 - 136.6
NT18	24	97.2	62.3 - 144.6	25	95.1	57.8 - 132.4
NT19	33	80.3	52.9 - 107.7	39	85.5	58.7 - 112.4

PNEUMONIA

Sex-Age specific mortality rate (1/100,000) of pneumonia in Hong Kong (1979–1983)

	Male		Female	
Age	No. of deaths	Mortality rate	No. of deaths	Mortality rate
0–4	197	18.68	134	13.54
5–9	90	8.48	78	7.91
10–14	40	3.49	29	2.71
15–19	33	2.31	21	1.58
20–24	40	2.61	21	1.51
25–29	38	2.88	23	1.98
30–34	42	3.81	18	1.96
35–39	39	5.40	14	2.52
40–44	100	14.21	25	4.52
45–49	163	22.60	49	8.10
50–54	263	38.28	83	13.61
55–59	361	63.46	112	20.94
60–64	497	108.77	205	44.94
65+	3268	479.34	4418	437.66
TOTAL	5171	39.22	5230	42.96

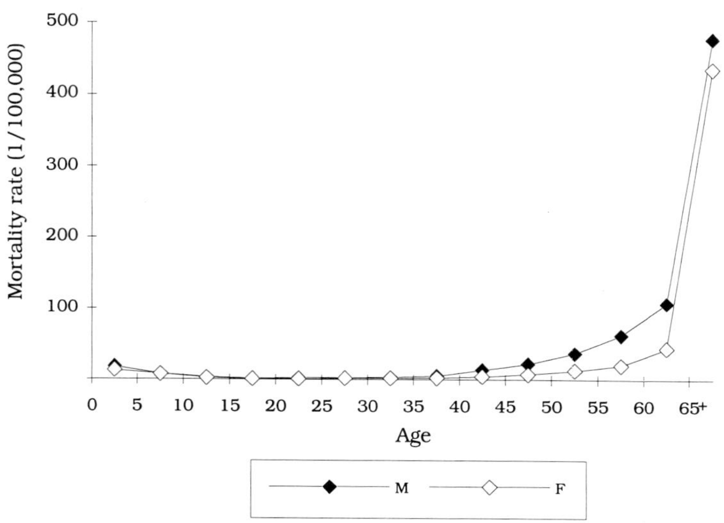

Number of communities on map by category based on standardized mortality ratio (SMR) during 1979–1983

Category	Number of communities Male	Female
SMR significantly high, in top 20%	8	10
SMR significantly high , not in top 20%	0	2
SMR not significantly high, in top 20%	5	3
SMR not significantly low, in bottom 20%	6	7
SMR significantly low, not in bottom 20%	3	4
SMR significantly low, in bottom 20%	7	6
other communities	36	33

Values of the standardized mortality ratio (SMR) which divide the 65 communities into quintile

Percentile	Male	Female
20th	72.13	66.34
40th	87.78	88.01
60th	99.42	101.58
80th	114.25	118.06
Lowest SMR	41.18	45.33
Highest SMR	172.75	176.64
No. of communities with zero death	0	0

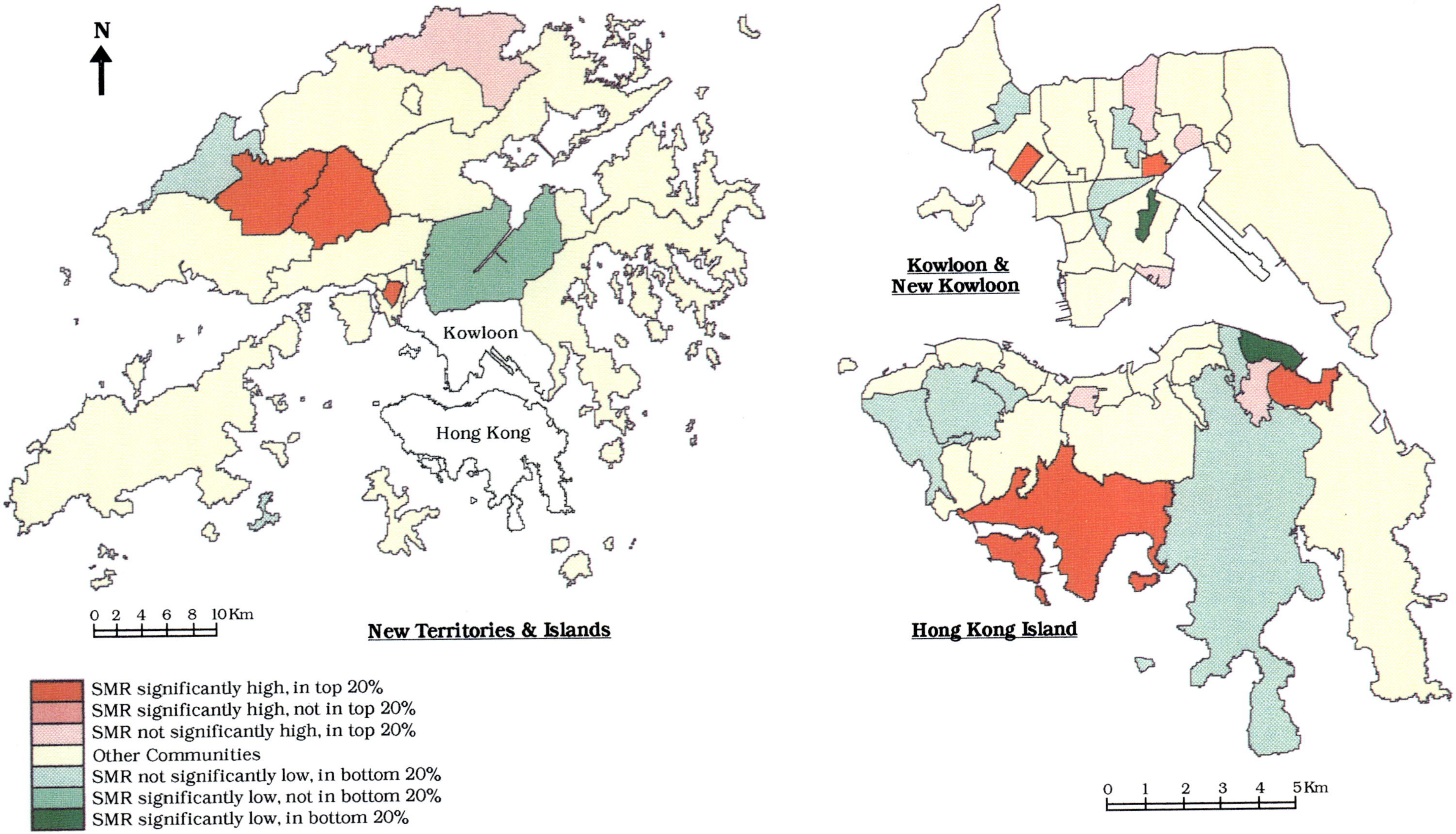

Pneumonia (Male, 1984 – 1988)

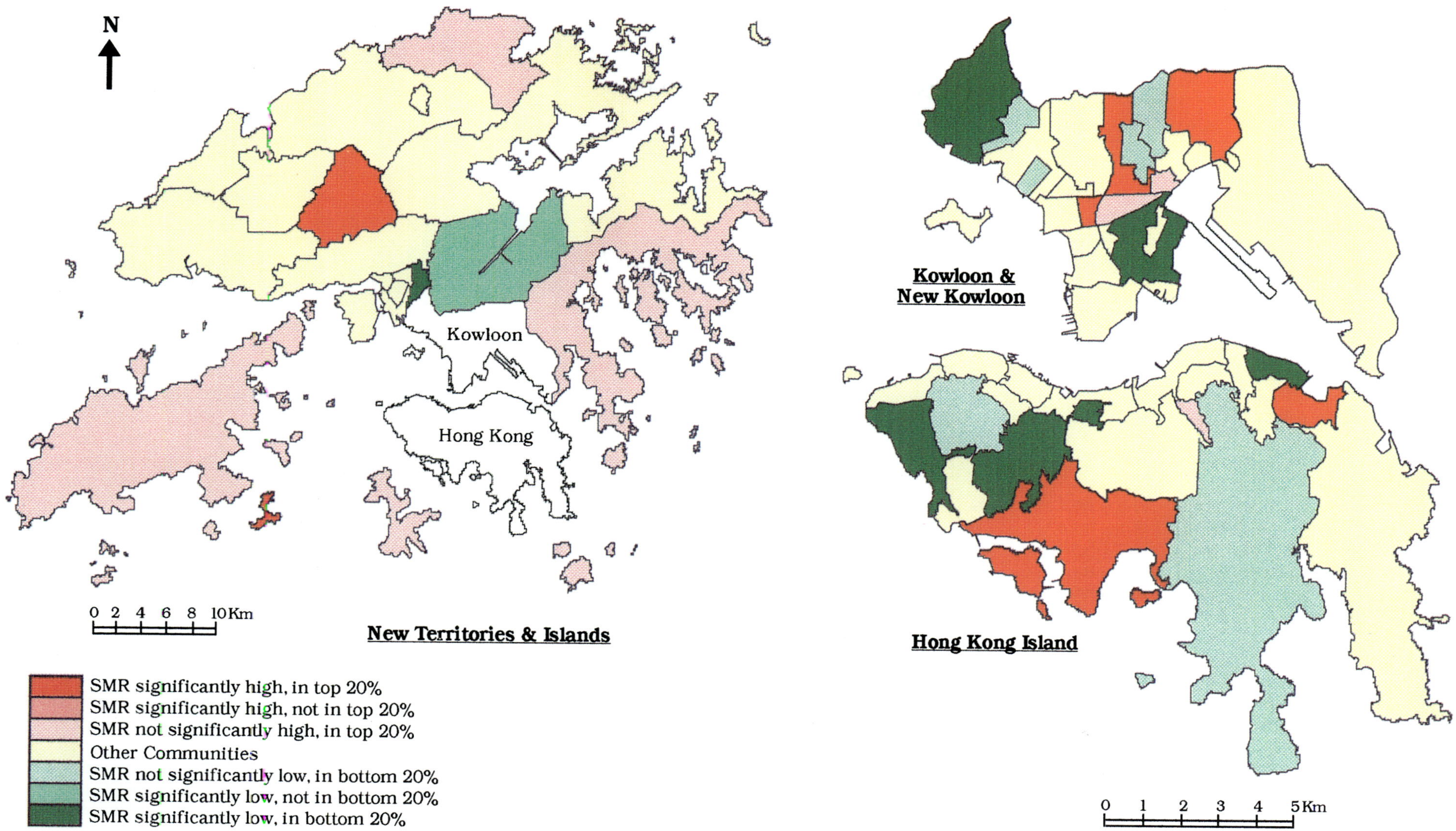

Pneumonia (Female, 1984 – 1988)

Number of Deaths, Standardised Mortality Ratio (SMR) and 95% Confidence Interval of Pneumonia by 65 Communities in 1984–1988

	Male			Female		
Community	Number of deaths	SMR	95% C.I.	Number of deaths	SMR	95% C.I.
HK1	58	82.3	61.1 - 103.5	68	102.6	78.2 - 127.0
HK2	106	105.0	85.0 - 125.0	92	95.5	76.0 - 115.0
HK3	30	80.3	51.5 - 109.0	32	100.7	65.8 - 135.6
HK4	65	108.5	82.1 - 134.9	58	100.9	75.0 - 126.9
HK5	68	131.1	99.9 - 162.3	40	74.2	51.2 - 97.2
HK6	44	79.9	56.3 - 103.5	63	94.9	71.4 - 118.3
HK7	8	70.3	30.3 - 138.5	9	69.2	31.8 - 131.4
HK8	12	58.3	30.1 - 101.8	22	94.5	59.1 - 143.2
HK9	7	83.1	33.4 - 171.4	4	35.6	9.7 - 91.1
HK10	154	102.6	86.4 - 118.7	173	101.1	86.0 - 116.1
HK11	11	84.2	42.1 - 150.7	12	123.1	63.4 - 214.8
HK12	12	98.8	50.9 - 172.5	13	95.8	51.0 - 163.8
HK13	14	77.6	42.4 - 130.3	15	94.3	52.7 - 155.6
HK14	32	56.9	37.2 - 76.6	37	60.4	40.9 - 79.8
HK15	26	152.7	99.8 - 223.9	21	103.9	64.1 - 158.9
HK16	96	126.3	101.0 - 151.5	98	133.1	106.8 - 159.5
HK17	116	111.8	91.5 - 132.2	99	100.5	80.7 - 120.2
HK18	5	43.6	14.1 - 101.8	6	43.6	16.0 - 95.1
HK19	45	96.8	68.5 - 125.0	50	105.1	76.0 - 134.3
HK20	152	141.8	119.3 - 164.4	158	153.9	129.9 - 177.9
HK21	8	66.1	28.5 - 130.2	8	60.1	25.9 - 118.3
KL1	51	95.0	68.9 - 121.1	45	92.7	65.6 - 119.8
KL2	111	112.3	91.4 - 133.2	109	110.9	90.1 - 131.7
KL3	26	80.8	49.7 - 111.9	49	140.6	101.2 - 180.0
KL4	94	99.6	79.4 - 119.7	87	103.3	81.6 - 125.0
KL5	66	93.2	70.7 - 115.7	59	91.5	68.1 - 114.8
KL6	16	76.8	43.9 - 124.6	37	146.2	99.1 - 193.3
KL7	10	68.1	32.7 - 125.2	17	116.5	67.7 - 186.3
KL8	30	63.7	40.9 - 86.5	38	81.2	55.4 - 107.0
KL9	177	93.5	79.7 - 107.2	146	77.7	65.1 - 90.3
KL10	25	134.7	86.9 - 198.6	16	80.7	46.1 - 131.0
KL11	49	85.9	61.9 - 110.0	40	69.4	47.9 - 90.9
KL12	11	71.9	35.9 - 128.6	8	55.1	23.7 - 108.4
KL13	166	98.0	83.1 - 113.0	171	104.3	88.7 - 119.9
KL14	144	105.9	88.6 - 123.2	105	89.5	72.4 - 106.6
KL15	33	162.6	111.7 - 228.6	15	66.6	37.2 - 109.9
KL16	40	92.6	63.9 - 121.3	33	83.4	55.0 - 111.9
KL17	20	90.5	55.2 - 139.9	49	141.1	101.6 - 180.6
KL18	3	38.7	8.0 - 113.1	5	64.0	20.7 - 149.6
KL19	175	98.6	84.0 - 113.2	204	118.3	102.1 - 134.5
KL20	56	129.2	95.4 - 163.1	35	77.7	52.0 - 103.4
KL21	86	110.4	87.1 - 133.8	79	117.0	91.2 - 142.8
KL22	18	120.9	71.5 - 190.9	16	110.7	63.3 - 179.7
KL23	57	149.2	110.4 - 187.9	47	132.4	94.6 - 170.3
KL24	31	89.8	58.2 - 121.5	29	103.3	65.7 - 140.8
KL25	512	93.2	85.2 - 101.3	520	99.6	91.0 - 108.1
NT1	35	110.6	74.0 - 147.3	34	106.4	70.6 - 142.1
NT2	34	87.1	57.8 - 116.4	28	79.4	50.0 - 108.8
NT3	71	104.4	80.1 - 128.7	44	82.5	58.1 - 106.8
NT4	59	108.7	80.9 - 136.4	52	91.5	66.7 - 116.4
NT5	146	121.0	101.3 - 140.6	110	100.4	81.6 - 119.2
NT6	71	98.5	75.6 - 121.4	42	65.0	45.3 - 84.6
NT7	30	84.1	54.0 - 114.2	29	95.9	61.0 - 130.8
NT8	124	94.3	77.7 - 110.8	157	115.2	97.2 - 133.3
NT9	16	70.0	40.0 - 113.7	20	82.5	50.3 - 127.5
NT10	138	121.0	100.8 - 141.2	116	114.1	93.4 - 134.9
NT11	31	157.2	106.8 - 223.3	32	152.3	104.1 - 215.3
NT12	102	102.4	82.5 - 122.3	99	98.0	78.7 - 117.3
NT13	29	109.4	69.6 - 149.3	23	109.3	69.2 - 164.1
NT14	22	134.8	84.2 - 204.2	21	125.7	77.6 - 192.2
NT15	91	98.7	78.4 - 119.0	107	106.4	86.2 - 126.5
NT16	157	81.9	69.1 - 94.8	181	80.4	68.7 - 92.2
NT17	35	85.2	57.0 - 113.4	46	120.3	85.5 - 155.0
NT18	16	77.9	44.5 - 126.4	32	152.6	104.2 - 215.6
NT19	32	103.5	67.7 - 139.4	38	125.3	85.4 - 165.1

PNEUMONIA

Sex-Age specific mortality rate (1/100,000) of pneumonia in Hong Kong (1984–1988)

	Male		Female	
Age	No. of deaths	Mortality rate	No. of deaths	Mortality rate
0–4	66	6.17	63	6.34
5–9	34	3.10	33	3.24
10–14	15	1.32	18	1.73
15–19	16	1.34	12	1.09
20–24	20	1.38	19	1.37
25–29	21	1.34	19	1.28
30–34	26	1.92	12	0.97
35–39	33	2.97	19	1.96
40–44	54	7.37	15	2.50
45–49	98	13.92	22	3.77
50–54	166	22.65	40	6.33
55–59	241	36.28	62	10.21
60–64	369	68.32	163	30.45
65+	3305	366.04	3801	307.97
TOTAL	4464	31.31	4298	32.02

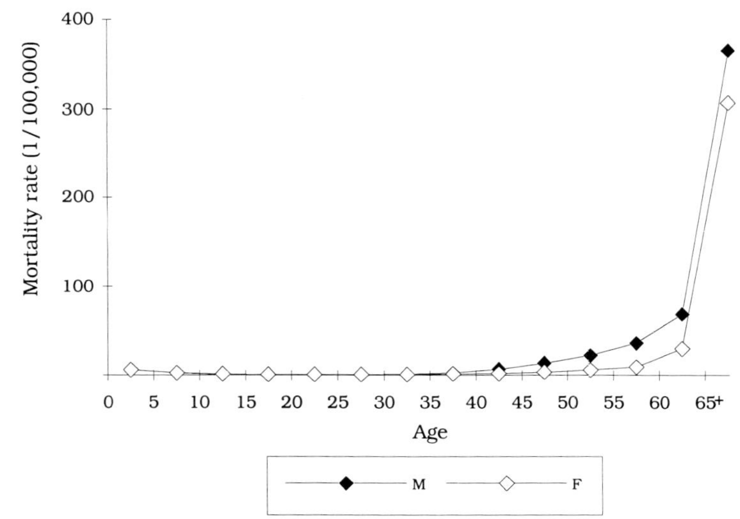

Number of communities on map by category based on standardized mortality ratio (SMR) during 1984–1988

Category	Number of communities Male	Number of communities Female
SMR significantly high, in top 20%	7	7
SMR significantly high , not in top 20%	0	0
SMR not significantly high, in top 20%	6	6
SMR not significantly low, in bottom 20%	11	6
SMR significantly low, not in bottom 20%	1	1
SMR significantly low, in bottom 20%	2	7
other communities	38	38

Values of the standardized mortality ratio (SMR) which divide the 65 communities into quintile

Percentile	Male	Female
20th	77.86	77.74
40th	90.49	94.51
60th	99.57	103.27
80th	112.29	116.99
Lowest SMR	38.68	35.64
Highest SMR	162.65	153.86
No. of communities with zero death	0	0

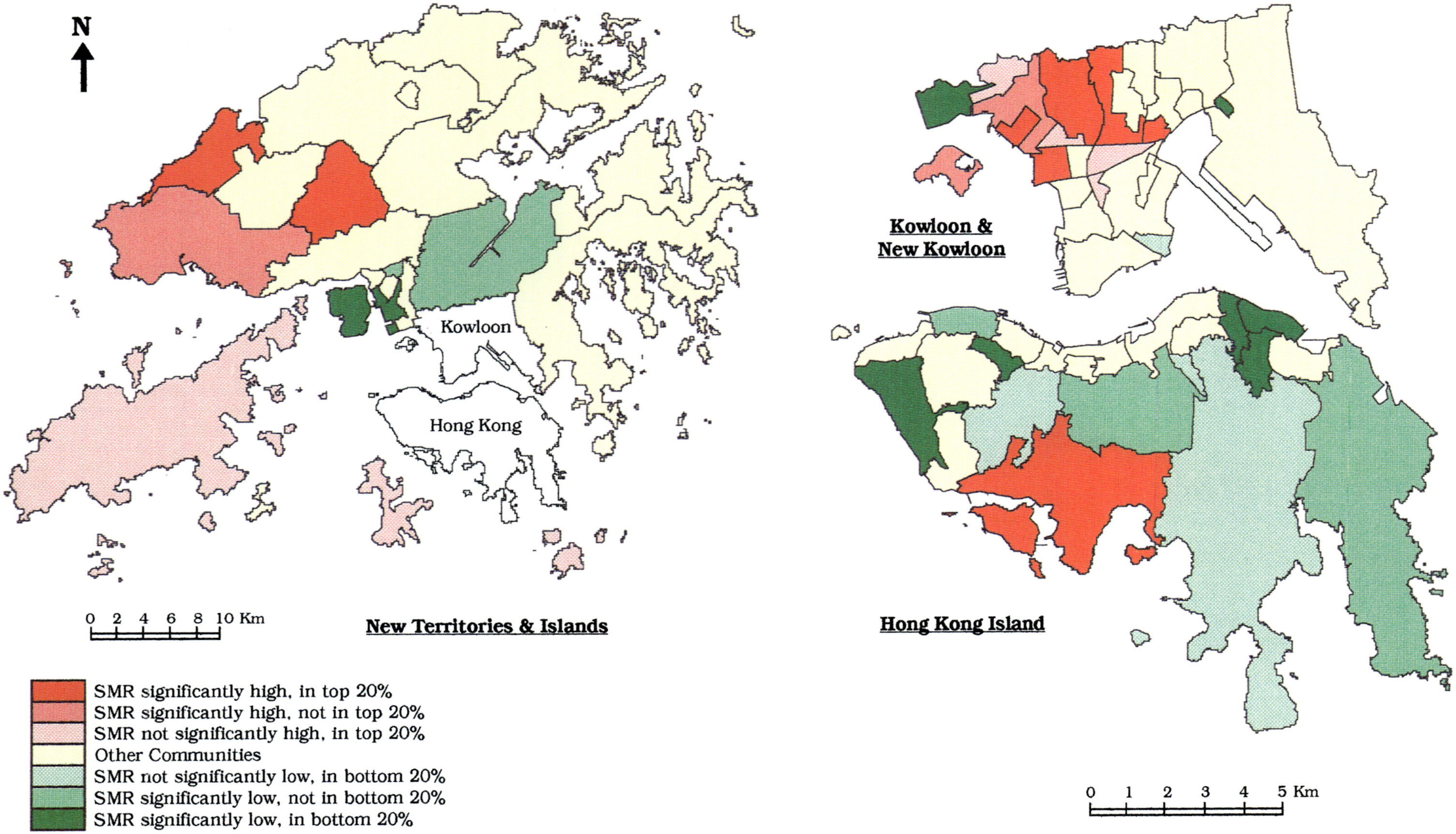

Pneumonia (Male, 1989 –1993)

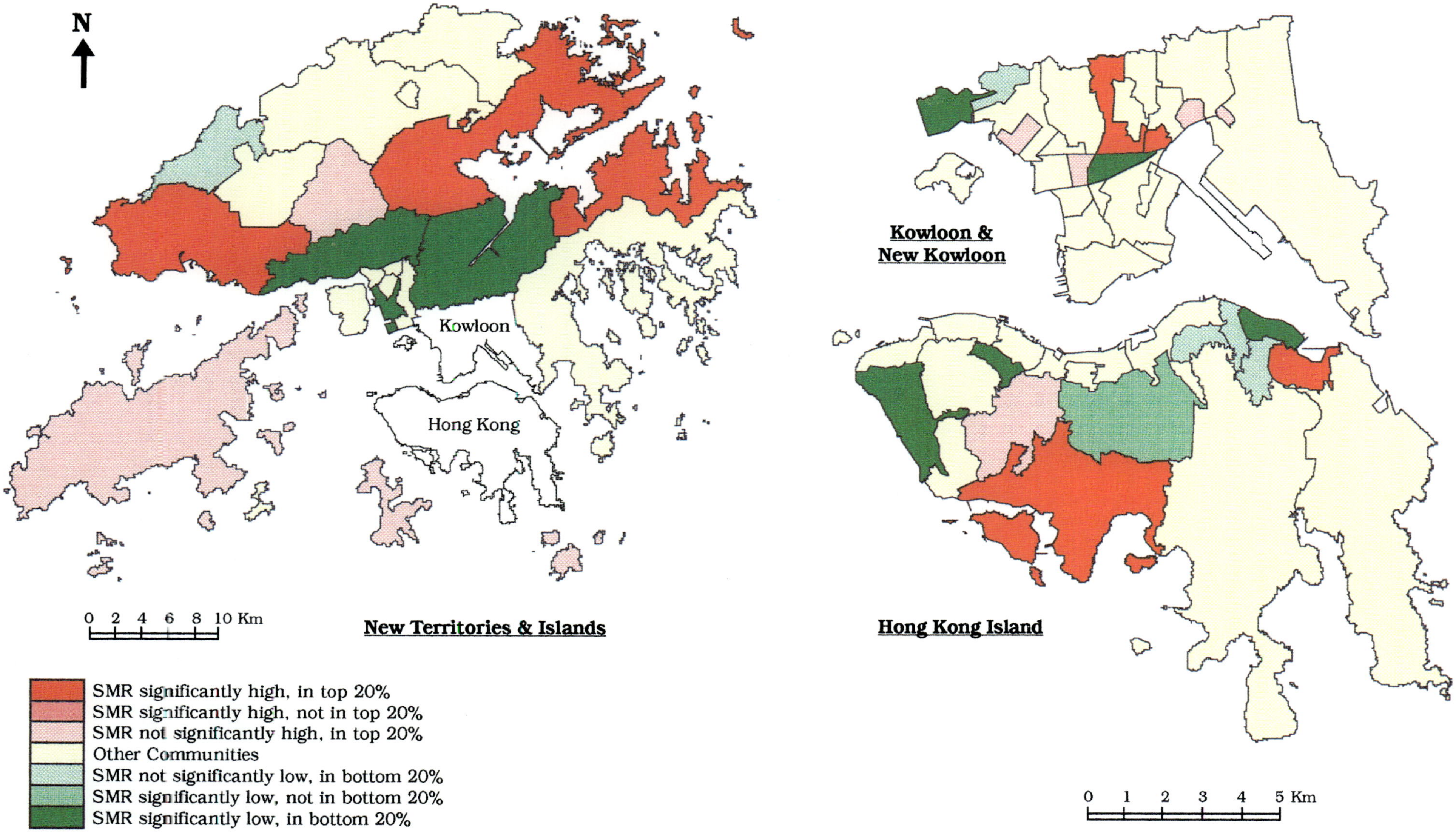

Pneumonia (Female, 1989 –1993)

Number of Deaths, Standardised Mortality Ratio (SMR) and 95% Confidence Interval of Pneumonia by 65 Communities in 1989–1993

Community	Male			Female		
	Number of deaths	SMR	95% C.I.	Number of deaths	SMR	95% C.I.
HK1	66	84.0	63.7 - 104.3	54	83.0	60.9 - 105.2
HK2	86	81.0	63.9 - 98.1	77	97.7	75.9 - 119.5
HK3	30	81.7	52.5 - 111.0	20	74.7	45.6 - 115.0
HK4	59	100.0	74.4 - 125.5	51	107.1	77.7 - 136.5
HK5	52	91.5	66.6 - 116.3	45	100.7	71.3 - 130.1
HK6	46	68.5	48.7 - 88.3	51	76.4	55.4 - 97.4
HK7	11	75.3	37.6 - 134.7	15	95.4	53.4 - 157.5
HK8	11	45.9	22.9 - 82.2	8	39.3	16.9 - 77.5
HK9	5	50.6	16.4 - 117.8	12	134.1	69.3 - 234.7
HK10	177	97.3	83.0 - 111.6	178	101.5	86.6 - 116.4
HK11	9	56.3	25.8 - 106.9	10	91.3	43.8 - 168.0
HK12	14	97.2	53.1 - 163.3	10	73.7	35.4 - 135.6
HK13	10	50.5	24.3 - 93.0	9	57.4	26.3 - 109.1
HK14	34	48.2	32.0 - 64.4	42	72.5	50.6 - 94.4
HK15	25	62.7	40.5 - 92.7	23	69.2	43.9 - 103.8
HK16	78	108.8	84.7 - 133.0	82	136.4	106.9 - 165.9
HK17	128	82.8	68.5 - 97.2	114	89.0	72.6 - 105.3
HK18	3	16.5	3.4 - 48.1	6	28.8	10.6 - 62.8
HK19	48	81.0	58.1 - 103.9	42	89.4	62.3 - 116.4
HK20	189	135.1	115.8 - 154.4	148	119.6	100.4 - 138.9
HK21	8	61.8	26.6 - 121.7	7	76.5	30.7 - 157.5
KL1	47	100.1	71.5 - 128.7	45	118.6	83.9 - 153.2
KL2	138	134.4	112.0 - 156.8	93	106.3	84.7 - 127.9
KL3	29	89.8	57.1 - 122.5	37	123.9	84.0 - 163.8
KL4	99	110.7	88.9 - 132.4	69	104.3	79.7 - 128.9
KL5	72	108.8	83.7 - 134.0	60	112.7	84.2 - 141.3
KL6	36	128.2	86.3 - 170.0	56	51.9	27.4 - 76.4
KL7	22	120.6	75.6 - 182.1	19	95.2	57.3 - 148.5
KL8	48	93.3	66.9 - 119.6	52	119.4	86.9 - 151.8
KL9	229	108.0	94.0 - 122.0	202	114.1	98.4 - 129.8
KL10	24	68.3	43.8 - 101.7	29	86.1	54.7 - 117.4
KL11	34	67.1	44.5 - 89.6	23	50.8	32.2 - 76.2
KL12	19	118.8	71.5 - 185.4	8	51.9	22.4 - 102.2
KL13	232	117.4	102.3 - 132.5	177	110.9	94.6 - 127.3
KL14	170	118.8	101.0 - 136.7	103	89.0	71.8 - 106.2
KL15	40	164.4	113.4 - 215.3	29	130.7	83.1 - 178.3
KL16	59	131.9	98.3 - 165.6	37	103.1	69.9 - 136.3
KL17	64	274.1	206.9 - 341.2	100	330.8	265.9 - 395.6
KL18	8	86.5	37.3 - 170.5	8	78.2	33.7 - 154.1
KL19	231	108.1	94.2 - 122.1	207	103.1	89.1 - 117.2
KL20	39	82.8	56.8 - 108.8	44	115.4	81.3 - 149.4
KL21	76	96.6	74.9 - 118.3	71	103.3	79.3 - 127.3
KL22	16	103.7	59.3 - 168.0	16	121.5	69.5 - 196.8
KL23	83	253.6	199.0 - 308.2	71	260.2	199.7 - 320.7
KL24	25	61.2	39.6 - 90.6	36	129.1	86.9 - 171.3
KL25	618	100.4	92.5 - 108.3	536	99.0	90.6 - 107.3
NT1	48	99.7	71.5 - 127.9	26	58.1	35.8 - 80.5
NT2	27	52.2	32.5 - 71.9	33	69.6	45.9 - 93.3
NT3	78	86.4	67.2 - 105.5	58	90.5	67.2 - 113.8
NT4	45	75.1	53.1 - 97.0	55	96.5	71.0 - 122.0
NT5	145	108.3	90.7 - 125.9	104	94.1	76.0 - 112.2
NT6	96	111.3	89.1 - 133.6	64	83.9	63.4 - 104.5
NT7	72	34.9	26.9 - 43.0	57	87.0	64.4 - 109.6
NT8	245	118.8	103.9 - 133.7	217	121.2	105.1 - 137.4
NT9	50	169.5	122.5 - 216.5	20	68.3	41.7 - 105.2
NT10	149	105.7	88.7 - 122.7	119	101.0	82.8 - 119.1
NT11	46	166.0	118.1 - 214.0	34	128.5	85.3 - 171.7
NT12	114	88.8	72.5 - 105.0	104	90.4	73.0 - 107.7
NT13	19	74.1	44.6 - 115.5	23	89.7	56.8 - 134.5
NT14	18	117.9	69.9 - 186.3	16	103.6	59.2 - 167.8
NT15	153	106.0	89.2 - 122.8	168	121.5	103.2 - 139.9
NT16	240	71.7	62.6 - 80.8	227	65.8	57.2 - 74.3
NT17	83	95.9	75.2 - 116.5	80	97.5	76.1 - 118.9
NT18	20	76.9	47.0 - 118.5	23	99.7	63.2 - 149.6
NT19	42	133.9	93.4 - 174.4	38	124.9	85.2 - 164.6

PNEUMONIA

Sex-Age specific mortality rate (1/100,000) of pneumonia in Hong Kong (1989–1993)

	Male		Female	
Age	No. of deaths	Mortality rate	No. of deaths	Mortality rate
0–4	39	4.09	41	4.64
5–9	24	2.27	22	2.25
10–14	15	1.37	5	0.50
15–19	19	1.74	17	1.70
20–24	19	1.66	10	0.88
25–29	25	1.73	14	0.95
30–34	41	2.63	17	1.12
35–39	43	3.21	17	1.35
40–44	62	5.63	23	2.37
45–49	64	8.76	22	3.68
50–54	132	19.03	32	5.62
55–59	272	38.92	65	10.67
60–64	390	63.18	134	23.19
65+	4092	369.41	4179	297.46
TOTAL	5237	35.81	4598	32.86

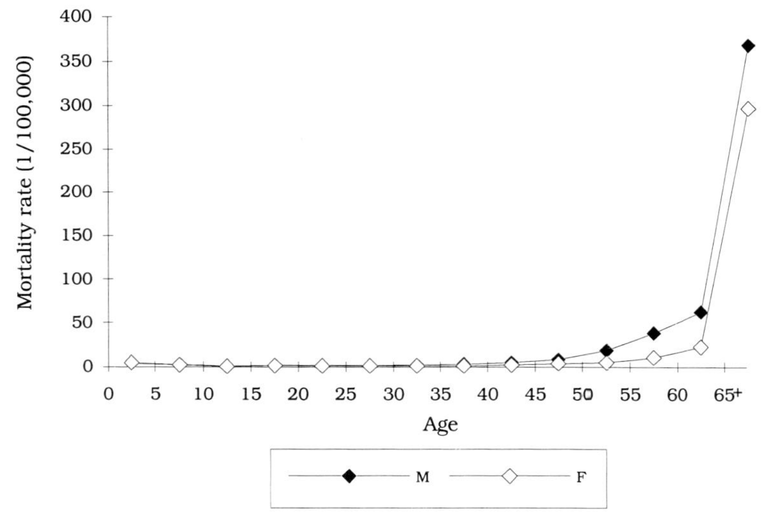

Number of communities on map by category based on standardized mortality ratio (SMR) during 1989–1993

Category	Number of communities Male	Female
SMR significantly high, in top 20%	8	6
SMR significantly high , not in top 20%	2	0
SMR not significantly high, in top 20%	5	7
SMR not significantly low, in bottom 20%	4	5
SMR significantly low, not in bottom 20%	5	1
SMR significantly low, in bottom 20%	9	8
other communities	32	38

Values of the standardized mortality ratio (SMR) which divide the 65 communities into quintile

Percentile	Male	Female
20th	68.27	73.68
40th	86.35	90.38
60th	100.41	101.47
80th	118.81	119.35
Lowest SMR	16.49	28.79
Highest SMR	274.09	330.77
No. of communities with zero cases	0	0

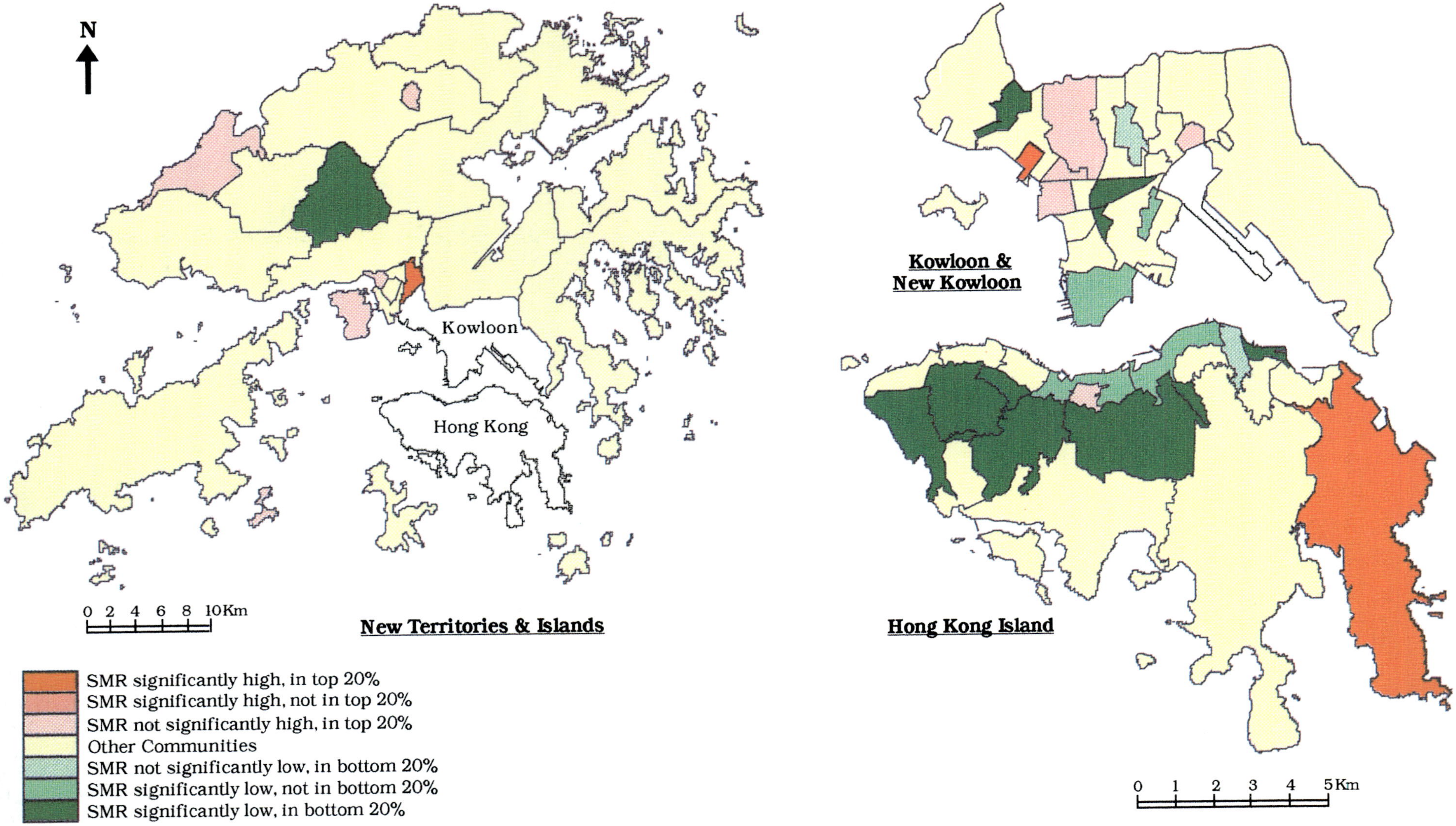

COAD (Male, 1979 – 1983)

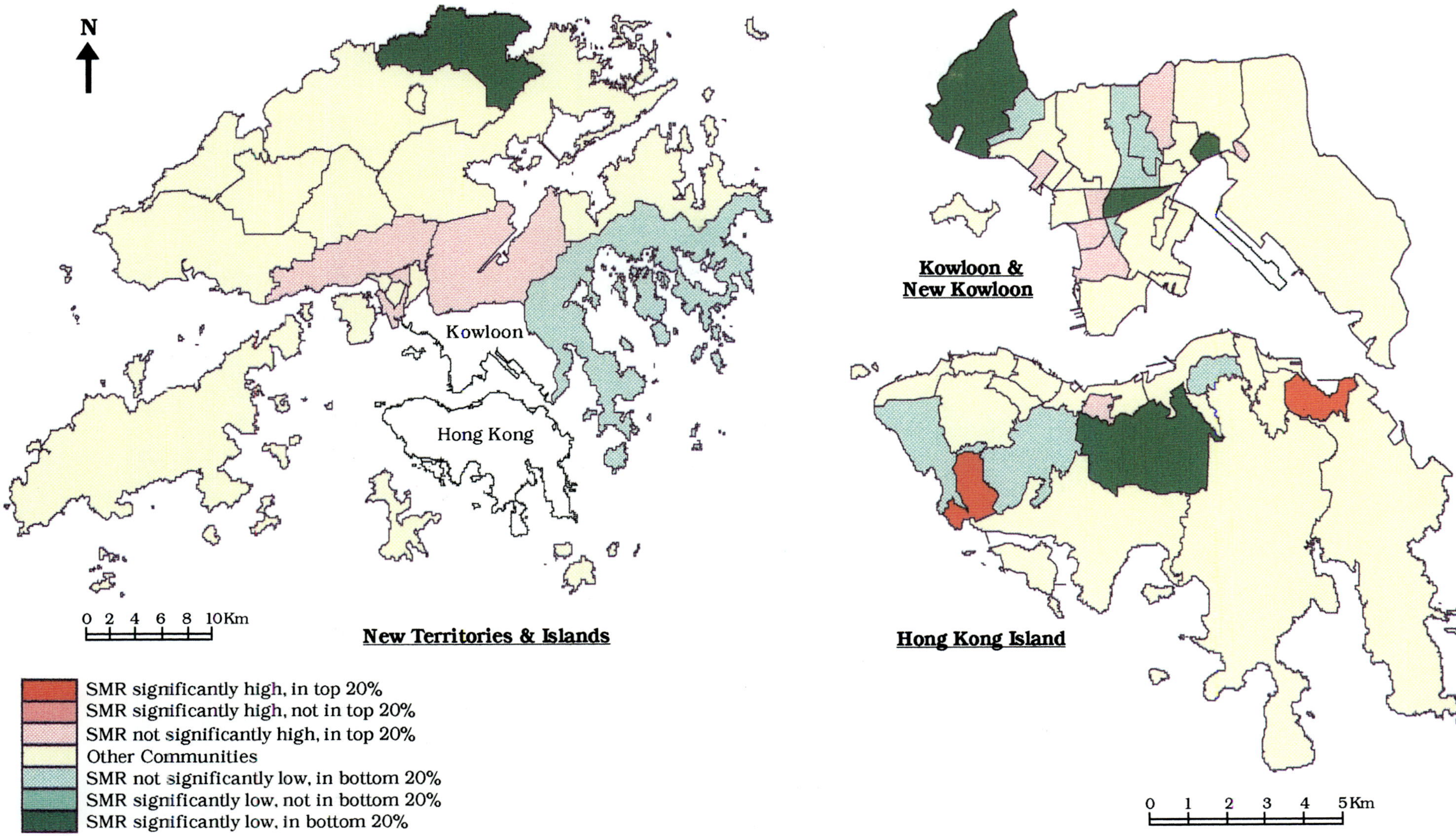

COAD (Female, 1979 – 1983)

Number of Deaths, Standardised Mortality Ratio (SMR) and 95% Confidence Interval of COAD by 65 Communities in 1979–1983

	Male			Female		
Community	Number of deaths	SMR	95% C.I.	Number of deaths	SMR	95% C.I.
HK1	86	100.8	79.5 - 122.1	52	102.2	74.4 - 130.0
HK2	155	110.8	93.3 - 128.2	84	111.1	87.3 - 134.8
HK3	49	88.5	63.7 - 113.3	29	102.3	65.1 - 139.5
HK4	64	77.0	58.1 - 95.8	44	91.7	64.6 - 118.8
HK5	100	122.1	98.2 - 146.0	55	118.8	87.4 - 150.2
HK6	33	49.5	32.6 - 66.3	32	60.3	39.4 - 81.3
HK7	5	37.5	12.2 - 87.7	9	84.4	38.7 - 160.2
HK8	16	60.2	34.4 - 97.8	18	82.0	48.5 - 129.6
HK9	3	25.9	5.3 - 75.6	5	53.9	17.4 - 125.8
HK10	130	70.9	58.7 - 83.1	119	92.0	75.5 - 108.5
HK11	8	50.7	21.9 - 99.9	10	116.4	56.0 - 214.0
HK12	9	69.9	32.1 - 132.7	4	33.5	9.1 - 85.7
HK13	12	57.3	29.6 - 100.1	9	63.9	29.3 - 121.3
HK14	27	52.1	32.5 - 71.8	26	76.9	47.3 - 106.4
HK15	17	83.7	48.7 - 133.9	12	85.5	44.1 - 149.3
HK16	95	97.4	77.9 - 117.0	81	145.2	113.5 - 176.8
HK17	135	124.6	103.6 - 145.7	62	99.5	74.7 - 124.3
HK18	7	46.6	18.7 - 96.1	6	55.7	20.4 - 121.4
HK19	48	98.2	70.4 - 125.9	47	148.7	106.2 - 191.2
HK20	121	107.0	88.0 - 126.1	61	93.6	70.1 - 117.1
HK21	10	76.4	36.7 - 140.4	8	110.8	47.8 - 218.2
KL1	54	75.7	55.5 - 95.8	42	103.5	72.2 - 134.8
KL2	168	115.9	98.4 - 133.5	102	116.0	93.5 - 138.5
KL3	39	90.9	62.3 - 119.4	35	121.5	81.2 - 161.8
KL4	136	114.8	95.5 - 134.1	84	122.3	96.2 - 148.5
KL5	115	113.9	93.1 - 134.7	68	120.7	92.0 - 149.3
KL6	12	46.2	23.8 - 80.7	10	45.2	21.7 - 83.0
KL7	8	43.1	18.6 - 84.9	9	60.5	27.8 - 114.8
KL8	43	70.0	49.1 - 90.9	33	81.0	53.4 - 108.6
KL9	221	96.9	84.1 - 109.6	168	112.1	95.1 - 129.0
KL10	23	101.5	64.2 - 152.4	15	94.5	52.8 - 155.9
KL11	58	90.8	67.4 - 114.1	27	61.1	38.1 - 84.2
KL12	8	40.2	17.3 - 79.1	6	52.5	19.2 - 114.3
KL13	231	96.7	84.2 - 109.1	144	102.2	85.5 - 118.9
KL14	175	117.2	99.8 - 134.6	87	112.4	88.8 - 136.0
KL15	21	191.3	118.1 - 292.6	10	142.8	68.6 - 262.4
KL16	67	118.4	90.0 - 146.7	37	103.2	70.0 - 136.5
KL17	12	74.3	38.3 - 129.7	9	59.4	27.2 - 112.7
KL18	5	50.0	16.2 - 116.7	3	40.8	8.4 - 119.3
KL19	223	108.0	93.8 - 122.2	143	106.6	89.1 - 124.1
KL20	76	102.1	79.1 - 125.0	54	119.8	87.8 - 151.7
KL21	124	101.4	83.6 - 119.3	79	107.0	83.4 - 130.6
KL22	25	124.2	75.5 - 172.9	4	36.7	10.0 - 93.9
KL23	65	103.7	78.5 - 128.9	32	88.2	57.6 - 118.7
KL24	31	84.7	54.9 - 114.5	29	135.8	86.4 - 185.2
KL25	595	105.7	97.2 - 114.2	347	101.1	90.4 - 111.7
NT1	26	89.9	55.4 - 124.5	23	119.2	75.4 - 179.0
NT2	38	93.2	63.5 - 122.8	29	122.0	77.6 - 166.4
NT3	101	122.0	98.2 - 145.8	37	88.5	60.0 - 117.0
NT4	42	99.5	69.4 - 129.6	34	117.6	78.1 - 157.1
NT5	180	113.4	96.8 - 130.0	97	101.5	81.3 - 121.6
NT6	98	129.1	103.6 - 154.7	57	116.2	86.1 - 146.4
NT7	32	123.0	80.4 - 165.7	10	64.6	31.1 - 118.8
NT8	101	114.7	92.4 - 137.1	46	91.2	64.9 - 117.6
NT9	39	136.5	93.6 - 179.3	13	83.0	44.1 - 141.8
NT10	116	98.2	80.4 - 116.1	53	82.5	60.3 - 104.7
NT11	13	52.7	28.0 - 90.1	10	78.3	37.7 - 144.0
NT12	131	115.9	96.1 - 135.8	62	97.0	72.8 - 121.1
NT13	31	147.0	95.2 - 198.7	14	109.9	60.1 - 184.5
NT14	15	75.4	42.1 - 124.4	5	37.4	12.1 - 87.3
NT15	76	97.0	75.2 - 118.8	38	77.1	52.6 - 101.6
NT16	86	94.1	74.2 - 113.9	70	117.0	89.6 - 144.5
NT17	49	104.5	75.3 - 133.8	18	63.5	37.6 - 100.3
NT18	28	119.2	75.1 - 163.4	17	114.0	66.3 - 182.5
NT19	33	83.3	54.9 - 111.7	21	81.5	50.3 - 124.7

COAD

Sex-Age specific mortality rate (1/100,000) of COAD in Hong Kong (1979–1983)

	Male		Female	
Age	No. of deaths	Mortality rate	No. of deaths	Mortality rate
0–4	6	0.57	4	0.40
5–9	2	0.19	3	0.30
10–14	9	0.79	6	0.56
15–19	10	0.70	11	0.83
20–24	11	0.72	8	0.57
25–29	21	1.59	6	0.52
30–34	25	2.27	16	1.75
35–39	19	2.63	8	1.44
40–44	52	7.39	17	3.07
45–49	136	18.85	40	6.61
50–54	307	44.69	64	10.49
55–59	487	85.62	160	29.92
60–64	729	159.54	312	68.40
65+	3086	452.65	2349	232.70
TOTAL	4900	37.16	3004	24.67

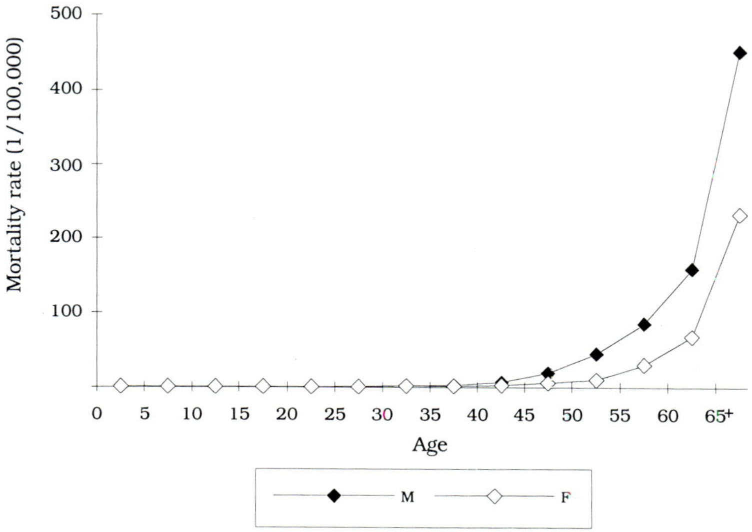

Number of communities on map by category based on standardized mortality ratio (SMR) during 1979–1983

Category	Number of communities Male	Female
SMR significantly high, in top 20%	3	2
SMR significantly high , not in top 20%	0	0
SMR not significantly high, in top 20%	10	11
SMR not significantly low, in bottom 20%	2	7
SMR significantly low, not in bottom 20%	4	0
SMR significantly low, in bottom 20%	11	6
other communities	35	39

Values of the standardized mortality ratio (SMR) which divide the 65 communities into quintile

Percentile	Male	Female
20th	60.24	63.49
40th	89.91	88.18
60th	101.45	102.31
80th	115.91	116.43
Lowest SMR	25.87	33.51
Highest SMR	191.34	148.71
No. of communities with zero death	0	0

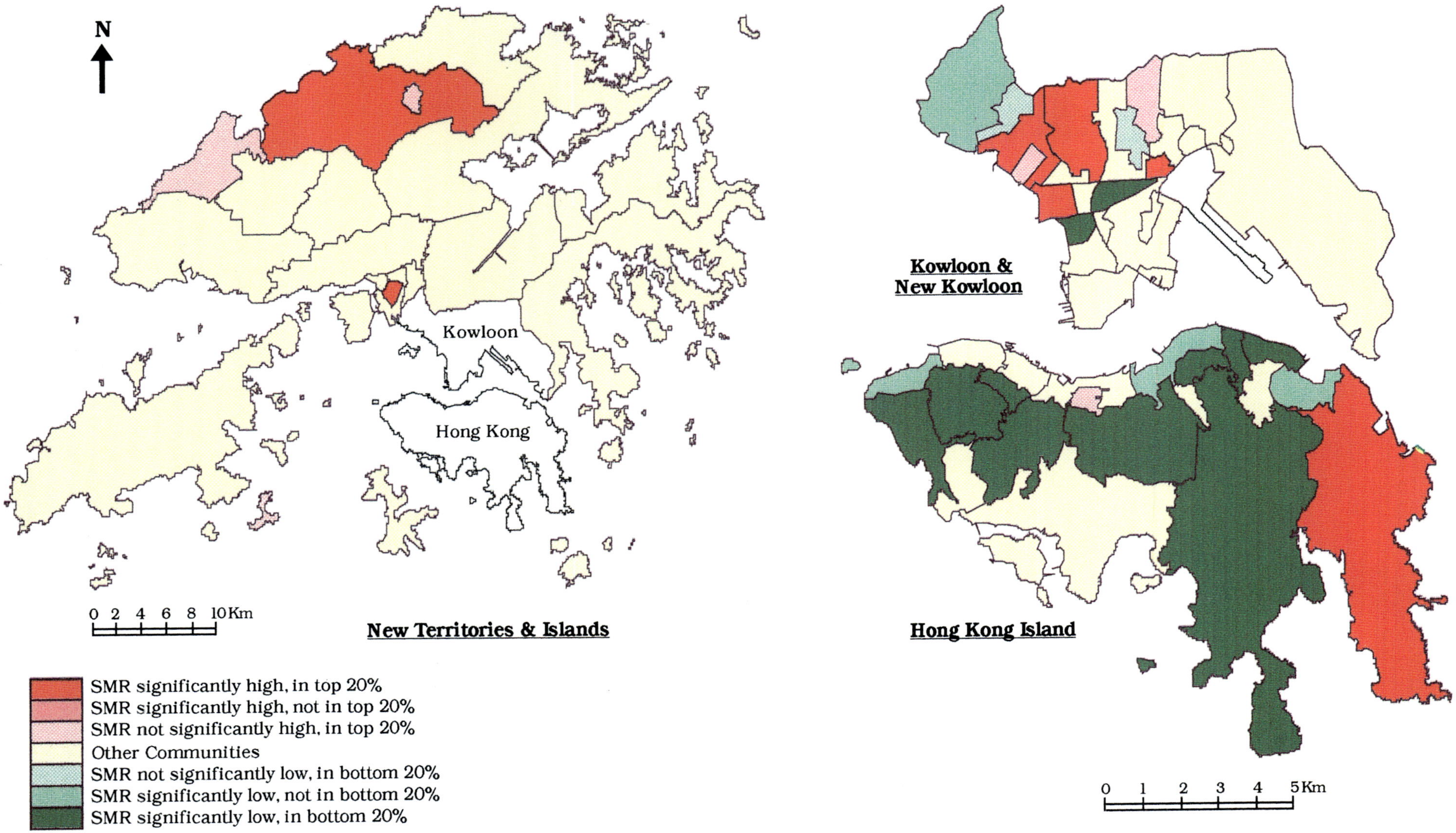

COAD (Male, 1984 – 1988)

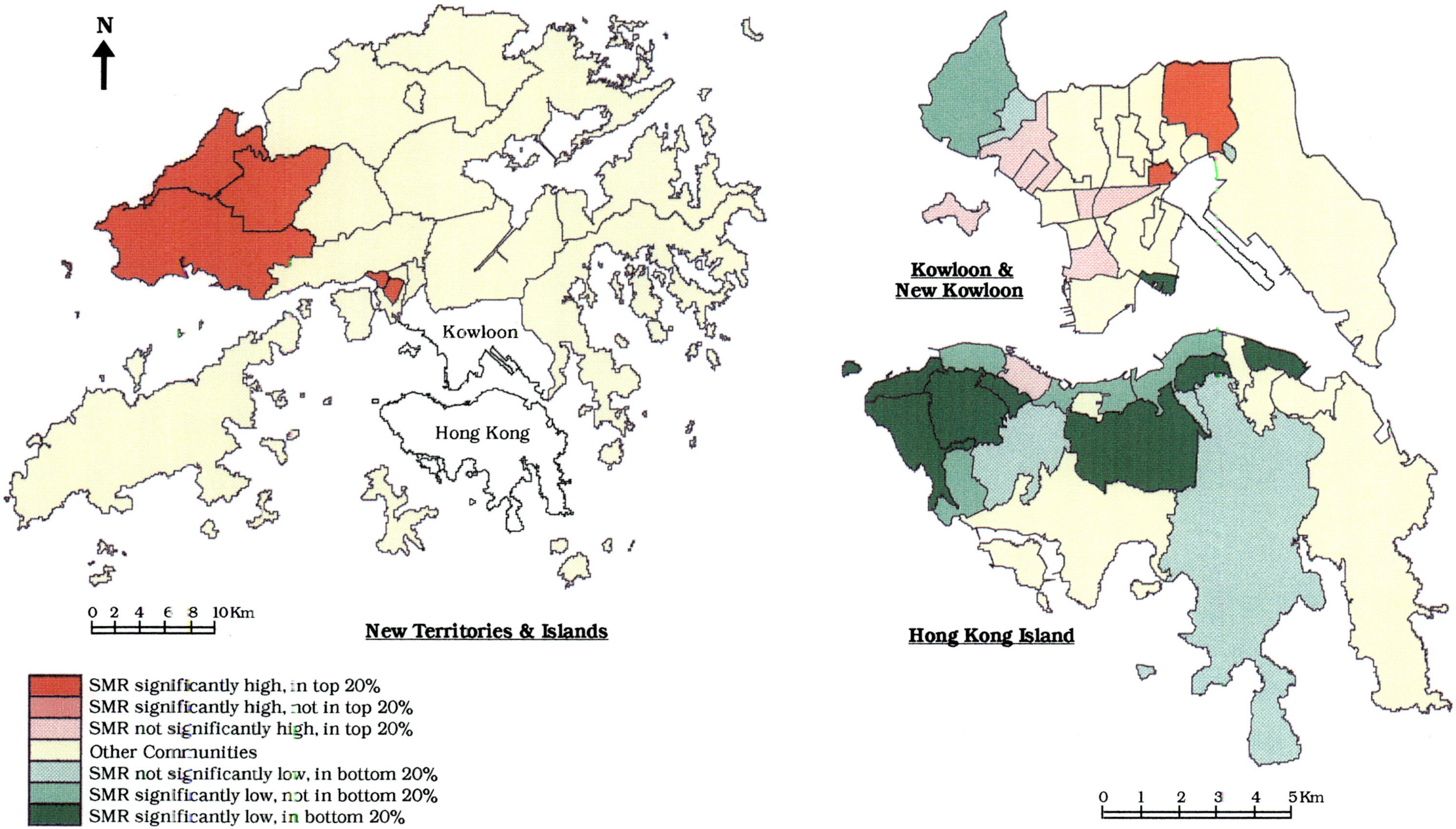

COAD (Female, 1984 – 1988)

Number of Deaths, Standardised Mortality Ratio (SMR) and 95% Confidence Interval of COAD by 65 Communities in 1984–1988

Community	Male			Female		
	Number of deaths	SMR	95% C.I.	Number of deaths	SMR	95% C.I.
HK1	87	82.1	64.8 - 99.3	40	68.0	46.9 - 89.0
HK2	133	87.9	72.9 - 102.8	60	70.5	52.7 - 88.4
HK3	55	96.9	71.3 - 122.5	33	116.6	76.8 - 156.4
HK4	74	82.3	63.5 - 101.0	38	74.5	50.8 - 98.2
HK5	96	120.8	96.7 - 145.0	48	100.1	71.8 - 128.4
HK6	42	51.3	35.8 - 66.8	29	49.3	31.4 - 67.3
HK7	8	47.7	20.6 - 94.0	4	34.7	9.5 - 88.7
HK8	18	58.7	31.6 - 85.8	9	43.3	19.9 - 82.2
HK9	0	0.0	...	4	39.9	10.9 - 102.2
HK10	171	76.6	65.1 - 88.1	120	78.8	64.7 - 93.0
HK11	18	89.8	53.2 - 141.9	6	66.4	24.3 - 144.7
HK12	5	27.8	9.0 - 64.9	3	25.0	5.2 - 73.2
HK13	16	58.7	29.9 - 87.5	14	98.7	53.9 - 165.6
HK14	39	47.2	32.4 - 62.0	27	49.8	31.0 - 68.6
HK15	24	95.2	57.1 - 133.3	15	83.9	46.9 - 138.5
HK16	84	73.8	58.0 - 89.6	71	109.2	83.8 - 134.6
HK17	203	131.0	113.0 - 149.0	78	89.3	69.5 - 109.1
HK18	8	48.3	20.8 - 95.0	4	33.6	9.2 - 86.0
HK19	74	106.2	82.0 - 130.4	30	71.2	45.7 - 96.7
HK20	153	96.1	80.9 - 111.3	101	112.1	90.2 - 133.9
HK21	8	44.9	19.3 - 88.3	6	51.8	19.0 - 112.9
KL1	71	88.2	67.6 - 108.7	33	76.3	50.3 - 102.4
KL2	190	126.7	108.7 - 144.7	79	90.8	70.8 - 110.9
KL3	44	91.9	64.8 - 119.1	37	120.3	81.5 - 159.1
KL4	75	52.3	40.5 - 64.2	64	86.1	65.0 - 107.2
KL5	103	96.2	77.6 - 114.8	69	120.4	92.0 - 148.8
KL6	19	60.9	33.5 - 88.3	31	138.0	93.8 - 196.1
KL7	16	74.0	42.3 - 120.1	14	108.1	59.1 - 181.5
KL8	62	86.5	65.0 - 108.1	44	106.0	74.6 - 137.3
KL9	258	90.4	79.4 - 101.5	177	105.7	90.1 - 121.2
KL10	21	76.7	43.9 - 109.5	9	51.6	23.6 - 97.8
KL11	59	69.8	52.0 - 87.7	37	72.7	49.3 - 96.2
KL12	15	64.4	36.0 - 106.3	8	62.6	27.0 - 123.3
KL13	316	122.7	109.2 - 136.2	166	114.0	96.6 - 131.3
KL14	270	133.6	117.7 - 149.6	104	99.5	80.4 - 118.7
KL15	36	116.0	78.1 - 153.9	25	125.7	81.1 - 185.4
KL16	60	92.8	69.3 - 116.3	37	105.8	71.7 - 139.9
KL17	26	81.2	50.0 - 112.4	28	91.9	57.9 - 126.0
KL18	8	69.3	29.9 - 136.5	7	102.2	41.0 - 210.7
KL19	285	106.1	93.7 - 118.4	183	119.0	101.7 - 136.2
KL20	76	114.9	89.1 - 140.7	31	77.2	50.0 - 104.3
KL21	120	101.9	83.7 - 120.1	65	107.2	81.2 - 133.3
KL22	18	79.5	47.0 - 125.5	12	94.1	48.5 - 164.2
KL23	100	175.1	140.8 - 209.4	67	214.1	162.8 - 265.4
KL24	56	103.0	76.0 - 129.9	18	70.1	37.7 - 102.5
KL25	809	97.9	91.2 - 104.7	448	96.8	87.9 - 105.8
NT1	37	81.1	55.0 - 107.3	26	94.3	58.0 - 130.5
NT2	54	93.5	68.6 - 118.5	35	112.5	75.2 - 149.8
NT3	110	107.9	87.8 - 128.1	66	139.3	105.7 - 172.9
NT4	77	93.7	72.8 - 114.6	46	92.4	65.7 - 119.1
NT5	223	121.6	105.6 - 137.5	148	152.0	127.5 - 176.4
NT6	95	87.4	69.8 - 105.0	59	102.7	76.5 - 128.9
NT7	54	104.1	76.3 - 131.8	29	111.7	71.0 - 152.3
NT8	203	110.5	95.3 - 125.7	137	120.3	100.2 - 140.5
NT9	45	131.2	92.9 - 169.5	33	156.3	107.4 - 219.8
NT10	187	110.8	94.9 - 126.7	132	148.2	122.9 - 173.5
NT11	31	105.5	68.4 - 142.7	19	103.3	62.3 - 161.5
NT12	193	131.6	113.0 - 150.1	95	108.0	86.2 - 129.7
NT13	43	111.7	78.3 - 145.0	18	98.7	58.4 - 156.0
NT14	23	93.7	59.3 - 140.8	13	88.5	47.1 - 151.3
NT15	142	106.5	89.0 - 124.0	85	98.0	77.2 - 118.8
NT16	299	107.5	95.3 - 119.7	197	101.3	87.2 - 115.5
NT17	57	95.0	70.3 - 119.6	37	110.6	74.9 - 146.2
NT18	41	136.0	94.4 - 177.7	16	87.2	49.8 - 141.5
NT19	45	98.6	69.8 - 127.4	23	86.2	51.0 - 121.5

COAD

Sex-Age specific mortality rate (1/100,000) of COAD in Hong Kong (1984–1988)

Age	Male: No. of deaths	Male: Mortality rate	Female: No. of deaths	Female: Mortality rate
0–4	0	0.00	1	0.10
5–9	6	0.55	3	0.29
10–14	10	0.88	4	0.38
15–19	9	0.75	8	0.73
20–24	12	0.83	14	1.01
25–29	18	1.15	8	0.54
30–34	21	1.55	5	0.40
35–39	27	2.43	11	1.13
40–44	57	7.78	16	2.67
45–49	111	15.77	28	4.80
50–54	300	40.93	62	9.82
55–59	525	79.04	107	17.61
60–64	816	151.08	232	43.34
65+	4608	510.36	3269	264.87
TOTAL	6520	45.72	3768	28.07

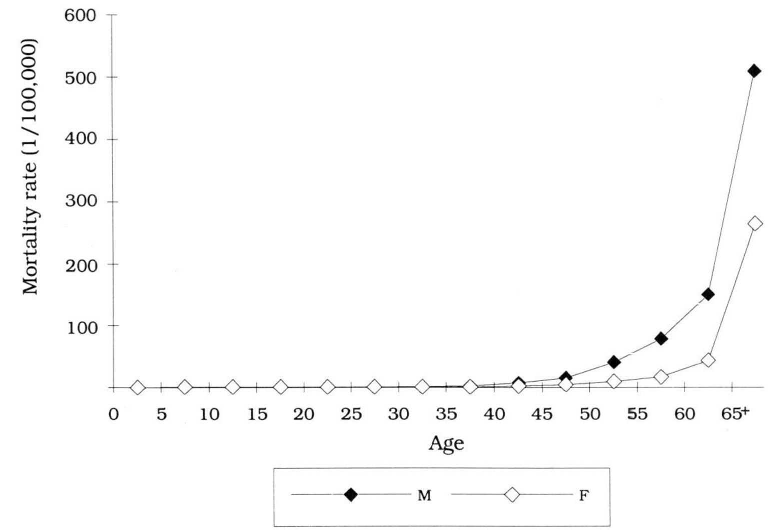

Number of communities on map by category based on standardized mortality ratio (SMR) during 1984–1988

Category	Number of communities: Male	Number of communities: Female
SMR significantly high, in top 20%	7	7
SMR significantly high , not in top 20%	0	0
SMR not significantly high, in top 20%	6	6
SMR not significantly low, in bottom 20%	2	5
SMR significantly low, not in bottom 20%	4	5
SMR significantly low, in bottom 20%	11	8
other communities	35	34

Values of the standardized mortality ratio (SMR) which divide the 65 communities into quintile

Percentile	Male	Female
20th	69.34	70.13
40th	87.86	89.33
60th	96.87	102.20
80th	110.80	112.50
Lowest SMR	0.00	25.03
Highest SMR	175.09	214.09
No. of communities with zero death	1	0

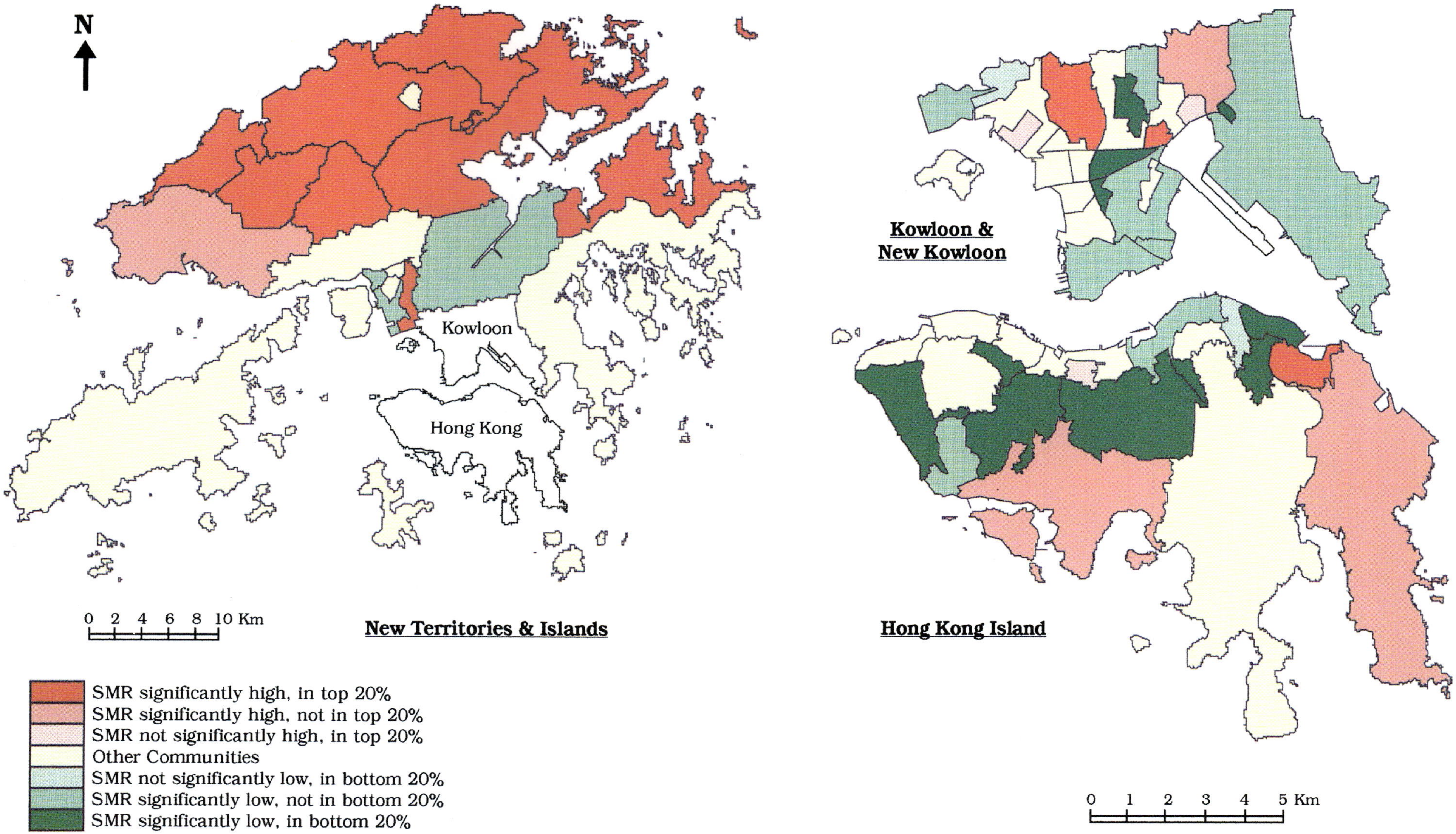

COAD (Male, 1989 -1993)

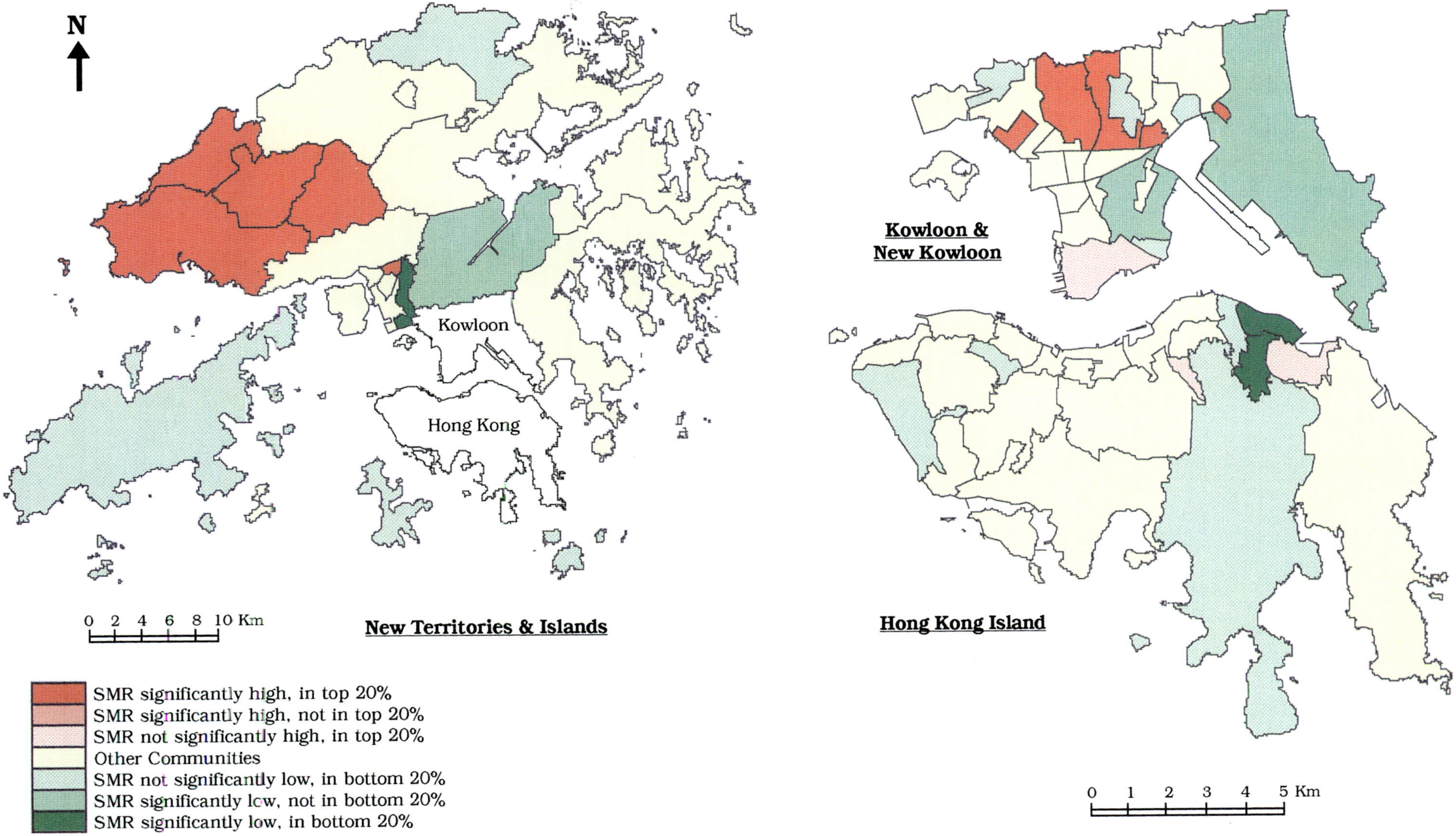

COAD (Female, 1989 -1993)

Number of Deaths, Standardised Mortality Ratio (SMR) and 95% Confidence Interval of COAD by 65 Communities in 1989–1993

Community	Male			Female		
	Number of deaths	SMR	95% C.I.	Number of deaths	SMR	95% C.I.
HK1	106	99.6	80.6 - 118.5	43	78.9	55.3 - 102.5
HK2	146	101.6	85.1 - 118.0	79	119.1	92.8 - 145.3
HK3	40	79.9	55.2 - 104.7	25	112.5	72.8 - 166.5
HK4	75	93.2	72.1 - 114.3	33	83.8	55.2 - 112.5
HK5	93	120.6	96.1 - 145.1	44	118.3	83.3 - 153.2
HK6	55	62.5	46.0 - 79.0	53	97.0	70.9 - 123.1
HK7	16	84.5	48.3 - 136.8	10	77.9	37.4 - 143.3
HK8	15	48.1	26.9 - 79.4	12	70.3	36.3 - 123.0
HK9	1	7.8	0.2 - 43.5	7	91.9	36.8 - 189.2
HK10	200	82.8	71.4 - 94.3	144	97.9	81.9 - 113.9
HK11	10	44.9	21.5 - 82.6	12	124.3	64.2 - 217.5
HK12	13	68.9	36.6 - 117.8	11	96.9	48.4 - 173.5
HK13	17	62.7	36.5 - 100.3	8	61.0	26.3 - 120.2
HK14	59	63.0	46.9 - 79.1	34	68.3	45.4 - 91.3
HK15	32	60.0	39.2 - 80.8	17	58.3	34.0 - 93.3
HK16	132	134.4	111.5 - 157.4	60	120.0	89.6 - 150.4
HK17	241	115.2	100.7 - 129.8	124	114.8	94.6 - 135.1
HK18	10	43.3	20.8 - 79.6	11	68.4	34.1 - 122.4
HK19	56	68.7	50.7 - 86.7	32	80.0	52.3 - 107.7
HK20	220	117.1	101.7 - 132.6	100	99.5	80.0 - 119.0
HK21	11	66.8	33.4 - 119.6	6	77.2	28.3 - 168.3
KL1	46	72.7	51.7 - 93.7	38	121.0	82.5 - 159.4
KL2	166	117.4	99.5 - 135.2	61	85.0	63.7 - 106.4
KL3	38	87.4	59.6 - 115.2	22	90.2	56.6 - 136.3
KL4	134	109.5	91.0 - 128.1	50	91.1	65.9 - 116.4
KL5	81	89.7	70.2 - 109.3	41	93.8	65.1 - 122.6
KL6	20	54.5	33.3 - 83.9	24	92.1	59.1 - 137.3
KL7	14	58.7	32.0 - 98.5	16	99.4	56.8 - 161.0
KL8	69	96.6	73.8 - 119.4	38	104.7	71.4 - 138.0
KL9	249	85.6	75.0 - 96.3	116	78.3	64.0 - 92.5
KL10	33	71.4	47.0 - 95.7	21	73.1	45.3 - 111.9
KL11	45	66.8	47.3 - 86.4	32	84.6	55.3 - 113.9
KL12	13	60.4	32.1 - 103.3	6	50.6	18.6 - 110.3
KL13	247	90.7	79.4 - 102.0	145	110.5	92.5 - 128.5
KL14	259	134.0	117.7 - 150.3	127	130.6	107.9 - 153.3
KL15	46	138.0	98.1 - 177.9	30	164.8	105.8 - 223.8
KL16	62	103.2	77.5 - 128.9	32	108.6	71.0 - 146.2
KL17	32	108.6	70.9 - 146.2	38	163.1	111.2 - 215.0
KL18	5	41.1	13.3 - 95.7	4	49.8	13.5 - 127.4
KL19	333	113.4	101.2 - 125.6	170	103.2	87.7 - 118.7
KL20	43	65.7	46.0 - 85.3	27	83.7	52.1 - 115.3
KL21	105	96.8	78.3 - 115.4	48	83.9	60.2 - 107.7
KL22	26	125.4	77.2 - 173.7	7	65.1	26.1 - 134.1
KL23	83	190.4	149.4 - 231.4	45	201.8	142.8 - 260.7
KL24	39	65.6	45.0 - 86.2	37	152.0	103.0 - 200.9
KL25	737	87.2	80.9 - 93.4	374	83.3	74.8 - 91.7
NT1	51	81.7	59.2 - 104.1	33	90.2	59.4 - 121.0
NT2	54	77.4	56.8 - 98.1	30	77.9	50.0 - 105.7
NT3	92	75.3	59.9 - 90.6	54	100.4	73.6 - 127.2
NT4	96	117.0	93.6 - 140.4	65	140.7	106.5 - 174.9
NT5	207	112.2	97.0 - 127.5	105	114.3	92.4 - 136.2
NT6	142	120.2	100.4 - 140.0	43	68.8	48.3 - 89.4
NT7	104	97.9	79.1 - 116.8	47	86.9	62.1 - 111.7
NT8	305	116.4	103.3 - 129.5	174	120.3	102.5 - 138.2
NT9	77	196.4	152.5 - 240.2	41	180.5	125.3 - 235.8
NT10	266	143.5	126.3 - 160.8	154	163.5	137.7 - 189.3
NT11	58	160.1	118.9 - 201.3	38	185.5	126.6 - 244.5
NT12	213	125.5	108.7 - 142.4	105	114.3	92.4 - 136.1
NT13	38	110.6	75.4 - 145.8	20	97.2	59.4 - 149.7
NT14	36	175.1	117.9 - 232.3	7	56.3	22.6 - 116.0
NT15	257	137.4	120.6 - 154.2	127	114.6	94.7 - 134.5
NT16	396	90.1	81.2 - 98.9	239	85.2	74.4 - 96.0
NT17	102	90.4	72.9 - 108.0	56	84.4	62.3 - 106.5
NT18	35	101.4	67.8 - 135.0	16	86.1	49.2 - 139.5
NT19	44	106.8	75.2 - 138.3	16	66.7	38.1 - 108.0

COAD

Sex-Age specific mortality rate (1/100,000) of COAD in Hong Kong (1989–1993)

	Male		Female	
Age	No. of deaths	Mortality rate	No. of deaths	Mortality rate
0–4	1	0.10	0	0.00
5–9	2	0.19	3	0.31
10–14	6	0.55	5	0.50
15–19	9	0.82	13	1.30
20–24	16	1.40	4	0.35
25–29	19	1.32	3	0.20
30–34	23	1.47	14	0.92
35–39	33	2.46	14	1.11
40–44	42	3.81	15	1.54
45–49	68	9.31	21	3.52
50–54	152	21.91	36	6.32
55–59	372	53.23	81	13.30
60–64	712	115.34	179	30.97
65+	5591	504.74	3396	241.73
TOTAL	7046	48.18	3784	27.04

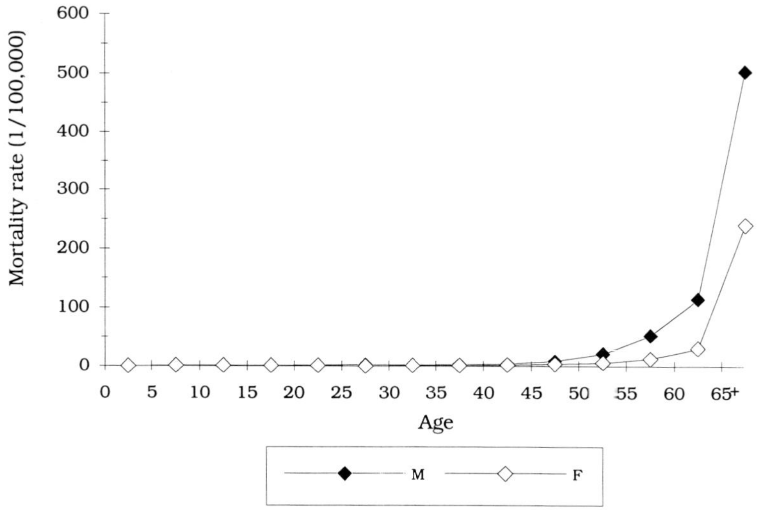

Number of communities on map by category based on standardized mortality ratio (SMR) during 1989–1993

Category	Number of communities Male	Female
SMR significantly high, in top 20%	10	10
SMR significantly high , not in top 20%	4	0
SMR not significantly high, in top 20%	3	3
SMR not significantly low, in bottom 20%	2	10
SMR significantly low, not in bottom 20%	11	3
SMR significantly low, in bottom 20%	11	3
other communities	24	36

Values of the standardized mortality ratio (SMR) which divide the 65 communities into quintile

Percentile	Male	Female
20th	65.60	77.22
40th	84.45	85.23
60th	101.43	99.33
80th	117.38	119.05
Lowest SMR	7.81	49.76
Highest SMR	196.38	201.79
No. of communities with zero cases	0	0

Appendices

Appendix 1: 65 Communities and TPUs in 1981 Census, 1986 By-Census and 1991 Census

Community	TPU by 1981 Census	TPU by 1986 By-census	TPU by 1991 Census	District
HK1	111, 116	111, 116	111, 116	West
HK2	112–13, 115	112–13, 115	112–13, 115	West/Sheung Wan
HK3	114, 121–23	114, 121–23	114, 121–23	Central/Sheung Wan
HK4	124, 132–35	124, 132–35	124, 132–35	Wan Chai
HK5	131	131	131	Wan Chai (southern)
HK6	140, 144–45, 149, 183–84, 190	140, 144–45, 149, 183–84, 190	140, 144–45, 149, 183–84, 190	Mid Level/Peak/Tai Hang
HK7	141, 181	141, 181	141, 181	Mid Level/Peak
HK8	142	142	142	Mid Level
HK9	143, 182	143, 182	143, 182	Mid Level/Peak
HK10	146–47, 151, 153	146–47, 151, 153	146, 151, 153	Tai Hang/North Point
HK11	148	148	148	Tai Hang
HK12	152	152	152	North Point
HK13	154	154	154	North Point (eastern)
HK14	155, 157	155, 157	155, 157	Quarry Bay
HK15	156	156	156	Quarry Bay
HK16	161	161	161	Shau Kei Wan
HK17	162–65, 196–97	162–65, 196–97	162–66, 196–97	Chai Wan
HK18	171	171	171	Pok Fu Lam
HK19	172	172	172	Pok Fu Lam (southern)
HK20	173–76, 191, 199	173–76, 191, 199	173–75, 191, 199	Aberdeen
HK21	192–95, 198	192–95, 198	192–95, 198	South
KL1	211–16	211–16	211–16	Tsim Sha Tsui

Appendix 1 (Continued)

Community	TPU by 1981 Census	TPU by 1986 By-census	TPU by 1991 Census	District
KL2	221	221	221	Mong Kok
KL3	222	222	222	Mong Kok
KL4	223–24	220, 227–29	220, 227–29	Mong Kok
KL5	225–26	225–26	225–26	Yau Ma Tei
KL6	231–33	231–33	231–33	Ho Man Tin (northern)
KL7	235	235	235	Ho Man Tin
KL8	241	241	241	Ho Man Tin
KL9	234, 236–37, 242–44, 246	234, 236–37, 242–44, 246	234, 236–37, 242–44, 246	Ho Man Tin/Hung Hom
KL10	245	245	245	Hung Hom
KL11	251, 253–57	251, 253–57	260	Lai Chi Kok/Tsuen Wan new town
KL12	261	261	261	Cheung Sha Wan (northern)
KL13	262, 264, 266, 269	262, 264, 266, 269	262, 264, 266, 269	Cheung Sha Wan/Sham Shui Po
KL14	263, 268	263, 268	263, 268	Shek Kip Mei
KL15	265	265	265	Cheung Sha Wan (southern)
KL16	267	267	267	Sham Shui Po
KL17	271	271	271	Kowloon Tong (western)
KL18	272	272	272	Kowloon Tong (eastern)
KL19	281	281	281	Tsz Wan Shan
KL20	282	282	282	Kowloon City/Wong Tai Sin
KL21	283	283	283	Kowloon City/Wong Tai Sin (central)
KL22	284	284	284	San Po Kong

Appendix 1 (Continued)

Community	TPU by 1981 Census	TPU by 1986 By-census	TPU by 1991 Census	District
KL23	285–86	285	285	Kowloon City/Wong Tai Sin (southern)
KL24	287	287	287	Ngau Chi Wan
KL25	280, 288–99	280, 288–99	280, 288–98	Kwun Tong/Jordan Valley/Ngau Chi Wan/Yau Tong
NT1	310, 321–23, 331–32, 340	310, 321–23, 331–32, 340	310, 321–23, 331–36, 340	Tsuen Wan new town & other area
NT2	320, 328	320, 328–29	320, 328–29	Tsuen Wan new town
NT3	324	324	324	Tsuen Wan new town (western)
NT4	325	325	325	Kwai Chung new town
NT5	326	326	326	Kwai Chung new town
NT6	327	327	327	Kwai Chung new town
NT7	350	350	350–51	Tsing Yi
NT8	413–14, 422–27, 431–32, 441–42	413–14, 421–28, 431–32, 441–42	412–16, 422–27, 432–33, 441–42	Tuen Mun new town/Tuen Mun other area
NT9	511–16	511–16	511–16	Yuen Long other area
NT10	517–19, 521–23,	517–19, 521–27	517–19, 521–29	Yuen Long new town & other area
NT11	531–33	531–33	531–33	Yuen Long other area
NT12	541–46, 610, 621–24, 626–29, 632–34	541–46, 610, 621–24, 626–29, 632–34	541–46, 610, 621–24, 626–29, 632–34	Yuen Long other area/Sheung Shui/Fanling new town & other area
NT13	625	625	625	Sheung Shui/Fanling new town
NT14	641–42, 651–52	641–42, 651–52	641–42, 651–52	Sheung Shui/Fanling other area

Appendix 1 (Continued)

Community	TPU by 1981 Census	TPU by 1986 By-census	TPU by 1991 Census	District
NT15	631, 653, 711–12, 720–29, 741–42, 751	631, 653, 711–12, 720–29, 741–42, 751	631, 653, 711, 720, 722–29, 741–42	Sheung Shui/Fanling other area/Tai Po new town & other area
NT16	732, 752–59, 761–62	732–33, 752–59, 761–62	732, 753–59, 761–62	Shatin new town & other area
NT17	811–15, 821–27, 831–34	811–15, 821–27, 831–34	811–15, 821–28, 831–39	Sai Kung
NT18	920	920	920	Cheung Chau
NT19	911–13, 931–76	911–13, 931–76	911, 931–76	Islands

Appendix 2: Diseases in the Top 20% of Each Community by Sex and Period

		Male		Female	
Community	Period	Number of diseases in the top 20%	Name of disease	Number of diseases in the top 20%	Name of disease
HK1	1979–83	1	Oesophageal CA	5	Oesophageal CA, Colorectal CA, **Gastric CA**, Lung CA, **Pneumonia**
	1984–88	1	NPC	3	Gastric CA, Cervical CA, IHD
	1989–93	0		3	**Colorectal CA**, Lung CA, Cervical CA
HK2	1979–83	3	Oesophageal CA, **CVA**, **Pneumonia**	5	Lung CA, Breast CA, Leukaemia, **CVA**, **Pneumonia**
	1984–88	1	Leukaemia	1	Lung CA
	1989–93	0		2	Oesophageal CA, Cervical CA
HK3	1979–83	3	Colorectal CA, **IHD**, **Pneumonia**	5	Colorectal CA, Liver CA, **Breast CA**, **IHD**, **CVA**
	1984–88	2	Oesophageal CA, IHD	2	NPC, COAD
	1989–93	0		3	NPC, Colorectal CA, Leukaemia
HK4	1979–83	0		0	
	1984–88	2	Liver CA, **IHD**	3	Lung CA, **Breast CA**, **Cervical CA**
	1989–93	2	Colorectal CA, Liver CA	4	Oesophageal CA, Gastric CA, Liver CA, **IHD**
HK5	1979–83	6	Gastric CA, **Liver CA**, **Lung CA**, CVA, **Pneumonia**, COAD, TB, Leukaemia	10	**Colorectal CA**, **Liver CA**, **Lung CA**, **Breast CA**, Cervical CA, **IHD**, **CVA**, **TB**, **Pneumonia**, COAD
	1984–88	5	**IHD**, CVA, TB, Pneumonia, COAD	2	Lung CA, CVA
	1989–93	5	Gastric CA, Colorectal CA, Liver CA, Leukaemia, COAD	4	Gastric CA, Lung CA, Leukaemia, Cervical CA

Diseases with significant difference ($p < 0.05$) are printed in bold.

Appendix 2 (Continued)

		Male		Female	
Community	Period	Number of diseases in the top 20%	Name of disease	Number of diseases in the top 20%	Name of disease
HK6	1979–83	1	**IHD**	1	Breast CA
	1984–88	1	IHD	1	Leukaemia
	1989–93	0		1	Leukaemia
HK7	1979–83	3	Colorectal CA, HBP, **IHD**	1	Colorectal CA
	1984–88	2	Oesophageal CA, **IHD**	2	Gastric CA, Lung CA
	1989–93	2	Gastric CA, Colorectal CA	2	Oesophageal CA, **Liver CA**
HK8	1979–83	2	**Colorectal CA**, **IHD**	2	Colorectal CA, Leukaemia
	1984–88	0		2	Breast CA, Leukaemia
	1989–93	2	Colorectal CA, IHD	1	Colorectal CA
HK9	1979–83	1	**IHD**	0	
	1984–88	1	IHD	1	Leukaemia
	1989–93	1	Leukaemia	5	Oesophageal CA, Breast CA, HBP, IHD, Pneumonia
HK10	1979–83	3	Gastric CA, **Colorectal CA**, **IHD**	1	**Breast CA**
	1984–88	1	**IHD**	2	Breast CA, **IHD**
	1989–93	1	**IHD**	0	
HK11	1979–83	5	Oesophageal CA, Gastric CA, Colorectal CA, Liver CA, Lung CA	4	Colorectal CA, Leukaemia, IHD, CVA
	1984–88	5	NPC, Gastric CA, Colorectal CA, Lung CA, **IHD**	8	NPC, Oesophageal CA, Gastric CA, Lung CA, Breast CA, Leukaemia, IHD, Pneumonia
	1989–93	1	Leukaemia	4	Leukaemia, Breast CA, CVA, COAD

Appendix 2 (Continued)

		Male		Female	
Community	Period	Number of diseases in the top 20%	Name of disease	Number of diseases in the top 20%	Name of disease
HK12	1979–83	3	Gastric CA, Colorectal CA, **IHD**	3	Gastric CA, Leukaemia, HBP
	1984–88	1	Gastric CA	3	Colorectal CA, Breast CA, Leukaemia
	1989–93	2	**Colorectal CA**, IHD	5	Colorectal CA, Leukaemia, **Breast CA**, Cervical CA, IHD
HK13	1979–83	0		2	Gastric CA, **IHD**
	1984–88	3	Colorectal CA, Leukaemia, HBP	5	Oesophageal CA, Gastric CA, **Colorectal CA**, Breast CA, IHD
	1989–93	1	Leukaemia	3	Colorectal CA, Liver CA, Cervical CA
HK14	1979–83	0		0	
	1984–88	0		1	Cervical CA
	1989–93	0		0	
HK15	1979–83	2	Colorectal CA, HBP	1	IHD
	1984–88	7	Gastric CA, Colorectal CA, Lung CA, Leukaemia, **IHD**, **CVA**, Pneumonia	5	Oesophageal CA, Colorectal CA, Liver CA, Lung CA, **IHD**
	1989–93	1	Leukaemia	2	**Oesophageal CA**, Gastric CA
HK16	1979–83	5	Oesophageal CA, **Lung CA**, Leukaemia, **CVA**, **Pneumonia**	7	Breast CA, Colorectal CA, **Liver CA**, **Lung CA**, **CVA**, **Pneumonia**, **COAD**
	1984–88	7	NPC, **Colorectal CA**, **Liver CA**, **Lung CA**, **IHD**, **CVA**, **Pneumonia**	3	NPC, TB, **Pneumonia**
	1989–93	3	Colorectal CA, **IHD**, **COAD**	8	Oesophageal CA, Lung CA, Leukaemia, **Breast CA**, HBP, **IHD**, **Pneumonia**, COAD

Appendix 2 (Continued)

Community	Period	Male: Number of diseases in the top 20%	Male: Name of disease	Female: Number of diseases in the top 20%	Female: Name of disease
HK17	1979–83	5	Oesophageal CA, Gastric CA, Lung CA, Leukaemia, **COAD**	4	Gastric CA, Lung CA, Leukaemia, IHD
	1984–88	5	**NPC**, Oesophageal CA, **Lung CA**, TB, **COAD**	2	Oesophageal CA, Lung CA
	1989–93	3	Oesophageal CA, Liver CA, **Lung CA**	0	
HK18	1979–83	0		1	Cervical CA
	1984–88	0		0	
	1989–93	0		0	
HK19	1979–83	3	Lung CA, Leukaemia, CVA	6	Colorectal CA, Liver CA, Lung CA, IHD, CVA, **COAD**
	1984–88	2	**Colorectal CA**, Lung CA	4	Colorectal CA, Lung CA, Breast CA, IHD
	1989–93	5	NPC, Oesophageal CA, Colorectal CA, Liver CA, CVA	3	Oesophageal CA, **Lung CA**, **CVA**
HK20	1979–83	7	NPC, **Gastric CA**, **Liver CA**, **Lung CA**, HBP, **CVA**, **Pneumonia**	6	NPC, Liver CA, Lung CA, **IHD**, **CVA**, **Pneumonia**
	1984–88	8	**NPC**, Oesophageal CA, Gastric CA, Liver CA, **Lung CA**, **IHD**, **CVA**, **Pneumonia**	5	Gastric CA, **Leukaemia**, **IHD**, **CVA**, **Pneumonia**
	1989–93	4	**Oesophageal CA**, Gastric CA, **CVA**, **Pneumonia**	3	**IHD**, **CVA**, **Pneumonia**
HK21	1979–83	3	HBP, IHD, Pneumonia	3	Oesophageal CA, IHD, Pneumonia
	1984–88	0		1	CVA
	1989–93	1	HBP	0	

Appendix 2 (Continued)

Community	Period	Male: Number of diseases in the top 20%	Male: Name of disease	Female: Number of diseases in the top 20%	Female: Name of disease
KL1	1979–83	3	Oesophageal CA, HBP, **IHD**	2	Cervical CA, **IHD**
	1984–88	4	Leukaemia, **HBP**, **IHD**, TB	5	Gastric CA, Colorectal CA, Breast CA, CVA, TB
	1989–93	3	Leukaemia, HBP, **IHD**	2	IHD, COAD
KL2	1979–83	1	COAD	2	**HBP**, TB
	1984–88	3	Lung CA, **TB**, **COAD**	2	NPC, Cervical CA
	1989–93	3	Colorectal CA, Liver CA, **Pneumonia**	1	Cervical CA
KL3	1979–83	3	Lung CA, Leukaemia, HBP	4	Cervical CA, HBP, TB, COAD
	1984–88	2	NPC, Liver CA	4	NPC, Breast CA, **Pneumonia**, COAD
	1989–93	0		5	**NPC**, Gastric CA, Breast CA, Cervical CA, Pneumonia
KL4	1979–83	2	**TB**, **Pneumonia**	4	Liver CA, Cervical CA, **Pneumonia**, COAD
	1984–88	0		1	Cervical CA
	1989–93	1	**IHD**	1	Lung CA
KL5	1979–83	3	Leukaemia, HBP, Pneumonia	6	NPC, **Lung CA**, **Cervical CA**, HBP, **Pneumonia**, COAD
	1984–88	1	Liver CA	5	NPC, **Liver CA**, Cervical CA, **HBP**, COAD
	1989–93	3	TB, **IHD**, **CVA**	3	Lung CA, Breast CA, HBP
KL6	1979–83	3	NPC, Colorectal CA, Leukaemia	0	
	1984–88	3	Leukaemia, HBP, CVA	6	Breast CA, HBP, **IHD**, CVA, Pneumonia, COAD
	1989–93	2	CVA, Pneumonia	2	Colorectal CA, CVA

Appendix 2 (Continued)

Community	Period	Male: Number of diseases in the top 20%	Male: Name of disease	Female: Number of diseases in the top 20%	Female: Name of disease
KL8	1979–83	0		1	Breast CA
	1984–88	2	Gastric CA, Colorectal CA	1	TB
	1989–93	2	Colorectal CA, HBP	2	Colorectal CA, TB
KL9	1979–83	1	Gastric CA	0	
	1984–88	1	Gastric CA	1	**HBP**
	1989–93	1	Gastric CA	0	
KL10	1979–83	4	NPC, Gastric CA, Colorectal CA, Leukaemia	3	NPC, Leukaemia, HBP
	1984–88	5	Gastric CA, Colorectal CA, Liver CA, HBP, Pneumonia	1	Liver CA
	1989–93	1	Leukaemia	1	Breast CA
KL11	1979–83	0		1	Liver CA
	1984–88	1	Leukaemia	2	Colorectal CA, Cervical CA
	1989–93	0		0	
KL12	1979–83	1	NPC	2	TB, HBP
	1984–88	0		2	NPC, Oesophageal CA
	1989–93	2	CVA, Pneumonia	0	
KL13	1979–83	0		1	TB
	1984–88	2	TB, **COAD**	1	COAD
	1989–93	1	**CVA**	1	TB

Appendix 2 (Continued)

Community	Period	Male: Number of diseases in the top 20%	Male: Name of disease	Female: Number of diseases in the top 20%	Female: Name of disease
KL14	1979–83	2	**TB**, COAD	5	NPC, Oesophageal CA, Cervical CA, Leukaemia,
	1984–88	3	Oesophageal CA, **TB**, **COAD**	1	TB
	1989–93	6	Oesophageal CA, Colorectal CA, Lung CA, TB, **Pneumonia**, **COAD**	5	Lung CA, Leukaemia, Cervical CA, TB, **COAD**
KL15	1979–83	6	Lung CA, **IHD**, **CVA**, TB, **Pneumonia**, **COAD**	12	NPC, Oesophageal CA, Colorectal CA, **Gastric CA**, Liver CA, Lung CA, **Cervical CA**, **IHD**, **CVA**, TB, **Pneumonia**, COAD
	1984–88	7	Oesophageal CA, Lung CA, Leukaemia, HBP, CVA, **Pneumonia**, COAD	7	NPC, Colorectal CA, **Liver CA**, Breast CA, Leukaemia, TB, COAD
	1989–93	11	NPC, **Oesophageal CA**, Gastric CA, Colorectal CA, **Liver CA**, **Lung CA**, TB, IHD, **CVA**, **Pneumonia**, COAD	9	Colorectal CA, Lung CA, **Leukaemia**, Breast CA, TB, HBP, CVA, Pneumonia, **COAD**
KL16	1979–83	7	NPC, Oesophageal CA, **Liver CA**, **Lung CA**, CVA, **Pneumonia**, COAD	10	**Colorectal CA**, Gastric CA, **Lung CA**, Breast CA, Cervical CA, Leukaemia, HBP, IHD, TB, **Pneumonia**
	1984–88	0		3	NPC, Liver CA, Cervical CA
	1989–93	5	NPC, **Lung CA**, TB, **IHD**, Pneumonia	3	NPC, TB, CVA
KL17	1979–83	3	Colorectal CA, **IHD**, Pneumonia	2	Gastric CA, Leukaemia
	1984–88	2	**Colorectal CA**, Leukaemia	2	HBP, **Pneumonia**
	1989–93	7	Colorectal CA, Liver CA, TB, HBP, **IHD**, **CVA**, **Pneumonia**	9	Lung CA, Breast CA, Cervical CA, TB, **HBP**, **IHD**, **CVA**, **Pneumonia**, **COAD**

Appendix 2 (Continued)

Community	Period	Male: Number of diseases in the top 20%	Male: Name of disease	Female: Number of diseases in the top 20%	Female: Name of disease
KL18	1979–83	2	IHD, TB	4	Breast CA, Leukaemia, HBP, IHD
	1984–88	2	NPC, Colorectal CA	3	Oesophageal CA, Gastric CA, Breast CA
	1989–93	0		1	NPC
KL19	1979–83	2	**Oesophageal CA**, Gastric CA	3	Oesophageal CA, **CVA**, TB
	1984–88	1	**Oesophageal CA**	4	Cervical CA, **HBP**, **Pneumonia**, **COAD**
	1989–93	2	**Oesophageal CA**, Lung CA	1	**Gastric CA**
KL20	1979–83	6	NPC, Oesophageal CA, **Liver CA**, Lung CA, Leukaemia, **TB**	3	Oesophageal CA, Leukaemia, COAD
	1984–88	4	**Oesophageal CA**, **Gastric CA**, Pneumonia, COAD	3	NPC, Cervical CA, **Leukaemia**
	1989–93	0		1	Oesophageal CA
KL21	1979–83	5	**Oesophageal CA**, Liver CA, **Gastric CA**, **CVA**, **TB**	2	NPC, Liver CA
	1984–88	3	**Oesophageal CA**, Lung CA, TB	5	Oesophageal CA, Colorectal CA, Liver CA, CVA, TB
	1989–93	6	NPC, **Oesophageal CA**, Lung CA, Leukaemia, **TB**, HBP	3	Gastric CA, Liver CA, **HBP**
KL22	1979–83	4	Oesophageal CA, Colorectal CA, Leukaemia, COAD	2	Oesophageal CA, HBP
	1984–88	3	HBP, TB, Pneumonia	2	**Oesophageal CA**, Colorectal CA
	1989–93	4	**Liver CA**, TB, HBP, COAD	4	Colorectal CA, Breast CA, CVA, Pneumonia

Appendix 2 (Continued)

Community	Period	Male: Number of diseases in the top 20%	Male: Name of disease	Female: Number of diseases in the top 20%	Female: Name of disease
KL23	1979–83	1	Oesophageal CA	3	Breast CA, HBP, TB
	1984–88	11	**NPC**, **Oesophageal CA**, Gastric CA, Colorectal CA, **Lung CA**, **HBP**, **IHD**, **CVA**, **TB**, **Pneumonia**, **COAD**	12	**Oesophageal CA**, Colorectal CA, Liver CA, **Lung CA**, **Breast CA**, Leukaemia, **HBP**, **IHD**, **CVA**, TB, Pneumonia, **COAD**
	1989–93	11	NPC, **Oesophageal CA**, **Gastric CA**, **Liver CA**, **Lung CA**, TB, **HBP**, **IHD**, **CVA**, **Pneumonia**, **COAD**	14	NPC, Oesophageal CA, **Colorectal CA**, **Liver CA**, Lung CA, Leukaemia, **Breast CA**, Cervical CA, TB, HBP, **IHD**, **CVA**, **Pneumonia**, **COAD**
KL24	1979–83	2	Liver CA, HBP	5	Liver CA, Lung CA, CVA, Pneumonia, COAD
	1984–88	1	Leukaemia	2	Leukaemia, CVA
	1989–93	2	NPC, Gastric CA	5	Lung CA, Leukaemia, TB, Pneumonia, **COAD**
KL25	1979–83	1	**Gastric CA**	1	**Oesophageal CA**
	1984–88	0		0	
	1989–93	1	Oesophageal CA	0	
NT1	1979–83	1	Pneumonia	2	Oesophageal CA, COAD
	1984–88	1	Gastric CA	4	Oesophageal CA, Gastric CA, Lung CA, TB
	1989–93	1	HBP	1	Liver CA
NT2	1979–83	4	NPC, Oesophageal CA, Gastric CA, CVA	4	Gastric CA, Lung CA, Leukaemia, COAD
	1984–88	0		3	Colorectal CA, Liver CA, Leukaemia
	1989–93	2	NPC, Leukaemia	4	Oesophageal CA, Gastric CA, **Leukaemia**, TB

Appendix 2 (Continued)

Community	Period	Male: Number of diseases in the top 20%	Male: Name of disease	Female: Number of diseases in the top 20%	Female: Name of disease
NT3	1979–83	2	TB, COAD	6	Oesophageal CA, Colorectal CA, Gastric CA, Breast CA, Cervical CA, CVA
	1984–88	1	Leukaemia	5	NPC, Gastric CA, IHD, **CVA**, **COAD**
	1989–93	1	TB	0	
NT4	1979–83	2	CVA, TB	4	**NPC**, Oesophageal CA, Lung CA, COAD
	1984–88	2	NPC, Liver CA	1	Gastric CA
	1989–93	3	NPC, **Gastric CA**, Colorectal CA	6	NPC, **Oesophageal CA**, Gastric CA, Liver CA, TB, **COAD**
NT5	1979–83	1	Gastric CA	0	
	1984–88	4	**Oesophageal CA**, Liver CA, **Pneumonia**, **COAD**	4	Colorectal CA, **Liver CA**, CVA, **COAD**
	1989–93	1	Gastric CA	4	**Liver CA**, Leukaemia, Cervical CA, **TB**
NT6	1979–83	1	**COAD**	1	**TB**
	1984–88	2	Gastric CA, Leukaemia	1	Gastric CA
	1989–93	1	**COAD**	3	NPC, Gastric CA, **IHD**
NT7	1979–83	6	**Liver CA**, Lung CA, Leukaemia, CVA, COAD, TB	2	Cervical CA, CVA
	1984–88	4	**NPC**, Liver CA, Lung CA, CVA	2	Lung CA, **TB**
	1989–93	0		1	Colorectal CA
NT8	1979–83	1	NPC	2	**Oesophageal CA**, Gastric CA
	1984–88	0		5	**Oesophageal CA**, **Liver CA**, **HBP**, TB, **COAD**
	1989–93	1	HBP	4	NPC, **Breast CA**, **Pneumonia**, **COAD**

Appendix 2 (Continued)

Community	Period	Male: Number of diseases in the top 20%	Male: Name of disease	Female: Number of diseases in the top 20%	Female: Name of disease
NT9	1979–83	4	Liver CA, Leukaemia, **HBP**, COAD	2	NPC, HBP
	1984–88	7	**NPC**, Oesophageal CA, **Lung CA**, **HBP**, **CVA**, **TB**, COAD	6	NPC, **Gastric CA**, Cervical CA, **IHD**, CVA, **COAD**
	1989–93	10	NPC, Gastric CA, Liver CA, **Lung CA**, **TB**, HBP, **IHD**, **CVA**, **Pneumonia**, **COAD**	8	NPC, Gastric CA, Colorectal CA, **Liver CA**, HBP, **IHD**, **CVA**, **COAD**
NT10	1979–83	0		1	**NPC**
	1984–88	3	**HBP**, **CVA**, **Pneumonia**	4	**HBP**, **IHD**, **CVA**, **COAD**
	1989–93	5	TB, **HBP**, **IHD**, **CVA**, **COAD**	8	Gastric CA, Leukaemia, Cervical CA, TB, **HBP**, **IHD**, **CVA**, **COAD**
NT11	1979–83	0		2	TB, NPC
	1984–88	6	Oesophageal CA, Colorectal CA, HBP, CVA, **TB**, **Pneumonia**	3	**HBP**, TB, **Pneumonia**
	1989–93	5	Oesophageal CA, Leukaemia, CVA, **Pneumonia**, **COAD**	8	NPC, Liver CA, Cervical CA, HBP, **IHD**, CVA, Pneumonia, **COAD**
NT12	1979–83	2	NPC, **TB**	0	
	1984–88	3	Liver CA, Leukaemia, **COAD**	0	
	1989–93	2	Lung CA, **COAD**	1	Gastric CA
NT13	1979–83	4	TB, Leukaemia, HBP, COAD	5	NPC, **Oesophageal CA**, **Liver CA**, Leukaemia, Pneumonia
	1984–88	3	Liver CA, TB, COAD	1	Leukaemia
	1989–93	3	**NPC**, Liver CA, Lung CA	2	Gastric CA, HBP

Appendix 2 (Continued)

Community	Period	Male: Number of diseases in the top 20%	Male: Name of disease	Female: Number of diseases in the top 20%	Female: Name of disease
NT14	1979–83	2	NPC, Colorectal CA	1	Gastric CA
	1984–88	1	Pneumonia	3	Oesophageal CA, **HBP**, Pneumonia
	1989–93	5	NPC, Oesophageal CA, Gastric CA, CVA, **COAD**	2	NPC, Liver CA
NT15	1979–83	4	**NPC**, **Liver CA**, HBP, Pneumonia	2	Gastric CA, CVA
	1984–88	4	Gastric CA, **Liver CA**, **HBP**, TB	3	Cervical CA, **HBP**, TB
	1989–93	4	Liver CA, **Lung CA**, **HBP**, **COAD**	3	Liver CA, **HBP**, **Pneumonia**
NT16	1979–83	3	**Lung CA**, HBP, **CVA**	6	NPC, **Colorectal CA**, Liver CA, HBP, **Pneumonia**, COAD
	1984–88	0		1	**Lung CA**
	1989–93	0		1	**HBP**
NT17	1979–83	4	NPC, Liver CA, HBP, **TB**	3	**Liver CA**, HBP, TB
	1984–88	1	Gastric CA	4	Liver CA, Leukaemia, TB, Pneumonia
	1989–93	1	TB	0	
NT18	1979–83	5	NPC, Liver CA, **Lung CA**, **CVA**, COAD	3	Gastric CA, Breast CA, Cervical CA
	1984–88	7	**NPC**, Colorectal CA, **Liver CA**, Leukaemia, HBP, CVA, COAD	9	NPC, Oesophageal CA, Gastric CA, Colorectal CA, Liver CA, Cervical CA, HBP, **CVA**, **Pneumonia**
	1989–93	7	**NPC**, Oesophageal CA, Gastric CA, **Liver CA**, Lung CA, Leukaemia, TB	4	**NPC**, Oesophageal CA, TB, **CVA**

Appendix 2 (Continued)

		Male		Female	
Community	Period	Number of diseases in the top 20%	Name of disease	Number of diseases in the top 20%	Name of disease
NT19	1979–83	1	Liver CA	1	Breast CA
	1984–88	2	Lung CA, CVA	2	Liver CA, Pneumonia
	1989–93	6	**NPC**, Oesophageal CA, **Gastric CA**, Lung CA, Leukaemia, Pneumonia	7	NPC, Oesophageal CA, Liver CA, Lung CA, **Breast CA**, IHD, Pneumonia

Appendix 3: Diseases in the Bottom 20% of Each Community by Sex and Period

		Male		Female	
Community	Period	Number of diseases in the bottom 20%	Name of disease	Number of diseases in the bottom 20%	Name of disease
HK1	1979–83	1	HBP	1	Cervical CA
	1984–88	1	**HBP**	1	**COAD**
	1989–93	1	HBP	0	
HK2	1979–83	0		0	
	1984–88	3	**NPC**, **Liver CA**, **HBP**	0	
	1989–93	1	**HBP**	3	**TB**, **HBP**, IHD
HK3	1979–83	0		0	
	1984–88	3	Gastric CA, Colorectal CA, **HBP**	3	Gastric CA, Breast CA, **HBP**
	1989–93	0		3	Liver CA, Lung CA, **HBP**
HK4	1979–83	3	NPC, Leukaemia, **CVA**	3	Liver CA, Cervical CA, **TB**
	1984–88	0		0	
	1989–93	1	**CVA**	1	Breast CA
HK5	1979–83	0		0	
	1984–88	0		3	Liver CA, **HBP**, **Pneumonia**
	1989–93	0		2	NPC, Colorectal CA
HK6	1979–83	4	**CVA**, **TB**, **Pneumonia**, **COAD**	9	NPC, **Oesophageal CA**, Gastric CA, Liver CA, **Cervical CA**, **HBP**, **CVA**, **TB**, **COAD**
	1984–88	5	**NPC**, **Lung CA**, Leukaemia, **TB**, **COAD**	4	**NPC**, **CVA**, **TB**, **COAD**
	1989–93	4	**Oesophageal CA**, **Liver CA**, **Lung CA**, **COAD**	2	Gastric CA, **Liver CA**

Diseases with significant difference ($p < 0.05$) are printed in bold.

Appendix 3 (Continued)

Community	Period	Male: Number of diseases in the bottom 20%	Male: Name of disease	Female: Number of diseases in the bottom 20%	Female: Name of disease
HK7	1979–83	5	Liver CA, Lung CA, TB, Pneumonia, **COAD**	3	Lung CA, HBP, IHD
	1984–88	4	Liver CA, HBP, Pneumonia, **COAD**	4	Breast CA, CVA, Pneumonia, **COAD**
	1989–93	2	Liver CA, Lung CA	2	HBP, **CVA**
HK8	1979–83	7	NPC, Liver CA, **Lung CA**, **CVA**, **TB**, **Pneumonia**, **COAD**	1	Liver CA
	1984–88	8	**NPC**, **Oesophageal CA**, **Liver CA**, **Lung CA**, **CVA**, TB, Pneumonia, **COAD**	4	Gastric CA, Liver CA, **CVA**, **COAD**
	1989–93	10	NPC, Oesophageal CA, Gastric CA, Liver CA, **Lung CA**, HBP, **CVA**, **TB**, **Pneumonia**, **COAD**	6	Gastric CA, Breast CA, HBP, CVA, **Pneumonia**, COAD
HK9	1979-83	7	NPC, Liver CA, **Lung CA**, HBP, **CVA**, **Pneumonia**, **COAD**	5	Lung CA, HBP, **CVA**, **Pneumonia**, COAD
	1984–88	4	**Liver CA**, **Lung CA**, **CVA**, **COAD**	7	Colorectal CA, Lung CA, HBP, IHD, **CVA**, **Pneumonia**, COAD
	1989–93	6	Colorectal CA, **Liver CA**, Lung CA, HBP, Pneumonia, **COAD**	4	Colorectal CA, Liver CA, Lung CA, CVA
HK10	1979–83	0		1	**TB**
	1984–88	2	**Lung CA**, **TB**	2	Leukaemia, **TB**
	1989–93	0		1	**Gastric CA**

Appendix 3 (Continued)

Community	Period	Male: Number of diseases in the bottom 20%	Male: Name of disease	Female: Number of diseases in the bottom 20%	Female: Name of disease
HK11	1979–83	1	**COAD**	1	HBP
	1984–88	4	Oesophageal CA, Liver CA, HBP, CVA	2	Colorectal CA, COAD
	1989–93	6	NPC, Colorectal CA, Lung CA, CVA, Pneumonia, **COAD**	2	Colorectal CA, IHD
HK12	1979–83	4	Lung CA, TB, CVA, Pneumonia	4	**Lung CA**, CVA, Pneumonia, COAD
	1984–88	6	NPC, Oesophageal CA, Colorectal CA, Lung CA, CVA, **COAD**	4	Lung CA, HBP, CVA, **COAD**
	1989–93	3	Oesophageal CA, **Lung CA**, **CVA**	3	HBP, **CVA**, Pneumonia
HK13	1979–83	6	Gastric CA, Colorectal CA, Liver CA, TB, HBP, COAD	2	**CVA**, **Pneumonia**
	1984–88	5	Lung CA, CVA, TB, Pneumonia, **COAD**	1	Liver CA
	1989–93	9	**Oesophageal CA**, Gastric CA, Colorectal CA, **Liver CA**, Lung CA, HBP, IHD, **Pneumonia**, COAD	5	Gastric CA, HBP. CVA, Pneumonia, COAD
HK14	1979–83	6	NPC, **Oesophageal CA**, HBP, TB, **Pneumonia**, **COAD**	2	NPC, HBP
	1984–88	9	**NPC**, **Oesophageal CA**, Liver CA, **Lung CA**, **HBP**, **CVA**, TB, **Pneumonia**, **COAD**	5	**HBP**, **CVA**, **TB**, **Pneumonia**, **COAD**
	1989–93	11	**NPC**, **Oesophageal CA**, Gastric CA, Colorectal CA, **Liver CA**, **Lung CA**, **HBP**, **IHD**, **CVA**, **Pneumonia**, **COAD**	7	NPC, **Liver CA**, Cervical CA, IHD, **CVA**, **Pneumonia**, **COAD**

Appendix 3 (Continued)

Community	Period	Male: Number of diseases in the bottom 20%	Male: Name of disease	Female: Number of diseases in the bottom 20%	Female: Name of disease
HK15	1979–83	2	Oesophageal CA, Gastric CA	0	
	1984–88	0		0	
	1989–93	5	NPC, Oesophageal CA, **TB**, **Pneumonia**, **COAD**	3	**Liver CA**, Pneumonia, **COAD**
HK16	1979–83	1	**NPC**	1	Leukaemia
	1984–88	0		0	
	1989–93	0		0	
HK17	1979–83	0		2	Colorectal CA, **TB**
	1984–88	0		3	**Cervical CA**, Leukaemia, **HBP**
	1989–93	0		0	
HK18	1979–83	9	NPC, Oesophageal CA, Colorectal CA, Liver CA, Lung CA, HBP, CVA, Pneumonia, **COAD**	4	Lung CA, HBP, Pneumonia, COAD
	1984–88	9	NPC, Colorectal CA, Liver CA, **Lung CA**, **HBP**, IHD, **CVA**, Pneumonia, **COAD**	6	Colorectal CA, **Lung CA**, **HBP**, **CVA**, **Pneumonia**, **COAD**
	1989–93	10	NPC, **Oesophageal CA**, Liver CA, **Lung CA**, HBP, **IHD**, **CVA**, TB, **Pneumonia**, **COAD**	9	Gastric CA, **Colorectal CA**, Lung CA, Breast CA, HBP, **IHD**, **CVA**, **Pneumonia**, COAD
HK19	1979–83	0		1	Breast CA
	1984–88	1	**HBP**	1	**HBP**
	1989–93	1	**HBP**	3	Gastric CA, HBP, TB

Appendix 3 (Continued)

Community	Period	Male: Number of diseases in the bottom 20%	Male: Name of disease	Female: Number of diseases in the bottom 20%	Female: Name of disease
HK20	1979–83	0		0	
	1984–88	1	**HBP**	1	**HBP**
	1989–93	1	HBP	0	
HK21	1979–83	4	NPC, Gastric CA, Colorectal CA, **Liver CA**	1	HBP
	1984–88	8	NPC, Oesophageal CA, Gastric CA, Colorectal CA, Liver CA, **Lung CA**, Pneumonia, **COAD**	7	Colorectal CA, Lung CA, Breast CA, HBP, IHD, Pneumonia, COAD
	1989–93	4	Gastric CA, Colorectal CA, Liver CA, Pneumonia	0	**Colorectal CA**, HBP, COAD
KL1	1979–83	0		0	
	1984–88	1	**Lung CA**	0	
	1989–93	2	NPC, Liver CA	1	**Lung CA**
KL2	1979–83	0		1	**Gastric CA**
	1984–88	2	Colorectal CA, **HBP**	1	**Oesophageal CA**
	1989–93	3	**Oesophageal CA**, **Gastric CA**, **HBP**	0	
KL3	1979–83	2	**Gastric CA**, Colorectal CA	1	Liver CA
	1984–88	0		2	Liver CA, Lung CA
	1989–93	1	Liver CA	1	**CVA**
KL4	1979–83	0		0	
	1984–88	4	**Colorectal CA**, **IHD**, **CVA**, **COAD**	3	Oesophageal CA, Colorectal CA, **CVA**
	1989–93	1	Leukaemia	1	Breast CA

Appendix 3 (Continued)

Community	Period	Male		Female	
		Number of diseases in the bottom 20%	Name of disease	Number of diseases in the bottom 20%	Name of disease
KL5	1979–83	0		0	
	1984–88	0		0	
	1989–93	0		0	
KL6	1979–83	7	Liver CA, **Lung CA**, HBP, **CVA**, **TB**, **Pneumonia**, **COAD**	6	Liver CA, Lung CA, Breast CA, Cervical CA, **CVA**, **COAD**
	1984–88	6	Oesophageal CA, Gastric CA, Liver CA, TB, Pneumonia, **COAD**	1	Liver CA
	1989–93	5	NPC, Gastric CA, **Lung CA**, TB, **COAD**	2	Liver CA, **Pneumonia**
KL7	1979–83	7	NPC, Gastric CA, Liver CA, Lung CA, **CVA**, Pneumonia, **COAD**	3	Gastric CA, **CVA**, COAD
	1984–88	6	Oesophageal CA, Gastric CA, IHD, **CVA**, TB, Pneumonia	2	Lung CA, **CVA**
	1989–93	5	**Oesophageal CA**, Gastric CA, CVA, TB, **COAD**	1	Breast CA
KL8	1979–83	0		0	
	1984–88	3	**Liver CA**, **CVA**, **Pneumonia**	2	Leukaemia, **IHD**
	1989–93	2	**Liver CA**, Leukaemia	2	NPC, IHD
KL9	1979–83	0		0	
	1984–88	0		2	**IHD**, **Pneumonia**
	1989–93	0		0	

Appendix 3 (Continued)

Community	Period	Male: Number of diseases in the bottom 20%	Male: Name of disease	Female: Number of diseases in the bottom 20%	Female: Name of disease
KL10	1979–83	3	**Lung CA**, TB, Pneumonia	3	Gastric CA, Lung CA, Pneumonia
	1984–88	1	**TB**	4	**Breast CA**, IHD, CVA, **COAD**
	1989–93	3	HBP, **CVA**, Pneumonia	5	Gastric CA, Colorectal CA, **Liver CA**, IHD, COAD
KL11	1979–83	2	NPC, **TB**	5	NPC, Breast CA, **CVA**, **Pneumonia**, **COAD**
	1984–88	3	NPC, **Lung CA**, **TB**	3	NPC, **CVA**, **Pneumonia**
	1989–93	6	**Gastric CA**, Colorectal CA, **Lung CA**, TB, HBP, **Pneumonia**	4	NPC, Gastric CA, CVA, **Pneumonia**
KL12	1979–83	6	Oesophageal CA, **Gastric CA**, Liver CA, HBP, **IHD**, **COAD**	3	Colorectal CA, **IHD**, COAD
	1984–88	5	NPC, HBP, IHD, Pneumonia, COAD	6	**Lung CA**, HBP, **IHD**, CVA, Pneumonia, COAD
	1989–93	6	NPC, Oesophageal CA, Gastric CA, Colorectal CA, IHD, COAD	6	Colorectal CA, Lung CA, HBP, CVA, Pneumonia, COAD
KL13	1979–83	1	**Gastric CA**	0	
	1984–88	0		2	**Gastric CA**, Leukaemia
	1989–93	0		0	
KL14	1979–83	0		0	
	1984–88	1	**IHD**	0	
	1989–93	0		0	

Appendix 3 (Continued)

Community	Period	Male: Number of diseases in the bottom 20%	Male: Name of disease	Female: Number of diseases in the bottom 20%	Female: Name of disease
KL15	1979–83	0		0	
	1984–88	1	Colorectal CA	3	Gastric CA, CVA, Pneumonia
	1989–93	0		0	
KL16	1979–83	0		0	
	1984–88	2	Leukaemia, **IHD**	0	
	1989–93	1	Oesophageal CA	0	
KL17	1979–83	6	NPC, Oesophageal CA, Gastric CA, Lung CA, **CVA**, TB	3	**CVA**, **Pneumonia**, COAD
	1984–88	3	Gastric CA, Liver CA, **Lung CA**	2	Liver CA, **Lung CA**
	1989–93	1	NPC	0	
KL18	1979–83	5	Liver CA, Lung CA, CVA, Pneumonia, COAD	4	Lung CA, CVA, Pneumonia, COAD
	1984–88	3	CVA, Pneumonia, COAD	3	HBP, IHD, Pneumonia
	1989–93	3	IHD, CVA, **COAD**	5	Lung CA, HBP, IHD, **CVA**, COAD
KL19	1979–83	1	**Colorectal CA**	0	
	1984–88	1	**IHD**	0	
	1989–93	0		0	

Appendix 3 (Continued)

Community	Period	Male: Number of diseases in the bottom 20%	Male: Name of disease	Female: Number of diseases in the bottom 20%	Female: Name of disease
KL20	1979–83	1	**IHD**	2	**Gastric CA**, **Cervical CA**
	1984–88	0		3	**Colorectal CA**, Breast CA, Pneumonia
	1989–93	3	Leukaemia, **IHD**, **CVA**	5	Liver CA, Lung CA, Breast CA, **IHD**, **CVA**
KL21	1979–83	1	**IHD**	0	
	1984–88	1	**IHD**	1	NPC
	1989–93	1	**IHD**	3	Colorectal CA, Lung CA, **IHD**
KL22	1979–83	3	NPC, Liver CA, TB	4	Colorectal CA, Lung CA, IHD, **COAD**
	1984–88	2	Oesophageal CA, Gastric CA	3	Lung CA, Breast CA, IHD
	1989–93	3	NPC, Colorectal CA, Lung CA	2	HBP, COAD
KL23	1979–83	2	Liver CA, HBP	2	**Colorectal CA**, **CVA**
	1984–88	1	Leukaemia	0	
	1989-93	0		0	
KL24	1979–83	1	Colorectal CA	2	NPC, Breast CA
	1984–88	3	Gastric CA, Liver CA, **CVA**	1	COAD
	1989–93	6	**Oesophageal CA**, **Lung CA**, **CVA**, **TB**, **Pneumonia**, **COAD**	1	Liver CA
KL25	1979–83	0		0	
	1984–88	0		0	
	1989–93	0		1	**IHD**

Appendix 3 (Continued)

Community	Period	Male: Number of diseases in the bottom 20%	Male: Name of disease	Female: Number of diseases in the bottom 20%	Female: Name of disease
NT1	1979–83	2	**NPC**, IHD	3	Colorectal CA, HBP, **Pneumonia**
	1984–88	4	Oesophageal CA, Colorectal CA, **Liver CA**, IHD	3	NPC, Colorectal CA, **IHD**
	1989–93	0		2	Colorectal CA, **Pneumonia**
NT2	1979–83	1	HBP	1	Colorectal CA
	1984–88	1	NPC	1	**Gastric CA**
	1989–93	6	Liver CA, **HBP**, **IHD**, **CVA**, TB, **Pneumonia**	5	Lung CA, Breast CA, HBP, IHD, **Pneumonia**
NT3	1979–83	1	Leukaemia	0	
	1984–88	1	**NPC**	1	**Lung CA**
	1989–93	2	Colorectal CA, **IHD**	3	Oesophageal CA, Leukaemia, **Breast CA**
NT4	1979–83	0		2	Leukaemia, HBP
	1984–88	1	**IHD**	0	
	1989–93	0		1	**Breast CA**
NT5	1979–83	0		0	
	1984–88	0		0	
	1989–93	0		1	Breast CA
NT6	1979–83	2	**HBP**, **IHD**	4	**Colorectal CA**, **Gastric CA**, Liver CA, **IHD**
	1984–88	0		2	**Breast CA**, **Pneumonia**
	1989–93	1	**Colorectal CA**	2	Colorectal CA, **COAD**

Appendix 3 (Continued)

		Male		Female	
Community	Period	Number of diseases in the bottom 20%	Name of disease	Number of diseases in the bottom 20%	Name of disease
NT7	1979–83	2	Colorectal CA, IHD	2	IHD, Pneumonia
	1984–88	1	Leukaemia	1	Breast CA
	1989–93	2	**TB**, **Pneumonia**	0	
NT8	1979–83	2	Colorectal CA, **IHD**	2	Liver CA, **IHD**
	1984–88	0		0	
	1989–93	0		0	
NT9	1979–83	4	Gastric CA, Lung CA, **IHD**, **Pneumonia**	5	Liver CA, Lung CA, Breast CA, **IHD**, **CVA**
	1984–88	2	**Colorectal CA**, Pneumonia	2	Colorectal CA, Lung CA
	1989–93	1	Colorectal CA	2	Lung CA, Pneumonia
NT10	1979–83	1	**Oesophageal CA**	4	**Breast CA**, Leukaemia, **IHD**, **Pneumonia**
	1984–88	0		1	**Colorectal CA**
	1989–93	0		0	
NT11	1979–83	7	**Oesophageal CA**, Colorectal CA, Lung CA, **IHD**, **CVA**, **Pneumonia**, **COAD**	5	Colorectal CA, **Lung CA**, **IHD**, **CVA**, Pneumonia
	1984–88	2	NPC, Gastric CA	4	Gastric CA, Colorectal CA, Liver CA, Breast CA
	1989–93	3	NPC, Gastric CA, **Colorectal CA**	2	Colorectal CA, Lung CA

Appendix 3 (Continued)

Community	Period	Male: Number of diseases in the bottom 20%	Male: Name of disease	Female: Number of diseases in the bottom 20%	Female: Name of disease
NT12	1979–83	1	**IHD**	6	**Gastric CA**, **Colorectal CA**, **Lung CA**, **Breast CA**, Cervical CA, Leukaemia
	1984–88	1	**IHD**	6	**Colorectal CA**, Liver CA, **Lung CA**, Breast CA, Leukaemia, **IHD**
	1989–93	1	Gastric CA	1	NPC
NT13	1979–83	4	NPC, Oesophageal, Colorectal CA, Gastric CA	2	Colorectal CA, **Lung CA**
	1984–88	2	Gastric CA, **IHD**	2	Gastric CA, IHD
	1989–93	1	**IHD**	6	Colorectal CA, Liver CA, Lung CA, Breast CA, IHD, **CVA**
NT14	1979–83	4	Oesophageal CA, Gastric CA, Liver CA, Lung CA	6	Lung CA, HBP, IHD, **CVA**, Pneumonia, **COAD**
	1984–88	6	Oesophageal CA, Gastric CA, Colorectal CA, Lung CA, **IHD**, CVA	3	Colorectal CA, Breast CA, IHD
	1989–93	0		2	Lung CA, COAD
NT15	1979–83	0		3	Colorectal CA, Leukaemia, **HBP**
	1984–88	0		0	
	1989–93	0		0	
NT16	1979–83	0		0	
	1984–88	0		0	
	1989–93	1	**IHD**	1	**Pneumonia**

Appendix 3 (Continued)

		Male		Female	
Community	Period	Number of diseases in the bottom 20%	Name of disease	Number of diseases in the bottom 20%	Name of disease
NT17	1979–83	3	Colorectal CA, **IHD**, **CVA**	3	Breast CA, **IHD**, COAD
	1984–88	0		2	Lung CA, IHD
	1989–93	0		1	Colorectal CA
NT18	1979–83	3	Colorectal CA, HBP, IHD	2	Colorectal CA, IHD
	1984–88	1	Pneumonia	0	
	1989–93	2	Colorectal CA, IHD	1	IHD
NT19	1979–83	5	Oesophageal CA, **HBP**, IHD, **CVA**, TB	4	**Gastric CA**, Cervical CA, HBP, **IHD**
	1984–88	3	Oesophageal CA, Colorectal CA, HBP	2	Gastric CA, HBP
	1989–93	1	**CVA**	1	COAD

Appendix 4.1: Spearman's Correlation Coefficients of SMR Ranks between Two Periods by Sex

Diseases	1979–83 vs 1984–88		1979–83 vs 1989–93		1984–88 vs 1989–93	
	Male	Female	Male	Female	Male	Female
All causes	0.6929**	0.4851**	0.6735**	0.5346**	0.6510**	0.6355**
All cancers	0.6501**	0.5280**	0.5215**	0.4136**	0.6443**	0.3678**
Nasopharyngeal cancer (NPC)	0.2699*	0.2899*	0.4022**	0.2669*	0.3583**	0.2318
Oesophageal cancer	0.3328**	0.1590	0.2666*	0.1093	0.4248**	0.1751
Gastric cancer	0.3782**	0.2228	0.2371	–0.1125	0.2724*	0.0098
Colorectal cancer	0.1955	0.1062	0.2903*	0.1559	0.0012	0.3173*
Liver cancer	0.3257**	0.0988	0.3177**	0.1236	0.4728**	0.2073
Lung cancer	0.3980**	0.3215**	0.4938**	0.4391**	0.6631**	0.2921*
Leukaemia	–0.0309	0.2321	–0.0007	0.1054	0.1188	0.2272
Hypertensive disease (HBP)	0.2347	0.2205	0.2816*	0.0500	0.4872**	0.5810**
Ischaemic heart disease (IHD)	0.4179**	0.2206	0.4637**	–0.0098	0.4613**	0.3833**
Cerebrovascular disease (CVA)	0.4329**	0.2764*	0.3412**	0.1962	0.5124**	0.5691**
Tuberculosis (TB)	0.5281**	0.3329**	0.3824**	0.1918	0.7319**	0.0530
Pneumonia	0.4555**	0.0185	0.2734*	0.2764*	0.3711**	0.4049**
Chronic obstructive airway disease (COAD)	0.6804**	0.1535	0.6587**	0.2460*	0.6068**	0.4183**
Breast cancer		0.2872*		0.1872		0.3119*
Cervical cancer		0.1509		0.0693		0.3048*

* $p \leq 0.05$

** $p \leq 0.01$

Appendix 4.2: Spearman's Correlation Coefficients of SMR Ranks in Two Quinquennia (1979–83 & 1984–88) by Sex and Region

Diseases	Hong Kong (21 communities)		Kowloon (25 communities)		New Territories (19 communities)	
	Male	Female	Male	Female	Male	Female
All causes	0.7766**	0.6429**	0.6500**	0.3069	0.3789	0.4649*
All cancers	0.7519**	0.2766	0.4546*	0.4700*	0.7333**	0.8018**
Nasopharyngeal cancer (NPC)	0.5740**	0.4240	–0.2592	0.1590	0.1860	–0.1018
Oesophageal cancer	0.2384	0.2053	0.4508*	0.2706	0.2474	0.0808
Gastric cancer	0.4404*	0.2766	0.3515	0.1531	0.1789	0.0930
Colorectal cancer	0.2558	0.1662	0.2854	0.1585	–0.1912	–0.1719
Liver cancer	0.5091**	0.2468	0.1154	0.2354	0.5263*	–0.0789
Lung cancer	0.7662**	0.3506	0.2146	0.1162	0.0825	0.4825*
Leukaemia	0.1020	0.3537	–0.1293	0.1215	–0.0597	0.3677
Hypertensive disease (HBP)	0.1831	0.2494	–0.0185	–0.2477	0.4772*	0.0386
Ischaemic heart disease (IHD)	0.2182	0.4377*	0.2731	0.1915	–0.1456	–0.3263
Cerebrovascular disease (CVA)	0.7844**	0.7169**	0.1946	–0.0654	0.1579	–0.0211
Tuberculosis (TB)	0.6476**	0.4179	0.2924	0.0964	0.2158	–0.0105
Pneumonia	0.5987**	0.3688	0.4992*	–0.0231	0.2386	–0.2912
Chronic obstructive airway disease (COAD)	0.7662**	0.5935**	0.5277**	0.0608	0.4702*	–0.0807
Breast cancer		–0.1584		0.5008*		0.4333
Cervical cancer		–0.2010		0.2719		0.3509

* $p \leq 0.05$
** $p \leq 0.01$

Appendix 4.3: Spearman's Correlation Coefficients of SMR Ranks in Two Quinquennia (1979–83 & 1989–93) by Sex and Region

Diseases	Hong Kong (21 communities)		Kowloon (25 communities)		New Territories (19 communities)	
	Male	Female	Male	Female	Male	Female
All causes	0.8636**	0.7610**	0.5723**	0.2962	0.4719*	0.2789
All cancers	0.7727**	0.5273*	0.5254**	0.3962*	0.1930	0.2596
Nasopharyngeal cancer (NPC)	0.5930**	0.2083	0.2977	0.0743	0.1526	0.1386
Oesophageal cancer	0.4755*	–0.0066	0.3000	0.4402*	–0.1579	–0.0123
Gastric cancer	0.4347*	0.1610	0.4777*	0.0108	–0.2211	–0.4544
Colorectal cancer	0.5857**	0.1935	–0.1596	–0.1346	0.1702	0.1596
Liver cancer	0.6208**	0.3247	–0.0577	0.3316	0.4702*	–0.1684
Lung cancer	0.7442**	0.4831*	0.6014**	0.4692*	0.0965	0.3509
Leukaemia	0.3395	0.1481	–0.2098	0.1947	–0.1124	–0.1282
Hypertensive disease (HBP)	0.5000*	–0.1039	–0.0337	–0.0947	0.4281	0.1105
Ischaemic heart disease (IHD)	0.5662**	0.0831	0.5500**	0.2492	–0.1825	–0.6912**
Cerebrovascular disease (CVA)	0.7844**	0.7065**	0.1200	–0.0162	0.0895	–0.3912
Tuberculosis (TB)	0.5488**	–0.0905	0.1715	0.1285	0.1140	0.2045
Pneumonia	0.6727**	0.4299	0.3823	0.4058	–0.0456	–0.2579
Chronic obstructive airway disease (COAD)	0.7701**	0.5455*	0.7600**	0.3115	–0.0333	–0.0404
Breast cancer		0.1922		0.0877		0.0982
Cervical cancer		0.0969		–0.0985		–0.0860

* $p \leq 0.05$

** $p \leq 0.01$

Appendix 4.4: Spearman's Correlation Coefficients of SMR Ranks in Two Quinquennia (1984–88 & 1989–93) by Sex and Region

Diseases	Hong Kong (21 communities)		Kowloon (25 communities)		New Territories (19 communities)	
	Male	Female	Male	Female	Male	Female
All causes	0.8273**	0.7532**	0.5738**	0.6392**	0.4193	0.3912
All cancers	0.8286**	0.6675**	0.3608	0.2600	0.5281*	0.0825
Nasopharyngeal cancer (NPC)	0.2910	0.3340	0.1431	0.0635	0.4281	0.3807
Oesophageal cancer	0.3558	0.2151	0.6000**	0.2411	0.0351	–0.0088
Gastric cancer	0.3891	0.2688	0.2131	–0.1315	0.1456	–0.1421
Colorectal cancer	0.0455	0.5403*	0.0369	0.1069	–0.2175	0.2912
Liver cancer	0.6688**	–0.1532	0.0154	0.5440**	0.5649*	–0.2211
Lung cancer	0.7675**	0.3987	0.4402*	0.1238	0.7596**	0.2632
Leukaemia	0.3610	0.1772	–0.2098	0.3374	0.1966	0.1878
Hypertensive disease (HBP)	0.2935	0.1909	0.5169**	0.4617*	0.3228	0.6982**
Ischaemic heart disease (IHD)	0.1312	0.1701	0.6169**	0.4392*	–0.0632	0.4088
Cerebrovascular disease (CVA)	0.6649**	0.6896**	0.4515*	0.4000*	0.2877	0.5386*
Tuberculosis (TB)	0.7018**	–0.0830	0.6586**	0.0565	0.5596*	–0.5529*
Pneumonia	0.7377**	0.3364	0.1631	0.2885	0.2842	0.7561**
Chronic obstructive airway disease (COAD)	0.4805*	0.3753	0.5608**	0.3738	0.2386	0.4649*
Breast cancer		0.4065		0.2369		–0.0386
Cervical cancer		0.2865		0.2717		–0.0193

* $p \leq 0.05$

** $p \leq 0.01$

Appendix 5: Spearman's Correlation Coefficients of F-Score and SMR Ranks in Three Periods by Sex

Diseases	1981		1986		1991	
	Male	Female	Male	Female	Male	Female
All causes	–0.6260**	–0.5736**	–0.5510**	–0.3852**	–0.6157**	–0.4201**
All cancers	–0.2997*	–0.0171	–0.4201**	–0.0221	–0.6184**	–0.2034
Nasopharyngeal cancer (NPC)	–0.4848**	–0.3347**	–0.3928**	–0.2959	–0.5370**	–0.2746*
Oesophageal cancer	–0.1520	–0.2889*	–0.4557**	–0.2894*	–0.4634**	–0.0589
Gastric cancer	–0.1702	–0.1750	–0.1651	0.0623	–0.3956**	–0.2698*
Colorectal cancer	0.3957**	0.3918**	0.1449	0.1415	0.1464	–0.0295
Liver cancer	–0.4013**	–0.1018	–0.4860**	–0.3460**	–0.5135**	–0.3075*
Lung cancer	–0.3023*	0.0259	–0.4355**	0.0130	–0.6560**	0.0068
Leukaemia	–0.1186	0.1279	0.0880	–0.0126	–0.0230	–0.1725
Hypertensive disease (HBP)	–0.1489	–0.1358	–0.1665	–0.3737**	–0.2276	–0.3690**
Ischaemic heart disease (IHD)	0.7087**	0.4146**	0.3858**	0.1753	0.1665	–0.0562
Cerebrovascular disease (CVA)	–0.3047*	–0.2289*	–0.3655**	–0.3155**	–0.5232**	–0.3589**
Tuberculosis (TB)	–0.5311**	–0.4291**	–0.7461**	–0.4393**	–0.6133**	–0.4038**
Pneumonia	–0.3199**	–0.2210	–0.4647**	–0.2518*	–0.4796**	–0.3114*
Chronic obstructive airway disease (COAD)	–0.6191**	–0.1575	–0.6726**	–0.4776**	–0.7209**	–0.2225
Breast cancer		0.1831		0.5225**		0.0617
Cervical cancer		–0.0042		0.3189**		–0.2191*

* $p \leq 0.05$

** $p \leq 0.01$